Rehabilitation

Gerald G. Hirschberg, M.D., F.A.C.P.
Clinical Professor of Physical Medicine and Rehabilitation,
California College of Medicine,
University of California, Irvine

Leon Lewis, M.D., F.A.C.P.
Physician in Charge,
Rehabilitation Center,
Contra Costa County Medical Services,
Martinez, California;
Formerly Director, Respiratory and Rehabilitation Center,
Fairmont Hospital of Alameda County, California

Patricia Vaughan, R.N., M.S.
Nurse Consultant, In-Service Education;
Organization Administration,
Kaiser Foundation International,
Oakland, California
Formerly Director of Education and Training,
French Hospital,
San Francisco, California
Formerly Nurse Consultant,
Regional Medical Program, Stroke Project,
University of California, San Francisco

Rehabilitation

SECOND EDITION

A Manual for the Care of the Disabled and Elderly

Gerald G. Hirschberg, M.D., F.A.C.P.

Leon Lewis, M.D., F.A.C.P.

Patricia Vaughan, R.N., M.S.

J. B. Lippincott Company

PHILADELPHIA

New York / San Jose / Toronto

Distributed in Great Britain by
Blackwell Scientific Publications, London,
Oxford and Edinburgh

ISBN 0-397-54195-3

Library of Congress Catalog Number 76-40316

Printed in the United States of America

3 5 7 9 8 6 4

Library of Congress Cataloging in Publication Data

Hirschberg, Gerald G
Rehabilitation.

Includes bibliographical references and index.
1. Physically handicapped—Rehabilitation.
2. Aged—Rehabilitation.   3. Geriatric nursing.
I. Lewis, Leon, joint author.   II. Vaughan,
Patricia, joint author.   [DNLM: 1. Handicapped.
2. Rehabilitation—In Old age.   WB460 H669r]
RM930.H57 1976   362.4   76-40316
ISBN 0-397-54195-3

**To the disabled,
who have been our teachers**

Acknowledgments

The authors are indebted to all their predecessors and colleagues who have contributed to knowledge in the field of rehabilitation. They are grateful for an enormous and informative literature from which they have gained knowledge and insight. Specifically, they acknowledge the support, the stimulation and the challenges of the following facilities, agencies and persons:

The Poliomyelitis Respiratory and Rehabilitation center at Fairmont Hospital, San Leandro, California, where, between 1953 and 1960, the authors were first stimulated to develop and teach simplified methods of rehabilitation. A nursing syllabus on rehabilitation and a manual for management of respiratory impairment developed by the authors while working as colleagues at the center provided much of the background for this text.

The staff of the Contra Costa County Hospital, Martinez, California, and particularly the personnel of the Rehabilitation Service who participated in working out and evaluating some of the material presented here. In addition to the nurses and therapists whose efforts in testing procedures were invaluable, special credit is due George Degnan, M.D., Medical Director, and Louie F. Girtman, M.D., Assistant Medical Director, for effectively supporting the study of new approaches to efficient rehabilitation of the disabled.

The National Foundation, Inc., for support and encouragement during the epoch of its achievements as the National Foundation for Infantile Paralysis, Inc. Dr. Kenneth S. Landauer, who was responsible for the unique respiratory center program, deserves special credit for his provocative leadership.

The California State Department of Social Welfare for a grant in support of a study of efficient and economical methods of rehabilitation.

The individuals without whose practical assistance this book would have remained unwritten:

The orthotists, prosthetists and appliance makers: Stewart A. Johnson, George B. Robinson, Michael Keropian, Matthew G. Laurence, and the staff of C. H. Hittenberger, Inc., whose talents and ingenuity have been freely exploited by the authors.

The artist Helen Gee, the photographers, George C. B. Tolleson and Dr. R. Leong who have made obvious and important contributions to the book.

Special acknowledgment is made to Dorothy Thomas who by her continued interest in the principles of rehabilitation has succeeded in maintaining the progressive growth of the large institution where she is now the Director of Nursing.

The manufacturers and distributors who were generous in providing illustrations of their products.

The publishers, for their patience, assistance and encouragement.

Preface to the Second Edition

Eleven years have passed since publication of the first edition of this book. During that time many new devices and techniques have been added to the armamentarium of physical restoration. The methods of rehabilitation described in this book continue to be based on common sense, efficiency and economy. None of the space in this limited volume is devoted to arguments to support its underlying philosophy, but the excellent reception of the book among the professionals for whom it is intended supports our view that readers understand precepts without having them forced upon them.

In the years between editions we have been actively engaged in the practice of rehabilitation medicine and in education. We have been constantly on the alert for innovations and have frequently tested new ideas and procedures to determine their usefulness, efficiency and economy. In addition, we have continued our interest in the perfection of methods of dealing with frequently encountered disabilities.

In addition to updating the material in the text, we have added several new chapters. The material on psychosocial aspects of patient care has been expanded into a completely new chapter entitled Economic, Social and Emotional Effects of Disability. We have also expanded the chapter on communication and have presented the management of aphasia in a more practical manner. In addition, Part Three of the book, consisting of four chapters dealing with the organization of rehabilitation, is new. The chapter on rehabilitation personnel contains a detailed discussion of the various functions of rehabilitation nurses and therapists. A new section on the treatment of the back with emphasis on the strictest possible protection of the intravertebral disc to allow it to heal is based on successful management of a large number of persons with clinically proven disc disease. The material on respiratory rehabilitation has been expanded into a chapter to include respiratory physiology and causes of respiratory disability. Finally, a new chapter on cardiac rehabilitation has been added.

In all these additions, the spirit of our basic philosophy has been maintained. It is our intention that this book will serve as a reference manual as well as a teaching tool. The index has been especially designed with this use in mind.

This book provides a wealth of information upon which to base clinical practice, including rationale, policies and procedures which are so much a part of the organization of patient care in institutions. The underlying philosophy with which the authors approach the subject of rehabilitation is especially important. All material presented in this book is based upon the belief that the elderly and disabled are entitled to function at their maximum capacity and that this basic concept is the foundation upon which policies, procedures, clinical practice and the educational process must be built.

Medicine and nursing are in a period of great and rapid change. The authors are committed to critical evaluation of each step in this change and will welcome the opportunity to discuss matters dealing with rehabilitation. We invite comments, inquiries and suggestions from our readers, addressed either directly to us or to the publisher.

Preface to the First Edition

Rehabilitation, by necessity, is a multidisciplinary endeavor. Physicians, nurses, social workers, therapists, orthotists, prosthetists, teachers, engineers and administrators are involved to some extent in the complex problems of medical rehabilitation. Although these facts have long been recognized, those in the disciplines involved have written mostly for others in the same field. There are texts on medical rehabilitation, manuals for nurses, articles on the role of social workers, textbooks of physical and occupational therapy and a large literature, much of which tends to perpetuate fragmentation of interest rather than unify the approach toward rehabilitation.

The authors are convinced that all personnel who work with disabled patients and have the common goal of rehabilitation must have a common knowledge of the principal medical, nursing, special therapeutic and social concepts of management of disabling conditions. Without such common knowledge, it is impossible for personnel with diverse backgrounds and methods to work together effectively, regardless of how competent they may be in their own limited fields. Accordingly, an attempt has been made to present both basic concepts and specific technics in plain language, hopefully understandable by any reasonably informed reader. If this attempt is successful, the text may provide a common avenue of communication among all rehabilitation personnel.

Most of this book is concerned with specific disabilities. In dealing with them there has been no attempt to present or discuss various methods of rehabilitation as practiced in different treatment centers. The authors have limited themselves to methods and procedures which they have tested and proved to be effective, economical and practical. The subject matter is presented with the objective of giving the reader the rationale of each rehabilitation procedure, not only in terms of applicability to the impairment treated but also in terms of maximum efficiency. This neither implies that there are no equally efficient methods nor that the authors regard the procedures described as the best that can be developed. Since they have participated in the rapid evolution of rehabilitation technology, they are well aware of the evanescence of what seemed at the moment to be the height of achievement.

Contents

Contents   xv

PART ONE

General Considerations

CHAPTER

1

Introduction

As everyone working in medical and allied fields knows, this is the age of specialization in the care of a patient. As specialties become more limited, there is an increasing danger of excessive fragmentation of services. In the course of multiple consultations the continuity of care may be lost. This is true especially in hospitals where there may be uncertainty about the responsibility of consultants, some of whom assume the role of clinical direction when their services were requested only for opinion or advice. Even when the battery of diagnostic and therapeutic services is well coordinated, often the patient is bewildered and inadequately informed. Elderly people, in particular, deal poorly with a multiplicity of clinical contacts. When they are shuttled about among doctors, therapists, psychologists, nurses, social workers and other experts, they frequently become confused and have a feeling of detachment from any authoritative and responsible person on whose therapeutic leadership they may rely.

The authors of this book are opposed to the current tendency toward overspecialization and fragmentation, and they hope to demonstrate that the rehabilitation of common severe disabilities can be accomplished with a minimum of personnel. Furthermore, the authors believe that simplicity of method leads to economy which can bring rehabilitation within the reach of the disabled who have modest means or are dependent on public or community funds.

This book is intended to be useful to all professional personnel concerned with the care of the disabled. The need for communication and close integration of effort is well known among workers in the field of rehabilitation. When everyone on the rehabilitation team knows how every other member plays his part, the chances of success are great. When the contrary situation prevails the chances for confusion and failure greatly outweigh those for success.

Medical rehabilitation, as it will be defined, is something both old and new. Throughout the ages, some aspects of medical rehabilitation have been an essential part of every form of medical care. Even if the ideas were not expressed, it seems to be obvious that the return of individuals to functional roles in society has been implicit in the endeavors of every clinician throughout history. Unfortunately, this basically social goal was often obscured by the traditional efforts to cure.

Deeply buried in the ancient heritage of medicine and in the folklore of various peoples is the notion of the eradication of disease. For thousands of years disease and deformity were regarded as divine retribution or the diabolical influence of some evil spirit or invading force, and exorcism was the principal method of treatment. Finally, incantations and concoctions were replaced by the specific antimicrobials and highly potent chemical armaments of the modern physician. However, even with the change in weaponry, the ancient ideas of eradication of disease have prevailed. In the search for restitution of a specific organ or part, the fate of the total organism has often been disregarded.

During the past three decades there has been growing concern about the prevention and the circumvention of disability. This is a result of a revolution in medical thought that has had its origin in diverse causes and historic events. One economic factor has been the growing cost of maintaining the handicapped and the institution-bound population of the aged. Another factor has been the rapid evolution of knowledge of bodily motion and function and the application of the physical and the engineering sciences to medical rehabilitation. A very powerful practical element was contributed almost by accident. Early ambulation after surgery, which is now one of the established dogmas of medical care, arose partly from the inadequacy of hospital facilities during World War II. While there were ideas and observations supporting early activity—some of them derived from studies of primitive people whose obstetric management involved little interruption of daily work—the principal motivation was necessity. When it was found that getting people out of bed the day after major surgical procedures or the very day of childbirth not only did no harm but led to speedy and healthy convalescence, the idea of early activation met almost universal acceptance.

Curiously enough, "early ambulation" ideas did not easily spread to the medical wards of hospitals. While otherwise healthy patients who had had their gallbladders removed one day were up walking on the next day, patients who entered hospitals with benign medical conditions continued to be bathed, fed, clothed and assisted in every act as though any use of muscle power might hamper the recovery processes of the body. The paradox of dynamic surgical convalescence versus devitalizing medical convalescence is explicable in part by the differences in population in medical and surgical wards.

For many medical patients, mobility and self-care are temporarily contraindicated or impossible because of acute illness. Their management requires knowledge and discretion and should not be based on tradition or ritual. Each problem requires careful analysis. For example, in the treatment of myocardial infarction it has long been assumed that energy is best spared by enforced bed rest. Yet, as long ago as 1950 the armchair was advocated for treatment of coronary thrombosis and heart failure because in the sitting position the work of the heart is eased, and the patient is not only better rested but also encouraged. In this situation the break with tradition leads to lesser physical activity but greater social participation and is beneficial on both counts.

In the case of management of the patient who has had a stroke, knowledge and discretion also oppose the traditional bed treatment. However, here, one usually deals with a patient who requires activity and benefits by it. The atmosphere in which such a patient should be treated differs greatly from the atmosphere appropriate for the treatment of the acutely ill, for example, the patient with heart failure.

These examples point out the rationale for segregation of patients according to the method of management needed at various phases of care. This principle is the basis for "progressive care" plans in hospitals that have established intensive care and rehabilitative care units.

GOALS OF REHABILITATION

The field of medical rehabilitation repels a great many health personnel because, by necessity, it has the qualities of a mission. It is a phase of medical practice that requires a zeal for social benefit. It is deeply rooted in ethics and rests on a primary postulate of human value. Like every other movement dependent on zeal, there is the danger of emotion prevailing over judgment. At times, the problems of the severely handicapped are treated in a ritualistic fashion without deep understanding and without realization of the degree of adaptation and change required to shift the outlook of the disabled person from one of depression and despair to an attitude of hopefulness, accompanied by the desire and the energy to make a new start in life.

The goal of medical rehabilitation as a technique is the prevention or the reversal of those biologic tendencies that cause the ill, the disabled and the elderly to withdraw from life, to deteriorate and to become dependent. The goal of rehabilitation as a movement is more complex. Its objectives are more than the achievement of individual rehabilitation; they include the education of all of the professions involved in medical and supportive care in order to focus endeavors on human values rather than on mere technical success. They include the orientation of the public toward a fair deal for the handicapped in opportunities to work and to share the joys of living.

The technical information in this manual may give the impression that standard routines are applicable to all types of disabilities and that success is assured if only the methods are applied carefully. Be assured that rehabilitation is not so simple. The endeavor is directed toward providing the person unable to function in standard or normal ways a chance to live a life which is acceptable, meaningful and in some measure contributory to the common good. However, the road to achievement is full of obstacles. These can be removed and the way made easier by understanding and skillful guidance and encouragement by those who are fortunate enough to play a part in the role of rebuilding a life for a fellow human being.

DEFINITION OF TERMS

Medical Rehabilitation. Medical rehabilitation is the clinical process by means of which the disabled person is restored to a state of optimal effectiveness and given an opportunity to enjoy a meaningful life. Although medical rehabilitation is especially concerned with the disabled, the concepts and the techniques of rehabilitation are also applicable in every phase of care of the acutely and the chronically ill. Before disability has occurred, the role of rehabilitation technology is preventive in nature. When disability exists, the role is both preventive and restorative, directed toward improvement of function.

It is important to distinguish the orientation of medicine and surgery in general from that of rehabilitation medicine. Medicine and surgery are oriented primarily toward organic pathology, and their objectives are the treatment and the reversal of pathology to achieve cure. In incurable diseases, the objective is the slowing down of the pathologic process and the prolongation of life. However, rehabilitation is concerned with the preservation and the restoration of function of any part of the individual or the individual as a whole. Functional disturbances can occur without organic pathology and can outlast the organic disorder even if it has been cured. The concept of disability as functional impairment is basic to the understanding of rehabilitation.

Disability. Terms used in medicine and especially in rehabilitation tend to be defined loosely and used in different ways by different people. There is great confusion between such words as "disability" and "impairment," both terms being used interchangeably in much of the literature dealing with the medical aspects of social welfare programs. An attempt is made to specify the precise use of the terms as follows.

Disability has three distinct technical meanings which depend on the context in which the term is used.

1. In medical rehabilitation, disability refers to anatomically defined functional loss or impairment.*

a. *Neurologic disabilities* are commonly expressed in functional terms, e.g., blindness for loss of vision, hemiplegia for loss of power of one side of the body, paraplegia for loss of power of both lower extremities.

b. *Musculoskeletal disabilities* are commonly expressed in anatomicopathologic terms, e.g., amputation for the loss of a limb (rather than loss of walking ability); ankylosed joint (rather than loss of a particular motion).

2. In the field of workmen's compensation, disability is expressed in terms of the percentage loss of bodily function or percentage loss of function of a part. In this sense, disability is a term of measurement based on systems of estimation of varying complexity and defined by statute.

3. In a nontechnical sense, disability may refer to inability to carry out any normal or ordinary function, e.g., inability to wash oneself, feed oneself, write or perform any other function. These functional losses, while described in such nontechnical terms, may be based on disabilities that can be defined technically, as indicated above. In other words, the nontechnical use of the term simply states a fact as an observed phenomenon but does not attempt to account for the cause.

Evaluation. Evaluation is the process of determining the functional status and the functional potential of the patient. It must be distinguished from diagnosis, which determines the pathologic status, and from prognosis, which estimates the course of the pathologic process. Obviously, evaluation cannot be divorced completely from diagnosis and prognosis, since the functional potential is often determined by the nature and the course of the disease. Evaluation requires all the basic information obtainable by general medical examination, i.e., history, physical examination and laboratory studies. In addition, careful

---

*Disability, in this sense, is sometimes called "impairment" to avoid confusion with the other meanings of the term. However, this distinction is not made consistently, even by its advocates. It is recommended that the term "impairment" should not be used synonymously with the term "disability." Either it should be used to qualify the nature of a disability (for example, impairment of vision), or it should be avoided entirely.

appraisal of strength, motor function, range of motion, self-care and communication abilities is necessary. Also, the individual must be assessed as a social being. His home, family, work and general environment must be considered. To this, a formal or informal assessment of personality, attitude and adaptability must be added to complete the evaluation. The way in which evaluation is achieved differs from case to case and depends largely on the complexity of the disability and the individual problem.

Experience in the process of evaluation and knowledge of the methods of rehabilitation lead to skill in estimating rehabilitation potential. Without this skill, waste and failure can be expected. From experience in the treatment of patients with hemiplegia, for example, the skilled physician can say that one individual will be ambulatory and able to return to his usual pursuits in 4 weeks, while another whose paralysis is complicated by pre-existing or concurrent disabilities other than hemiplegia will require treatment for 10 to 12 weeks. Accuracy in evaluation allows for proper timing of the various aspects of a rehabilitation program; it allows responsible agencies or families to plan the use of economic and other resources; it leads to a satisfactory outcome based on realism and honesty, rather than frustration caused by lack of knowledge or by wishful thinking.

CAUSES OF DISABILITY

Primary and Secondary Disabilities

It is important to distinguish between disabilities caused directly by disease or injury and those which occur as a result of a primary disability. The latter are called "secondary disabilities." Their importance in rehabilitation is considerable because they can frequently be avoided by proper care or corrected by rehabilitation measures. The causes of secondary disability are discussed in Chapter 3.

Causes of Primary Disabilities

Primary disability is the direct result of a pathologic process. It results from (1) congenital disorder, (2) disease or (3) injury. Pathology in any system of the body may lead to disability. However, the most common and most prolonged disabilities are caused by involvement of the nervous system, the musculoskeletal system and the cardiopulmonary system.

The major disabilities due to impairment of the nervous system are various types of paralyses, disorders of communication and disturbances of intellect. The causes of these disabilities are discussed in detail in Chapter 13. The most common cause of musculoskeletal disability is arthritis, particularly rheumatoid arthritis and osteoarthritis. Other musculoskeletal disabilities are caused by fractures and amputations.

Cardiopulmonary disorders are disabling because of either prescribed or forced restriction of activity. For example, in the treatment of tuberculosis before the introduction of antibiotics, total inactivity was prescribed as the principal method of medical treatment. The management of acute myocardial infarction is still based on prescribed maximal inactivity for at least 2 weeks. For individuals with extreme breathlessness due to pulmonary emphysema, pulmonary fibrosis or cardiac decompensation, inactivity is forced. Pain, for example, in angina pectoris and intermittent claudication, may also require reduced activity in cardiovascular disease.

Frequently, a single cause may lead to multiple disabilities. For example, a stroke may cause paralysis, disorientation and aphasia. A single injury may lead to amputation, paralysis, respiratory insufficiency and serious psychological disturbances. Not only may complex disabilities result from a single cause, but also multiple causes may produce multiple disabilities, particularly in elderly people. In fact, it is almost the rule for the elderly disabled person to have disorders of several systems. Both the stroke patient and the amputee commonly have cardiovascular disease or diabetes, or both.

While rehabilitation deals with disability and is not concerned primarily with causes, nevertheless, it is important to know the nature of the condition causing disability. From the standpoint of therapy, the condition may be amenable to medical or surgical treatment that would result in reversal of the disability, as in the case of surgical removal of a spinal cord tumor. Furthermore, medical management of the cause of disability may help to prevent aggravation, progression or recurrence. For instance, control of high blood pressure may prevent recurrent stroke. From the standpoint of prognosis, knowledge of the pathology of disabling conditions makes it possible to predict whether the disability will remain stationary or will progress or regress spontaneously. This knowledge is fundamental for establishment of a rehabilitation plan.

MANAGEMENT OF THE DISABLED

The disabled patient has many more problems than the patient who is just ill and in need of medical care. The disability may interfere with such vital functions as breathing, food intake and elimination, temperature regulation, and personal hygiene. Furthermore, primary disabilities lead to secondary disabilities which in turn have a tendency to snowball and lead to more secondary disabilities. Finally the severely disabled patient nearly invariably becomes a victim of great social, economic, and emotional upheaval. The management of the disabled therefore consists of three basic tasks which are:

1. Maintenance of vital functions (Chap. 2).
2. Prevention of secondary disabilities (Chap. 3).
3. Support of the patient's motivation by attention to his economic, social and emotional problems (Chap. 4).

The specific goal of rehabilitation requires two additional tasks:

1. Training in activities of daily living (Chaps. 5 through 8).
2. Vocational rehabilitation.

REFERENCES

1. Bonner, C. D.: Homburger and Bonner's Medical Care and Rehabilitation of the Aged and Chronically Ill, 3rd Ed. Boston: Little, Brown and Co., 1974.
2. Brunner, L. S. and Suddarth, D. S.: Chap. 1, "Rehabilitation Concepts," in The Lippincott Manual of Nursing Practice. Philadelphia: J. B. Lippincott Co., 1974.
3. Dean, R. J. N.: New Life for Millions: Rehabilitation for America's Disabled. New York: Hastings House, 1972.
4. Krusen, F. H., Kottke, F. J. and Ellwood, P. M. Jr.: Handbook of Physical Medicine and Rehabilitation, 2nd Ed. Philadelphia: W. B. Saunders Co., 1971.
5. Larson, C. B. and Gould, M.: Orthopedic Nursing, 8th Ed. St. Louis: The C. V. Mosby Co., 1974.
6. Licht, S.: Physical Medicine Library, Vol. 10; Rehabilitation and Medicine. New Haven: Elizabeth Licht, 1968.
7. Long, J. M.: Caring for and Caring About Elderly People. Philadelphia: J. B. Lippincott Co., 1974.
8. Rudd, J. L.: Rehabilitation Medicine. Medford, Mass.: WEST, 1969.
9. Rusk, H. A.: Rehabilitation Medicine, 3rd Ed. St. Louis: The C. V. Mosby Co., 1971.
10. Stryker, R. P.: Rehabilitative Aspects of Acute and Chronic Nursing Care. Philadelphia: W. B. Saunders Co., 1972.

2

Maintenance of Vital Functions

Severe disability may strike some vital organs directly. Myocardial infarction or respiratory paralysis may jeopardize circulation or respiration. Bulbar paralysis may prevent swallowing, while bladder and bowel paralysis may interfere with elimination. Severe disability also affects vital functions indirectly because the patient is unable to move. While the heart seems to continue to pump faithfully unless it is directly affected, respiration, nutrition and bladder and bowel function need special attention in the comatose or the paralyzed patient and in those with many other disabilities.

This chapter will deal with the maintenance of nutrition and bladder and bowel function in the severely disabled patient. A detailed discussion of the maintenance of respiratory function is presented in Chapter 17.

NUTRITION

Patients with severely disabling conditions often experience extreme disturbances in nutrition during the early phase of medical management. The survival of many patients with severe strokes, traumatic injuries of the spine or the brain, fractures of the hip or pelvis, amputations, paralyses due to neurotropic virus infections, as well as those with cardiorespiratory decompensation, often depends on intravenously administered fluids. Later, many of these patients require feeding by nasogastric tube, a measure which may have to be continued for weeks. Occasionally, a gastrostomy is substituted for the nasogastric tube, and a liquid or pureed diet is continued by this route. The daily requirement in calories, proteins, fat, carbohydrates, minerals, vitamins, and fluids must be administered. We favor the addition of a potent vitamin supplement, and if the current trend toward the administration of roughage is borne out by further investigation, an adequate amount of roughage should also be blended into this tube-feeding diet.

One would anticipate that in paralyzed patients, who always have an accompanying osteoporosis, the problem of calcium balance would be important. However, the literature on calcium metabolism is confusing and does not support a simple appraisal of calcium needs. For the time being, it is probably best to encourage the patient to stand and exercise as soon as possible when muscle function permits, and to administer a standard calcium diet to paralyzed patients without immediate concern for the formation of kidney stones. The chemical formula of the most common renal stones has changed in the past few years. The most common calcium stone is now calcium oxalate, whereas 20 years ago most renal stones were primarily composed of calcium phosphate.[3] Further information about stones in the urinary tract may be found in Chapter 3 (p. 30), which deals with secondary disabilities, and in Chapter 15 (p. 317), which deals specifically with quadriplegia and paraplegia.

While the maintenance of nutrition is vital during acute and subacute care of severely disabled patients, the major problem encountered in rehabilitation is neither undernourishment nor the difficulty of maintaining nutrition. Far outweighing these is the frequently superimposed handicap of obesity. Weight reduction is a great challenge, especially since it is important to bring about prompt weight loss whenever rehabilitation requires improvement of strength.

Maintenance of Nutrition During the Acute Phase

Fluid administration to maintain electrolyte and water balance is a universal problem in acute medical care that can now be solved with a wide variety of safe, well-controlled solutions, and a well-established technology of biochemical control. The use of intravenous fluids, salts and nutriments for acute phase management of the severely disabled patient is no longer a special problem.

When in the course of acute medical management there is no longer danger of vomiting or aspirating the gastric content, and when there has been sufficient improvement to warrant the use of food, nasogastric intubation may be necessary, because impaired swallowing, esophageal dysfunction or disturbed states of consciousness make ordinary feeding impossible. Most hospital formularies or nursing guides list gastric feeding formulae that are used routinely.

Fortunately, there is a fair variety of these preparations now available. They may be based principally on milk, liquified meat, tomato juice or soy milk. Although they are all nutritionally satisfactory, they may not be equally well tolerated. Diarrhea is a common problem among patients fed with formulae by nasogastric and gastrostomy tubes and a shift in the basic formula may often be indicated. Stools and blood count should be examined and even a blood culture should be obtained in order to be sure that a serious infection is not at the root of the problem. During this investigation, it may be advisable to borrow from folklore and to administer rice water in place of ordinary water, and to add rice or pureed rice to the diet.

Dietary Management in Paralytic Disorders and Forced Immobilization

Immobilization, whether the result of paralysis, enforced bed rest or extensive casting in plaster of Paris, invariably results in osteoporosis, which is a disturbance of the total volume of skeletal bone without change in its composition. It causes atrophy of both the protein matrix and the osseous content of bone. Evidently, the integrity of bone is normally maintained by a combination of weight-bearing and tension on the origins and insertions of muscles which result from motion and activity. In paralytic disorders, weight-bearing in itself is not enough to prevent osteoporosis. Placing paraplegic patients in parallel bars or placing quadriplegics on tilt tables does not significantly diminish calcium loss from bone. Only restoration of muscle strength or the presence of muscle pull due to spasticity (in upper motoneuron paralysis) can arrest osteoporosis caused by disuse. In the course of time the osteoporotic process slows gradually, and calcium loss diminishes. Curiously, even those patients with poliomyelitis who were fortunate enough to become ambulatory soon after the bulbar paralysis subsided continued to lose calcium for some weeks until homeostasis was restored.

Management of Obesity

Obesity is a relative term. In the severely disabled, even a small amount of excess weight may interfere with progress. Since motor strength is used for the movement of a part or all of the body, it is obvious that loss of weight may be equivalent to gain of strength if the weight that is lost represents useless tissue. Of course, it is highly desirable to avoid loss of muscle mass. Such loss results from lower motoneuron paralysis and also from the disuse of innervated muscles. Muscle mass increases as a result of active exercise, and the efficiency of muscle activity is heightened if adipose tissue is diminished to a minimum. Therefore, it is essential to start weight reduction in the obese patient at once, not only to attain normal weight according to standard tables but, in addition, to eliminate all useless adipose tissue. When there is lower motoneuron paralysis, standard tables of normal weight no longer apply. Muscle tissue that has become denervated disappears and is replaced to a considerable degree by fat, which may produce normal-appearing limbs but increases the handicap.

Theoretically, thermodynamic laws should make the management of obesity easy. The intake of foodstuffs is measurable, and can be calculated. Metabolic activities and exercise can be estimated in terms of energy expenditure, and it should be possible to equate the intake and the output to maintain a fixed nutritional balance or to shift the balance toward reduction or gain of weight.

Interestingly, if this theory is put to the test in metabolic experiments, there appears to be no deviation from thermodynamic laws. People who eat less in terms of calories lose weight and those who eat more gain weight. There have been endless speculations about differences in metabolism—"hollow legs" versus "solid legs," "easy keepers" versus "hard keepers," and so forth. Actually, when the experiments are done under controlled circumstances,[1] the deviations disappear. We must therefore assume that the person who gains weight despite a strictly ordered regimen is violating that regimen through the usual devices of snacks, candies and other foods brought by friends. Control of diet is made especially difficult when there are entertainments on the ward and when each person's birthday is celebrated by the usual high carbohydrate foods. Always the staff asks, "Can't she have just a little more today?" an exception that seems to be the rule for not only today but for every day.

Imposition of a stringent reducing diet requires tact and sometimes extreme caution. Patients can become acutely depressed when they are deprived of food, but usually the negative influences of dietary restriction are overcome by the positive effects of an advancing rehabilitation program. In general, however, there is little problem in supervising weight reduction if it is done with full understanding on the part of the patient and with rigorous control on the part of the nursing staff. First, the cooperation of family and friends must be assured by explaining to them the objectives of the program and obtaining their cooperation in avoiding gifts of sweets or other food supplements.

Since lessened activity of the disabled diminishes the need for energy, often it is found that limitation of caloric intake to the usual 1000- or 800-calorie level, which is effective in normal ambulatory individuals, fails to cause weight loss. The elderly disabled, in particular, often seem to require remarkably little food to meet their energy requirements. Accordingly, the diet must be diminished progressively to the 600- or 400-calorie level before daily weighings prove that weight loss is occurring.

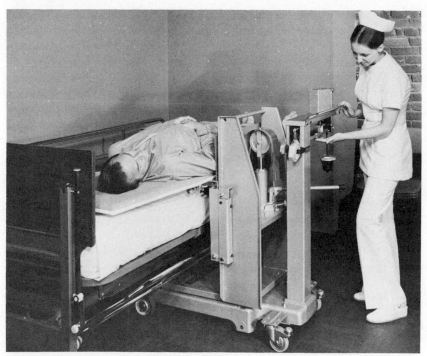

Fig. 2-1. In-Bed Scale. Weighing can be done with a platform scale for those who can stand. Bed patients and those who cannot stand should be weighed with the In-Bed Scale. (Acme Scale Co.)

There is no place for salt restriction or the use of diuretics simply for the removal of excess water from the body in a weight reduction program, unless there is edema (or cardiac disorder). This procedure may produce a psychological boost, but prompt regain of weight is discouraging, and the objective of losing excess adipose tissue is not attained by this means. Fortunately, it is possible to carry out very stringent weight reduction programs in institutions, especially if a regimen of exercise and self-care keeps patients busy enough to prevent boredom and is effective enough to heighten morale. The appetite becomes sharply diminished after the first few days on a 400- to 600-calorie diet, and patients make a much better adjustment to this program than is usually anticipated. Even with such low caloric intake, some patients fail to show daily weight loss. In all probability, fluid retention plays a part; but it is advisable to maintain the best possible balanced diet in terms of protein, carbohydrate and salt, with the expectation that diuresis will occur spontaneously. Of course, intake of sodium chloride should be determined by the patient's cardiorenal status. Frequently, it is necessary to limit sodium chloride intake.

Fasting was in vogue for a time as a dramatic means of losing weight rapidly. The enthusiasm for this method waned very quickly when metabolic studies demonstrated that protein loss was common and that fasting is at times not only dangerous but lethal.

The question often arises as to whether or not it is possible to exercise while undergoing a stringent weight reduction program. There is a prevailing belief that people promptly lose strength if they are maintained on a very low food intake. This belief is not well founded. Continuing exercise is a more important preventive measure than maintaining nutrition, since individuals who continue physical activity apparently do not lose strength, and the depletion of nitrogen that ordinarily occurs with markedly restricted diets can be largely prevented by properly planned low calorie diets. Weak muscles become strong during exercise whether or not the person is receiving food replacement for energy expended.

Low calorie diets that have been effective in weight reduction programs include the following:

Low Calorie Diets

	400 CALORIES	600 CALORIES	800 CALORIES	1,000 CALORIES
Liquid skimmed milk*	1 cup	2 cups	2 cups	2 cups
Low calorie cottage cheese	3 tablespoons	½ cup	¾ cup†	¾ cup†
Low fat meats	1½ oz.	2 oz.	3 oz.†	3 oz.†
Regular meats	1 oz.	. . .	2 oz.	2 oz.
Oil (cotton, corn, safflower)	1 tsp.	. . .	2 tsp.	3 tsp.
Walnuts	. . .	. . .	. . .	6 nuts
Cereal or bread	¼ cup or ½ slice	½ cup or 1 slice	½ cup or 1 slice	½ cup or 1 slice
7% vegetable	¼ cup	½ cup	½ cup	½ cup
3% vegetable	As desired	As desired	As desired	As desired
10% fruit	½ cup	1 cup	1 cup	1½ cups

*For 2 cups skimmed milk, one may substitute 2 oz. of low fat meats.
†For 800 to 1,000 calorie diets, give either ¾ cup cottage cheese or 3 oz. low fat meats.

400 Calorie Diet
Carbohydrate: 10 Gm., Fat: 25 Gm., Protein: 35 Gm.

Breakfast	Lunch	Dinner
1 soft-cooked or poached egg	2 ounces lean meat	2 ounces lean meat
Coffee or tea (no cream or sugar)	Vegetable from List 2	Vegetable from List 2
	Salad (from Vegetable List 2)	Salad (from Vegetable List 2)
	Unsweetened gelatin (D'Zerta)	1 serving fruit from List 1
	Coffee or tea (no cream or sugar)	Coffee or tea (no cream or sugar)

400 Calorie Diet—All Protein
Carbohydrate: 0, Fat: 11 Gm., Protein: 75 Gm.

Eat *only* the following foods:

Breakfast	Lunch	Dinner
2 hard-cooked egg whites	2 ounces white meat of chicken or turkey or white fish	3 ounces white meat of chicken or turkey or white fish
Coffee (no cream or sugar	1 hard-cooked egg white	1 hard-cooked egg white
D'Zerta—if desired	D'Zerta	D'Zerta
	Coffee or tea (no cream or sugar)	Coffee or tea (no cream or sugar)

Meat or fish should be boiled, baked or broiled. Do not add fat in cooking. Coffee or tea may be used as desired. Salt and spices may be used. Do not use sugar. Sugar substitute may be used.

The 400 calorie diet is inadequate in minerals and vitamins. Therapeutic multiple vitamins and minerals should be prescribed.

600 Calorie Diet

Breakfast	Lunch	Dinner
1 serving fruit	1 serving meat (2 oz.)	Clear broth
1 egg (boiled or poached)	Any amount of Vegetable List 2 (raw or cooked)	1 serving meat (2 oz.)
1 cup skimmed milk	1 cup skimmed milk	Any amount of Vegetable List 2 (raw or cooked)
Coffee or tea (no cream or sugar)	Coffee or tea (no cream or sugar)	1 cup skimmed milk
		Coffee or tea (no cream or sugar)

FOOD GROUPS

1. *Fruit List* (Equivalent food values)

Fruits should be fresh or frozen, canned or cooked without sugar. Include at least 1 serving of citrus fruits, such as orange or grapefruit, daily.

Apple	1 small	Grapefruit	½
Applesauce	½ cup	Grapefruit juice	½ cup
Apricots	2 whole	Grapes	12
Bananas	½ small	Grape juice	¼ cup
Blackberries	1 cup	Orange	1 small
Raspberries	1 cup	Orange juice	½ cup
Strawberries	1 cup	Peach	1 small
Blueberries	⅔ cup	Pear	1 small
Cantaloupe	¼ medium	Pineapple	2 slices
Honeydew melon	⅓ medium	Pineapple juice	⅓ cup
Watermelon	1 cup diced	Plums	2
Cherries	10	Raisins	2 tbsp.
Figs	2		

2. *Vegetable List*

Include 1 leafy green and 1 yellow vegetable daily. Do not add fat in preparation.

Asparagus	Sauerkraut
Broccoli	String beans
Brussels sprouts	Wax beans
Cabbage	Summer squashes
Cauliflower	Tomatoes
Celery	Tomato juice
Chicory	Watercress
Cucumbers	*Greens:*
Escarole	Spinach
Eggplant	Beet greens
Lettuce	Chard
Mushrooms	Collard
Okra	Kale
Peppers	Mustard greens
Radish	Turnip greens

3. *Meat, Fish and Poultry List*

Prepare meats without added fat by broiling, roasting or boiling. Canned meats and fish may be used if canned without added oil.

Beef	Turkey	Veal	Game
Chicken	Lamb	Any fish	Liver

The following foods may be substituted for meat:

Cottage Cheese	¼ cup for each ounce of meat
Cheddar Cheese	1 ounce for each ounce of meat
Egg	1 for each ounce of meat

18   *General Considerations*

4. *Miscellaneous*
The following foods may be used as desired:
Gelatin desserts made without sugar (D'Zerta)
Coffee, tea, Sanka, Postum
Herbs, spices, vinegar, catsup, mustard
Horseradish
Unsweetened pickles
Broths and bouillons without fat
Cranberries and rhubarb cooked without sugar (may use
artificial sweetener).

Avoid for low salt diets:
1. Salt or baking soda in preparation of food and at the table
2. Broths and bouillons prepared with salt. Bouillon cubes
3. Smoked, canned, salted or cured meats and fish. Salted cheeses
4. Seasonings which contain salt
5. Read labels to determine if salt or sodium has been added to packaged
   foods.

Whenever a stringent weight reduction program is carried out, a vitamin supplement should be used. This should insure at least the minimal daily requirements and should be continued as long as the weight reduction program is in effect. When optimal weight has been achieved, the diet should be liberalized, especially with respect to protein intake. Fortunately, the habit of eating smaller meals is fairly easy to establish by very limited diet, particularly among patients who become well motivated and stimulated by an obvious improvement in their status. Successful rehabilitation has the advantage of promoting physical and psychological reactions in which the improvement of physical strength and function can cause a psychological stimulation which can help the patient to overcome such unpleasant aspects as dietary restriction.

While there may be no serious contraindication to the use of many so-called appetite suppressants, our experience with the use of these drugs is that they have very transient effects and that they are not worth the trouble of procuring and prescribing. They are inadequate "crutches" and are no substitute for motivation or the discipline required for weight reduction.

Management of Undernutrition

While emphasis has been properly placed on the overweight person, there can be no question that occasionally one deals with a patient whose disability seems to be associated with progressive weight loss. In almost all such cases, the ultimate cause is a serious disease. Since many patients who become rehabilitation candidates are elderly and ill, there is a good deal of undiagnosed cancer, tuberculosis, pancreatitis and liver disease among them. Some persons fail to gain weight simply because they cannot swallow or eat, and others may be so severely depressed that they will not eat or drink. Although such problems are much less common than obesity, they are important and must be dealt with completely and carefully by appropriate diagnostic tests, by consultation and by attempted hyperalimentation.

In almost all instances, patients with spontaneous weight loss regain weight and strength when they become involved in a rehabilitation program. This does not mean that one need not be acutely aware of the possibility of multiple disorders, including some that produce weight loss.

Summary

1. Each phase of treatment of severe disabling conditions requires appropriate nutritional management. Initially, parenteral fluids may be required. If swallowing function or mental incompetence prevents normal feeding, nutritional fluid should be administered by nasogastric tube as soon as possible.

2. Liquid or pureed diet administered via nasogastric tube or gastrostomy should be well balanced and contain all of the essential nutrients, including sufficient fluid, to maintain normal metabolic balance. The question of calcium balance is left in abeyance at this time, since factual data are uncertain and contradictory. There are suitable commercial feedings available for most circumstances. Consideration of the addition of roughage may be warranted.

3. Overweight is the most important nutritional problem in rehabilitation. It must be dealt with promptly and effectively. Prompt weight reduction can be achieved by prescription of very low caloric diets.

4. Weight loss is a less common problem than overweight, yet it requires diagnosis and careful observation with consideration of the possibility of complicating disease.

BOWEL FUNCTION

Although the incessant barrage of radio and television advertising for cathartics may suggest that the human race is generally afflicted with constipation, it is probable that most people have well-established and satisfactory habits of defecation. These habits are easily interrupted by change of environment, by modification of diet and by illness or acute disabling conditions. Since most disabilities have their onset in some illness that causes disruption of all life habits, it is not surprising that management of bowel function becomes extremely important in rehabilitation. It is especially difficult to establish satisfactory bowel habits in people who have been constipated for a long time or are dependent on laxatives and enemas. Although less difficult to manage, those who have had normal bowel habits are also prone to develop acute and long-lasting difficulties of elimination.

Impaction

Acute disabling conditions often are accompanied by both diminution of oral intake and dehydration due to failure to supply adequate parenteral fluid. As a consequence, impaction of feces is very common. In some paralytic disorders, the impaction may occur relatively high in the large intestine, but in most instances the inspissated feces gradually fill the rectum and often distend it.

Impaction may not be suspected in some instances because after a few days of constipation some patients begin to pass liquid or pasty feces, and constipation is assumed to have been relieved. Actually, such fecal material may be expressed around the impaction that grows in size despite frequent bowel movements. Therefore, it is mandatory to perform digital examinations of the rectum every 2 or 3 days during the acute phase management of a recently disabled patient. In this way, impactions can be prevented by appropriate use of enemata or by breaking up firm fecal masses with the examining finger. When a high impaction descends to fill the rectal ampulla it becomes necessary to break up the impaction, to use oil retention enemas if necessary and to evacuate the rectal contents by repeated simple enemata. At times, it may be advisable to delay complete removal of the impaction to avoid exhausting the patient. Sometimes 2 or 3 days of repeated attempts may be necessary before the rectum is thoroughly emptied.

Prevention of Constipation

Measures that can be taken to avoid troublesome constipation and fecal impaction are the relatively simple ones of assuring adequate fluid intake, using wetting agents to maintain a soft stool and, rarely, resorting to bulk-producing agents when food intake is limited or impossible. If intravenous fluid is the only means of providing nutrition during acute phase care, constipation should be anticipated. Unfortunately, the intestinal contents present before the disabling illness may eventually become quite dehydrated and result in impaction. Therefore, it is advisable to replace parenteral feedings with oral or nasogastric feeding as soon as possible, in order to provide liquid and some bulk to the intestinal tract and to nourish the patient by these normal or more nearly normal routes. Tube feedings are by nature low residue diets; therefore, it is unrealistic to expect daily bowel movements. As a matter of fact, it is sometimes advisable purposely to delay defecation in order to avoid physical strain. A week or more of apparent constipation is not harmful unless impaction is allowed to occur.

Adequate fluid intake is the best assurance of satisfactory bowel function both in health and in disease. Adequacy is difficult to define, but in the presence of normal renal function, a fluid intake that assures at least 1500 ml. daily urinary output usually also provides an adequate amount for satisfactory intestinal function. The total amount of fluid, including all soups, beverages, juices and water, should be at least 2 liters daily, assuming that there is additional water content in foods. Often, the disabled person has difficulty in reaching a water bottle or in otherwise procuring fluids. For the severely disabled, it is highly advisable to arrange a plastic bottle with a drinking tube fixed in place, through which frequent sips of water can be taken. To make the water more agreeable, it is advisable to fill the water bottle only to the 1-inch level and place it in a freezer, so as to provide a layer of ice to which water can be added before the bottle is attached at the bedside. It goes without saying that good intake and output measurements are essential, at least until the patient's independence is reestablished and his bowel habits are restored.

Treatment of Constipation

Bowel training is discussed in some detail in Chapter 15. At this point, it is necessary only to state that patience and persistence are the prime requisites for reestablishing bowel habits. As soon as possible, the patient should be encouraged to use the commode in order to achieve a satisfactory posture for defecation. The bedpan should be used for the shortest possible period of time in the management of any illness or disability. A sunken bedpan (Fig. 16-16; p.368) is indicated when motion is painful or effort must be avoided.

Timing is a factor in establishing habit. Most people experience peristalsis soon after a meal. It is advisable, therefore, to provide a commode soon after breakfast, at first without the use of any aids to bowel function. If defecation does not occur, a glycerin suppository may be inserted after the patient returns to bed, and 15 to 30 minutes later he may be placed on the commode again. If fatigue occurs, it is well to wait until the next day, assuming that no impaction is found on rectal examination. If a glycerin suppository does not succeed in starting bowel action, a suppository of bisacodyl (Dulcolax) may be used. Usually, this agent stimulates bowel evacuation after approximately 20 minutes; it may be used safely every other day for a time, after which glycerin suppositories may be tried again and, eventually, ability to evacuate without any stimulation should be tested. To be effective,the Dulcolax suppository must be inserted in such a way that it comes in contact with the rectal wall, not the fecal mass.

During hospitalization, it is advisable to give most patients a wetting agent. The least expensive one is dioctyl sodium sulfosuccinate. It should be administered twice daily in doses of 100 or 250 mg., depending upon the individual patient. Most people do well on 250 mg. twice daily. If a laxative seems indicated and is better tolerated than repeated suppositories, the one which is most successful and least likely to require an increase in dosage, once the amount needed has been determined, is a preparation of senna. A standardized senna concentrate (Senokot) is available in tablet, granule and syrup forms. The appropriate dose can be arrived at by changing it, within the manufacturer's prescribed limits, to find the effective amount. Once established, this preparation may be used every second or third day without change of dose. It is best administered about 1 hour after the evening meal to assure a bowel movement in the morning. A Senokot suppository is also available which is more effective than the glycerin suppository but less certain in its effect than Dulcolax. The use of a laxative is not usually satisfactory in patients with paraplegia or quadriplegia. They are better served by the use of suppositories or the establishment of an enema program.

Patients with paraplegia and some with severe paralysis due to poliomyelitis may be dependent upon bowel stimulation for effective evacuation for years or for life. Patients with hemiplegia and with disabilities that may result in periods of inactivity can almost invariably reestablish normal bowel habits within a relatively short time.

Fecal Incontinence

Fecal incontinence is an unfortunate complication in some patients with paraplegia or quadriplegia. However, this problem always subsides with time, if the general rehabilitation program is successful. Persistent fecal as well as urinary incontinence in patients other than paraplegics is often an indication of psychological deterioration, and in many instances may be traced to inadequate medical and nursing care. Of course, it is true that in patients with severe brain damage, the best conceivable medical and nursing methods are frustrated by irreversible and uncontrollable pathology. Since such intractable brain damage may not be proved clinically, it is always well to give the severely disabled patient the advantage of a trial rehabilitation, including attempts at restoration of bowel function, before accepting the unfavorable prognosis that may eventually be inescapable. All too often failure of method is attributed to nonexistent severe pathology rather than to the faulty procedures and methods used.

Summary

1. Constipation and impaction are common occurrences following disabling injuries or illnesses. Impaction should be suspected even when bowel movements occur; digital examination of the rectum is necessary to prove that stool is not being expressed around impacted feces.

2. Bowel function can be managed by taking advantage of the physiologic effects of fluid intake, by timing the use of the commode to periods of peristaltic activity, and by judiciously using suppositories, stool softeners and senna as a laxative to stimulate bowel evacuation.

3. In all patients except those with severe mental impairment or severe spinal injuries, the reestablishment of a satisfactory bowel routine can be confidently expected if the program is developed with patience, persistence and optimism.

4. Strokes are not a cause of bowel or bladder paralysis.

BLADDER FUNCTION

Bladder function must be closely observed in the severely disabled patient. There are several possible causes of bladder dysfunction, including rupture of the bladder, urinary retention, urinary incontinence and urinary tract infection.

Rupture of the Bladder

In the injured patient first admitted to the hospital, one must always consider the possibility of rupture of the bladder, particularly in patients with fracture of the pelvis. The diagnosis and treatment of this condition are matters of emergency care.

Urinary Retention

Urinary retention occurs in some patients with neurogenic bladder, as in posterior column disease and in the early stages of spinal cord injury. Urinary retention is also seen in disabled elderly males with large prostates. Careful charting of urinary output and checking for abdominal distension help make the diagnosis. Patients with urinary retention require an indwelling catheter; some male patients may require a prostatectomy.

Urinary Incontinence

Urinary incontinence is common in severely disabled patients. However, it is most often due to a lack of communication, and rarely does one deal with true incontinence.

Urinary Incontinence Due to Lack of Communication

Communication is of course impossible with the unconscious patient, and an indwelling catheter is frequently used to keep the patient dry and to obtain urine specimens. If unconsciousness is not likely to be prolonged, however, intermittent catheterization for 2 or 3 days may be used. In a male patient, it is possible to use an external urine-collecting system, such as the condom-drainage tube combination (see Neurogenic Bladder, p. 312).

The obtunded or confused patient is frequently unable to call for the urinal or bedpan in time. But even the physically disabled patient who is mentally alert is frequently unable to get a urinal or bedpan at the proper time. It often takes a long time before the disabled person's call is answered and additional time before he receives the bedpan or urinal. Therefore, many disabled patients simply give up worrying about their bladder function and become functionally incontinent. The patient who can reach for a urinal himself or go to the bathroom usually does not become incontinent.

Disabled patients, whether alert, obtunded or confused, need not be incontinent if a proper method of bladder training is instituted. The word "training" is not entirely appropriate, since patients were already trained as children. The program actually consists of giving patients the assurance that they will have the ability to empty their bladders when they need to do so. This is done by offering them a bedpan or urinal every 2 hours initially, and if it is found that they can stand longer intervals, every 3 hours. Some explanation of the program is needed along with persistent encouragement to use the bedpan when it has been received.

True Incontinence

True incontinence exists among the disabled, particularly those with spinal cord injuries and neurogenic bladder. Their management is described in Chapter 15. It should be pointed out that the stroke patient does not have a neurogenic bladder; he may be incontinent for 2 or 3 days because he is obtunded. During this period he should be allowed either to be incontinent or, if possible, managed by bladder training as described above. He does not require an indwelling catheter and usually becomes continent within a few days of proper bladder training.

Urinary Tract Infection

Urinary tract infection is very common in the disabled. It is, of course, most common in those with a neurogenic bladder because of the use of a catheter and/or the frequent presence of a large amount of residual urine in the bladder. It is also common in the disabled patient without a neurogenic bladder because of immobility and the occasional use of catheterization. Urinalysis and a urine culture should be taken frequently on all patients; however, treatment is best reserved for those patients with symptoms of urinary tract infection (fever, chills and dysuria) except in the care of those with Pseudomonas and Proteus infections. Tests of sensitivity are essential for treatment.

In our opinion, attempts to prevent infection by long-term administration of antimicrobial drugs are not advisable. Since an awareness of urinary tract infection is essential in the care of the patient with a neurogenic bladder, a further discussion of the subject will be found in Chapter 15.

REFERENCES

1. Bell, J. D., Calloway, D. H. and Margen, S. M.: "Ketosis, Weight Loss, Uric Acid and Nitrogen Balance in Obese Women Fed Single Nutrients at Low Calorie Level." Metabolism, 18:193, 1969.
2. Bergstrom, D. A. and Grendahl, B.: Care of Patients with Bowel and Bladder Problems. Minneapolis: American Rehabilitation Foundation, 1968.
3. Elliot, J. S.: "A Comparison of the Chemical Composition of Urine of Normal Subjects and in Patients with Calcium Oxalate Urinary Calculi." Urinary Calculi, Int. Symp. Renal Stone Res. Madrid, 1972. (Karger, Basle, 1973).

3

Prevention of Secondary Disabilities

CAUSES OF SECONDARY DISABILITIES

The secondary disabilities of a patient arise either from inactivity or from contraindicated and injurious activity. The first category, disability due to inactivity, is termed *disuse syndromes*. The second category may be called *misuse syndromes*. In general, both types of secondary disability are preventable. This requires awareness of the specific secondary disabilities that may arise in different conditions and the application of specific means of prevention. Obviously, such preventive practice must begin immediately in the care of all disabled patients; otherwise, a disproportionate amount of effort is expended in dealing with secondary disabilities, many of which cannot be reversed. Unfortunately, at the present stage of rehabilitation medicine, this is the situation which prevails. For example, the expected disability of uncomplicated hemiplegia is paralysis of the extremities and the lower face on one side of the body. If a hemiplegic is neglected and does not start a program of adaptive and rehabilitative therapy, in all likelihood, in the course of weeks he will develop such complicating disorders as bed sores, urinary tract infection, painful and contracted joints, deformity of the leg and the foot, constipation and bowel impaction and urinary incontinence. These disorders are much more disabling than the hemiplegia. Depression and lack of motivation accompany the physical deterioration due to disuse.

Causes of Disuse

Disuse is caused by restrictions or conditions imposed on a person because of the existence of *disease* or disorder, or as a consequence of a particular habit or *way of life*. In extreme situations, for example, the binding of female infants' feet to satisfy an esthetic standard among the ancient Chinese, secondary disabilities may be imposed willfully. In our culture, more subtle but very disabling conditions result from our way of life. Our esthetic standards prescribe footwear that leads to heel cord shortening due to high heels; corns and calluses due to tight shoes; and bunions and toe deformities due to improper shape of shoes. Technologic development which has eliminated the need for most strenuous physical activities is responsible for muscular weakness, overweight, limited range of motion and deconditioning of the cardiorespiratory system. The consequence of inactivity is popularly known as impairment of physical fitness.

In sickness disuse may be due to a number of causes. The principal ones are:

1. Enforced rest, in bed or chair, during illness or convalescence.
2. Restricted activity because of vocational or cultural habits.
3. Mental disorders that cause immobilization, e.g., catatonia.
4. Immobilization as a result of braces, casts or corsets. Here, only the immobilized parts may suffer disuse.
5. Paralysis.
6. Joint stiffness.
7. Pain. Painful disorders of the joints and the surrounding soft tissues lead to protective limitation of motion and produce local disuse effects. If the involvement is generalized, the disuse effects may be systemic.
8. Loss of sensation. Normally, change of position is stimulated by discomfort. In the absence of sensory stimuli, a position may be maintained for too long a time with resulting damage.

All chronic and disabling diseases and conditions result in one or several of the above listed causes of disuse. Disuse syndromes are the most common and the most serious complications of chronic illness. Not only are there physical aspects that increase disability, but there are always parallel mental changes that may become dominant in any syndrome. It is important to realize that often the primary disability is greatly overshadowed by the unanticipated effects of disuse.

Each of the disuse phenomena leads to further inactivity and thereby aggravation and extension of disuse. The chronically ill patient with weakness, pressure sores, contractures, osteoporosis, incontinence, etc., all combined, is too common a sight in nursing homes and chronic-disease hospitals. Frequently, the initial disease state is negligible as a cause of disability as compared with the deteriorative effects of disuse.

Causes of Misuse

As the name implies the secondary disabilities due to misuse are caused by inappropriate activities. Though this is much less common than inactivity or disuse, misuse disabilities do occur in the later stages

General Considerations

of rehabilitation. The patient rarely suffers damage in an activity he should not do at all. Often misuse disability is due to lack of protection such as an injury during a transfer or during ambulation. Frequently it is due to the lack of adequate support to a body part, such as a painful shoulder in the hemiplegic patient or an unstable knee in the arthritic patient.

DISUSE SYNDROMES

Atrophy of Skeletal Muscle

If a muscle or a muscle group is not used for relatively strenuous exercise at fairly regular intervals, the muscle mass diminishes in volume. This is seen, for example, in the shrinkage of a limb after application of a cast. There is diminution in muscle strength as well as size.

Denervation Atrophy. The greatest disuse occurs in denervated muscle, that is, muscle that has lost its nerve supply. Moreover, this type of atrophy cannot be reversed by exercise, because voluntary movement of such muscle is not possible.

Disuse Atrophy. Muscle fibers that have not been contracted for some time gradually diminish in size, and the proportion of muscle fiber and connective tissue in a particular muscle changes so that there is more and more fibrous tissue and less and less muscle mass. If the muscle is exercised, the size of the muscle fibers increases again. Muscular atrophy of an innervated muscle is reversible.

Muscle atrophy generates additional weakness and therefore adds to the individual's overall disuse. This establishes a vicious cycle that leads to physical and psychological deterioration.

Contractures of Joints

A contracture is a limitation of the range of motion caused by shortening of soft tissue structures around a joint. As a disuse phenomenon this disability occurs whenever a joint is not moved frequently through its range of motion. Contracture may also occur as a primary disability, e.g., from scars, Dupuytren's contracture, etc.

Clinically, limitation of range of motion due to contracture is detected when one attempts to move a joint passively through its full range. There is either sensation of resistance that blocks further motion without any special discomfort to the patient, or there is pain and active resistance by the patient. In true contracture, there is limitation of motion even when the patient is anesthetized.

The most common and most disabling contractures are hip flexion contractures, knee flexion contractures and contractures of the shoulder. Knee and hip flexion contractures develop commonly in the patient who is confined to a chair or a wheelchair or lies on his side or in Fowler's position in bed. In these positions full extension of the hips and the knees never occurs. Knee and hip flexion contractures also result from spastic paraplegia. In this case, the spasticity of the flexor muscles maintains the patient's knees and hips in a flexed position. Pain or paralysis around the shoulder girdle predisposes to contracture. If severe, it is called "frozen shoulder." Plantar flexion contractures of the feet and the toes may arise from pressure of tight bed covers and also from a combination of paralysis and the pull of gravity.

Any joint of the body may become contracted. Frequently, contractures tend to get worse, particularly if they are painful. Reversal of contractures can be effected by stretching, casting or surgical procedures. The prognosis for reversing contracture in an elderly patient is poor.

Metabolic Disturbances

Osteoporosis. Osteoporosis is a wasting of bone, characterized by simultaneous loss of bone matrix and minerals. This occurs whenever a skeletal part is immobilized and muscular pull against bone is absent or diminished. Osteoporosis occurs also as a primary disorder in hyperparathyroidism and Cushing's disease and often after menopause. This condition is recognized on x-ray pictures by diminished density or opacity of bone.

Osteoporosis is disabling for the following reasons: (1) it may cause pain; (2) it leads to fractures; and (3) it leads to excessive excretion of calcium and may lead to the formation of stones in the urinary tract.

Stones in the Urinary Tract. *Causes of Stone Formation.* Many disuse factors may contribute to stone formation, including: (1) increased calcium excretion through the kidneys (hypercalciuria) because of demineralization of bones, (2) stagnation of urine in the kidney pelvis or the bladder because of supine position or inadequate change of position, (3) urinary tract infections that are common in the severely disabled, especially in those who have residual urine, and (4) alkaline urine due to diet or infection with urea-splitting organisms which favors precipitation of calcium salts.

Types of Stones. Kidney stones are often silent. Ureteral stones give rise to renal colic, and bladder stones may cause suprapubic discomfort. Irrespective of the location, stones lead to persistence of infection of the urinary tract. Dilatation of the ureters and the kidney pelves, impairment of function, and finally, destruction of the kidney may result from partial ureteral obstruction and chronic infection.

Hypercalciuria and the threat of stone formation can be diminished by activity and proper attention to infections of the urinary tract. (See Chapter 15.)

Circulatory Disturbances

Orthostatic Hypotension. This disorder is defined as the rapid fall of blood pressure when a recumbent patient is placed in an upright position. It is seen in patients who have been bedridden or have not been in upright position for a prolonged period. It is especially marked in patients who have had a lumbar sympathectomy and in paraplegics or quadriplegics. The patient faints when the blood pressure is inadequate to supply blood to the brain. If the patient is maintained in an upright position, brain damage and even death may result.

Fall of blood pressure in this case is caused by dilatation of the blood vessels in the abdomen and the lower extremities under the weight of the blood volume accumulating in the lower portions of the body when the patient is upright. Normally, the blood vessels have enough power to contract reflexly under this pressure and reduce the volume. However, in paralysis and prolonged disuse the blood vessels have lost the power of reflex contraction. They will regain it if subjected to greater pressures by a program of gradual adaptation to the upright position.

Phlebothrombosis. Fixed position and lack of motion in the lower extremities may lead to venous thrombosis. This in turn may cause pulmonary embolism, which is often fatal. Radioisotope scans of the lungs have shown pulmonary embolism to be very frequent.

Hypostatic Pneumonia. The supine position during bed rest, or prolonged rest on one side, often leads to lung congestion and pneumonia.

Pressure Sores. Pressure sores or ulcers are defined as areas of necrosis caused by excessive and prolonged pressure. They may involve skin, muscle, fascia and bone. They must be distinguished from other sores that can develop in a bedridden patient, such as (1) superficial abrasions of the skin due to irritation and maceration by sweat or urine, (2) lacerations that result from injury when, because of lack of muscular control, the patient's limb strikes a hard object and (3) furuncles or pustules that break down and leave a temporarily ulcerated area. To a certain extent these types of ulceration can be prevented by protection and cleanliness. However, contrary to what is commonly taught, true pressure sores cannot be prevented simply by keeping the patient clean and dry. It is pressure that causes true pressure sores, and it does so whether the skin is dry or wet, clean or soiled.

Pressure sores occur where a bony prominence is separated from the bed by only a thin layer of tissue. For this reason, the common sites of pressure sores are the sacrum, the greater trochanter and the ischial tuberosities.

Sacral pressure sores occur in patients maintained in the back-lying position. Usually these ulcers become rather wide because of the large area of the sacrum that compresses the soft tissue.

Trochanteric pressure sores result from prolonged lying on either side and are caused by compression of tissue between the greater trochanter of the femur and the bed. Trochanteric pressure sores tend to be round and small.

Ischial pressure sores result from prolonged sitting and the compression of tissues between the ischial tuberosities and the underlying surface.

Whatever the location, true pressure sores undergo a characteristic clinical evolution. The skin first becomes red and may develop a large blister. The discolored area darkens gradually and becomes black and hard. Over a period of weeks, the necrotic tissue is sloughed off gradually, leaving a deep ulcer. If no further pressure is exerted, this area will gradually fill in with granulation tissue over a period of weeks or months; finally, skin will grow over it.

Though the development of the ulcer may take several weeks because of the delay in sloughing of dead tissue, a pressure ulcer frequently is caused by one period of continued pressure. The damage may occur following as little as an hour of immobility and pressure! The only way to prevent this damage is to ensure frequent change of position.

Sphincter Disturbances

Constipation and also bladder and bowel incontinence are disuse phenomena. The patient, unable to go to the toilet, readily becomes constipated. Inability to obtain a bedpan or a urinal when needed also leads to incontinence. The latter goes hand in hand with the general psychological deterioration of the disabled patient.

Psychological Deterioration

After prolonged inactivity and subjection to a hospital regimen, the disabled patient shows loss of interest and initiative and develops personality changes characterized by dependence, aggression or withdrawal. Often, the basic psychological change is manifested by loss of appetite, incontinence and increasing loss of ability to communicate. These apparently organic disturbances are almost always attributed erroneously to advancing pathology.

Most of the above described disuse phenomena result principally in secondary disability. However, some of them contribute to morbidity and may cause death—for example, hypostatic pneumonia, phlebothrombosis, embolism, etc.

Prevention of Disuse Syndromes

Most of the disuse syndromes listed, and many other morbid effects of inactivity, can be prevented effectively by three therapeutic measures. These measures are simple. In fact, they are so simple that commonly they are ignored. They become a problem only because there is time involved in carrying them out. It is important to remember that a normal person does not lie still, even for as long as ½ hour at a time, whether awake or asleep. However, the paralyzed or immobilized patient or the patient in pain or under the influence of narcotics or anesthetics is likely to spend long periods of time without moving.

The total amount of activity sufficient to prevent physical disuse phenomena need not exceed 2 hours in a 24-hour period. However, it must be interspersed, among other scheduled events, in such a way that the patient does not remain inactive for more than 1 hour at a time. Pressure sores, it is emphasized, may develop if a change of position is not effected within an hour.

The three measures to prevent physical disuse are: (1) active exercise, (2) passive mobilization and (3) frequent change of position. For these measures to be carried out effectively the patient must have a proper bed with a firm smooth mattress and adequate foot room and a suitable chair.

Active Exercises

The prescribed exercise must be strenuous, and, though it need last for only a few minutes, it should be repeated several times daily. Turning from side to side, from back to abdomen and moving up and down on the bed are excellent exercises for a bedridden patient. Such a program will counteract most of the disuse syndromes described.

Passive Mobilization

Moving all joints through their full range of motion is necessary whenever active motion is not possible. If the patient has enough strength, he should be instructed in the technique of mobilizing his paralyzed limbs himself by using his nonparalyzed parts. Where paralysis is extensive, passive mobilization will have to be done by a nurse or therapist. It is important to ascertain that the range of motion performed is complete. This program prevents formation of contractures. It must be carried out with extreme care to prevent injury to joints, especially in those with sensory defects. In hemiplegia, the degree of passive mobilization of the shoulder may be restricted initially to prevent injury.

Frequent Change of Position

There are several positions in which a patient may be placed: standing, sitting, face-lying, back-lying and side-lying. Each patient should be given the advantage of all these positions insofar as this is possible. No one should be kept in any one of these positions for more than 1 hour, preferably not over ½ hour, without some change of position. If the patient stays in one position for ½ hour, he should relieve pressure over the areas of support for at least 60 seconds. In

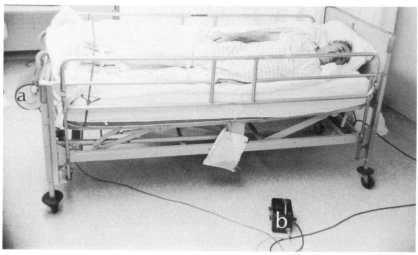

Fig. 3-1. "Cloud Nine" mattress. The patient is turned at regular intervals by alternately inflating the right or the left half of the mattress with air. The pump (a) is at the foot of the bed. A control box (b) permits the operator to select an automatic rate of turning of from 1- to 60-minute intervals.

standing position this can be done by shifting the weight from one foot to the other. In a sitting position it is done by the patient pushing himself up with both arms and staying off his seat for 60 seconds. In the lying position the change can be made by shifting temporarily from the side to the back for 60 seconds, or vice versa. If this cannot be done by the patient, he should be turned. Change of position, it is re-emphasized, is essential in the prevention of pressure sores. If it is done actively, it also counteracts muscle atrophy, contractures and demineralization of bones. A mechanical method of turning the patient from side to side is provided by the "Cloud Nine" mattress. The patient lies on two plastic bags which are inflated alternately at intervals from 5- to 6-minutes by an air pump (Fig. 3-1). Since positioning is limited to two side-lying positions, it must be supplemented by other methods.

Often, the use of the face-lying position is neglected. Yet it is the optimum position for drainage of the bronchial tree, and it is valuable for stretching the trunk and the extremity muscles.

Another important position is the standing position. It can be assumed easily by the patient who is able to stand. Patients who cannot stand by themselves have to be placed in upright position with the aid of a tilt table or a standing board. If the patient has orthostatic hypotension, he must wear a tight scultetus abdominal binder for this procedure, and his blood pressure should be observed closely while he is first being brought to a standing position. Weight-bearing in an upright position helps to prevent many of the above-mentioned disuse syndromes. It is effective against orthostatic hypotension and helpful in preventing demineralization of bones and the development of urinary tract stones.

Special Pads and Mattresses for Prevention of Pressure Sores. The search for a special device or mattress to help prevent pressure ulceration has continued for years. However, none of the current devices replaces vigilant personal care. Sheepskin pads have been so popular that a false sheepskin has been fabricated. Since sheepskin was supposed to have special merit because of the lanolin in the wool it is obvious that the ersatz variety must be credited with a psychosomatic effect. Alternating pressure pads have come and gone. A variety of useful seat pads has been developed for wheelchairs but here too the patient must have respite from sitting.

Water beds of various kinds have been credited with virtues that have yet to be subjected to scientific study.

Summary

Disuse Phenomena

Condition	Cause	Prevention
1. Muscle atrophy (weakness)	Lack of exercise	Exercise
2. Joint contracture (limited range)	Lack of joint motion	Passive range of motion and splinting
3. Metabolic disturbances:		
a. Osteoporosis	Lack of weight-bearing and muscle pull	Tilt table and stand-up exercises
b. Stones of the urinary tract	Demineralization of bone	Mobilization
	Urinary tract infection	Avoidance of urinary tract infection
		Minimal use of catheter
4. Circulatory disturbances:		
a. Orthostatic hypotension	Recumbent position	Tilt table and stand-up exercises
b. Venous thrombosis	Slowed venous flow	Change of position and exercise
		Anticoagulants
c. Hypostatic pneumonia	Lack of chest expansion, poor position	Change of position and exercise, especially face-lying position
d. Pressure sores	Prolonged pressure	Change of position
		Special pads and mattresses
5. Sphincter disturbances:		
a. Urinary incontinence	Lack of opportunity	Urinal or bedpan instead of indwelling catheter
b. Constipation	Improper diet	Regular use of toilet or bedside commode
	Lack of activity	
	Lack of opportunity	Adequate fluids; diet
		Medication
6. Psychological deterioration	Inactivity	Maximal activity
	Isolation	Liberal visiting and social privileges
	Separation from accustomed environment	Flexible program
	Institutional routine	Active participation in planning program

MISUSE SYNDROMES

The disorders due to misuse that are commonly seen in the severely disabled are due either to injury or to undue stress to a paralyzed or damaged part, most frequently a joint. The three major misuse syndromes that will be discussed are the painful shoulder syndrome following shoulder girdle paralysis, the hyperextended knee (back knee) associated with paralysis and the progressively unstable joint in arthritis.

Paralyzed Painful Shoulder

More than 50 per cent of stroke patients develop shoulder pain in the hemiplegic arm. In other types of paralysis, e.g., poliomyelitis and traumatic quadriplegia, painful shoulder occurs even more frequently. While the cause of shoulder pain associated with paralysis has not been established, it can be assumed that injury to structures of the shoulder joint is often responsible. The weight of the arm alone is sufficient to injure a joint that is dependent entirely on weak ligaments for support. In addition, handling the extremity during bathing, turning and dressing imposes greater stresses on the joint structures. When there is sensory loss associated with paralysis, even careful range of motion exercises may cause unremarked injury. Careless handling, especially in emergency transportation or in transfer to litter, operating table or x-ray table, almost invariably causes damage.

While it is customary to provide a paralyzed upper extremity with a sling support when the patient is out of bed, lack of support during bed nursing procedures is sufficient to account for injury. Therefore, it would be advisable to protect the paralyzed upper extremity against injury at all times. Unfortunately, a satisfactory method of immobilization has not yet been developed. Under the circumstances, it would seem to be advisable to apply a sling before the patient is moved rather than afterward. Those who are assigned to assist in the care of persons with paralyzed upper extremities must be fully informed of the need to be careful and gentle at all times.

Back Knee Deformity

Back knee deformity is commonly observed following paralysis of the quadriceps, the hamstrings or the gastrocnemius muscles. A completely paralyzed lower extremity can bear weight if the knee is hyperextended and locked. The danger of the back knee position is progressive relaxation of the ligaments of the knee joint that leads to instability and pain.

To prevent progressive back knee deformity, patients with marked quadriceps weakness must be provided with a long leg brace before being permitted to ambulate. If a patient with adequate quadriceps strength shows a tendency to back knee, first an attempt should be made to instruct him to walk with the knee slightly flexed. If he cannot avoid hyperextending the knee, he too will have to be braced.

The fact that a few people tolerate back knee deformity for years without discomfort is no argument against using proper protective bracing. As the asymptomatic person becomes older, the threat of instability and injury increases. By the time the deformity is a true handicap, it is often impossible to apply adequate protective devices.

The Progressively Unstable Joint

Serious disability, much of it preventable, occurs when weight-bearing joints are unprotected while the joint is actively inflamed or after mechanical defect has developed. The most vulnerable of the weight-bearing joints are the knees. Whether the initial pathologic disorder is in the cartilage or the ligaments, damage to either of these structures sets up a cycle of progressive instability. Usually, this leads to valgus (knock knee) deformity with additional mechanical disadvantage and further destruction. Often, people with knee instability of advanced degree have to walk with crutches with their knees constantly in contact for stability. Corticosteroid medication contributes to destruction of unprotected joints by relieving pain that might otherwise restrict weight-bearing and also by causing osteoporosis.

Of the non-weight-bearing joints, the fingers in rheumatoid arthritis are most likely to become unstable. Frequently, the interphalangeal joints and the metacarpophalangeal joints become dislocated. Obviously, in the management of disorders of these delicate structures, both excessive use of the hands in work and vigorous physical therapy are contraindicated. Unfortunately, patients with rheumatoid arthritis tolerate splints poorly, even when they are fully aware that support is the only means to prevent progressive deformity.

REFERENCES

1. Bergstrom, D. and Coles, C. H.: Basic Positioning Procedures. Minneapolis: Kenny Rehabilitation Institute, 1971.
2. Ellwood, P. M., Jr.: "Bed Positioning," in Krusen, F. H., Kottke, F. J. and Ellwood, P. M. Jr.: Handbook of Physical Medicine and Rehabilitation, 2nd Ed. Philadelphia: W. B. Saunders Co., 1971.

3. Kosiac, M.: "Etiology of Decubitus Ulcers," APMR, 42:19, 1961.
4. Kosiac, M.: "Decubitus Ulcers," in Krusen, F. H., Kottke, F. J. and Ellwood, P. M., Jr.: Handbook of Physical Medicine and Rehabilitation, 2nd Ed. Philadelphia: W. B. Saunders Co., 1971.
5. Toohey, P. and Larson, C. W.: Range of Motion Exercises: Key to Joint Mobility. Minneapolis: Kenny Rehabilitation Institute, 1968.

CHAPTER

4

Economic, Social, and Emotional Effects of Disability

Definitions. The word *economic* in this chapter refers solely to the financial effect of disability upon the patient. The cost of disability to the economy of the country is not within the scope of this book.

The word *social* as used here refers to the disabled person's function and role in society. This includes the attitudes of society toward the disabled. The word social may also refer to special care for the underprivileged, as used in social welfare and social legislation. Since this is provided essentially in monetary awards, it should logically be dealt with under economic aspects of disability.

Emotional response requires little definition. We shall describe the varieties of emotional reactions and resulting behavior related to disability.

The interplay of economic, social and emotional factors is great. The economic status of a person has an effect upon his social role in society and his associations. A drastic change in social status may have a profound effect upon his emotional reactions.

ECONOMIC EFFECTS OF DISABILITY
Minimal or No Effects

There are two groups of people whose economic status is only minimally affected by permanent disability: The very rich, who do not have to work for a living and for whom the additional cost resulting from their disability makes only a small dent into their fortunes, and the very poor who were supported by welfare programs prior to the disability. Other people whose economic status may not be seriously affected by disability are those who require relatively short-term care for the illness or injury causing the disability, have adequate insurance for medical costs and rehabilitation care, possibly have income protection insurance or continued wages or salaries and are capable of resuming their former occupations despite or without permanent disability.[6]

Awareness of the economic impact of disability on the patient early in the rehabilitation program may prevent severe economic losses to the disabled. An example is the case of a 40-year-old woman who suffered a cerebral vascular accident, with resulting right hemiplegia. At the time, she was employed as a bookkeeper in a bank. She was evaluated in a rehabilitation center within a few days after her stroke. The evaluation revealed that she would be completely independent and self-caring and able to walk and drive a car. However it was rather unlikely that she would recover enough function in her right arm to be able to write with it. For this reason, the physician insisted that she immediately start practicing left-handed writing for several hours a day in addition to her physical rehabilitation program. The patient accepted this reluctantly. After 3 weeks she was independent in all activities of daily living, and after 6 weeks she was able to drive her car with her left hand. She was then advised to have an interview with her employer to discuss resumption of her former job. She was told that there was no objection to her left-handed writing, but that she would have to be ready to return to work within 2 weeks. Since she had already been practicing left-handed writing, the patient was soon ready to resume her job as a bookkeeper. *Had she not started to practice left-handed writing immediately* after her stroke, she would have lost her job and as a hemiplegic she might never have found another one. This would, of course, have entailed a great economic loss to her. This case may serve as an example of how an efficient and foresighted rehabilitation program may prevent economic loss to the disabled.

Untoward Effects of Disability

The vast majority of the severely disabled patients suffer great economic losses because of their permanent disabilities. Like death, disability can be a great social leveler, at least among those below the level of great wealth. The successful businessman, the high-level executive, the professional with an above-average income as well as the average earner may all ultimately join the poor on the welfare rolls if struck by severe disability. With adequate medical and vocational rehabilitation services, however, a large number of the severely disabled may achieve a certain level of economic self-sufficiency.

The untoward economic effects of disability vary according to whether the disabled person is self-employed, employed, or retired.

The Self-employed Person

The self-employed businessman or professional person is very likely to lose a considerable amount of money during the phase of his medical and rehabilitative care. Not only does he suffer a loss of income during that period, but his business expenses may continue. An early full rehabilitation evaluation is important, so that the patient can be advised of what permanent disability he can expect. He can then decide whether it will be possible for him to continue his business or profession with such a disability. If this is not the case, it would be economically best for him to sell or liquidate his business as quickly as possible in order to reduce his expenses. The owner of a successful business can turn the direction over to capable subordinates, but a small businessman whose physical labor is needed to support the business may have to give it up.

In general, the self-employed person has a better chance to return to his former occupation than the employed person because he is not dependent upon the prejudices of the employer. The following two illustrations of a successfully rehabilitated physician and a similarly rehabilitated lawyer point to the truth of this statement.

One example of a self-made rehabilitatee is that of a physician who was practicing in a medium-sized California town and was a popular and much sought after general practitioner, when he developed poliomyelitis in 1948. The disease rendered him quadriplegic, with respiratory paralysis, and to this day he has not spent a night outside an iron lung. With precious little help, he learned how to adjust to auxiliary breathing devices, he mastered glossopharyngeal breathing and he undertook the study of dermatology and allergy, since these specialties would not require much mobility and would permit him to practice largely in an office. He set up his home and office on adjacent properties, and in time, built a charming garden between the two houses. With the assistance of a capable nursing staff he has developed a huge practice which permits him to treat large numbers of patients with allergies and skin diseases.

Many tales could be told about this man. He has, for example, traveled widely in a specially built van which holds his iron lung. One Monday morning he reported that he had just returned from Kings Canyon National Park, some 300 miles from his residence. He has succeeded not only in developing a medical practice, but he and his working wife have educated their four children, and a fifth child who is a relative. They are now the proud parents of a young physician and four other college educated children.

The ingenuity of the severely disabled is further illustrated by the case history of a practicing lawyer who was also paralyzed by poliomyelitis. He had a stormy convalescence, but eventually returned to his practice by designing an automobile to meet his needs. Confined to a wheelchair and dependent upon a portable respirator, he was able to lower the right front portion of his car, swing out a ramp, swing into position, strap himself into an operator's seat, start the car and travel with the security of a triple brake system. He thus became entirely independent on the road, which permitted him to go to court, carry out legal investigations and conduct a thriving law practice.

The Employed Person

Compared to the self-employed person, the employed individual suffers a minor economic loss during the initial phase of the medical care and rehabilitation. His medical cost is usually covered by insurance, and his income is at least partially substituted either by sick-leave pay or similar compensation in combination with state or private insurance for disability. If he becomes ill or is injured during and as a result of his employment, his medical expenses, rehabilitation costs, and income may all be supplied by Workmen's Compensation Insurance. However, the resources available to the injured salaried person, or the wage earner, are usually at subsistence level and do not provide an adequate income.

No attempt will be made to analyze all the various sources of benefits available to the injured or ill person. Some attempt will be made, however, to classify the principal resources because of the great amount of confusion that exists concerning the avenues open to an injured or ill employed person.

Nonwork-connected Disability. If an employed person suffers work loss because of illness or disability, he should immediately apply for benefits from the state agency or private insurance company which pays for sickness disability. Titles of the agencies vary from state to state, as do rules about alternate insurance coverage. Usually, the state agency is affiliated with the department of employment and the insurance is closely related to unemployment insurance. In most jurisdictions, payment is made for a maximum of 26 weeks and the amount of the weekly benefits depends partially upon wage and partially upon the limits set by the jurisdiction in charge. During periods of excessive unemployment, both unemployment insurance and sickness disability insurance may be extended for an additional 13 weeks or so. This insurance carries with it only a minimal time limit for the partial payment for hospitalization, usually up to 10 days. No other medical benefits are provided. So-called health insurance, which is actually medical insurance, is often written for groups of employees and may be a union fringe benefit. This pays part of hospital and medical costs and has a limitation which is imposed by the contract.

Work-connected Disability. If a person sustains an injury (sickness or accident) arising out of and in the course of his employment, he is, depending upon the restrictions listed in the laws of various jurisdictions, entitled to *partial income replacement, medical care* and *rehabilitation costs* on the basis of Workmen's Compensation Insurance. If he is in doubt about his eligibility for this insurance, he may receive sickness disability benefits, provided he signs a lien against the possibility of payments by Workmen's Compensation, which will reimburse the agency paying the benefits.

The permanently disabled employed person may have great difficulty in finding employment again, either because he is physically handicapped for his job, or merely because of the attitude of employers (see Attitudes of Employers, p. 47). If he has the intellectual ability, he may be retrained in another trade or profession with assistance from the Social Rehabilitation Service (SRS), an agency financed jointly by state and federal government. The tendency of this organization has been to train the disabled person in skills which allow him to be more or less self-employed, such as in accounting or clinical psychology. However, the severely disabled laborer invariably remains unemployed for the rest of his life, and is ultimately meagerly supported by welfare. Some may be eligible for small additional benefits, such as veterans' disability benefits, Social Security or Workmen's Compensation permanent disability benefits if their disability is work-connected. Even with several of such benefits, the disabled person is usually impoverished in relation to his predisability income.

Retired Person with Savings

Disability can create one of the worst economic catastrophes for the retired person who has managed to save money to have a reasonably comfortable and independent old age. Such financial loss due to disability was more severe before the enactment of the Medicare law, because an older person's savings were often used to pay for medical care, his sickness insurance had ended with his job or with his age and he had no resources to pay adequately for medical care or rehabilitation. The extent to which Medicare has alleviated his plight depends partly upon the patient's understanding of the law, partly upon the aggressive nature of his physicians and principally upon the precise compliance of the rehabilitation center or activity with the bureaucratic determinations of those who determine eligibility.

The retired person usually stands a very good chance at becoming a recipient of welfare benefits. If he is significantly disabled, he may well have to give up his home and family and spend the rest of his life in a so-called convalescent hospital. His fate is at best unpredictable.

Beneficial Economic Effects of Disability

It can be stated categorically that disability is practically never economically beneficial. It can also be said, with almost equal authority, that the economic benefits of disability when added to the disability itself usually end on the negative side of the ledger. Even in those few instances of benefit, the amount of money is relatively small as, for example, in the case of a welfare client. On "general relief," he may receive $90 a month (1974 California), while on the "Aid to the Disabled" program he may receive $120 a month.

Though true economic benefit from disability is nil or nonexistent, the desire of some patients to benefit may greatly prolong or aggravate a disability, or even make it permanent. This is sometimes seen in workmen's compensation cases or in other forms of litigation. It must be pointed out that these cases represent only a very small number of the total, but because of their very protracted course and the frustration they create for physicians, lawyers and agencies, they constitute an impressive problem.

SOCIAL EFFECTS OF DISABILITY

The social life and social role of the disabled are markedly affected by two factors: the *physical limitation* imposed by illness and disability, and the *attitude* that prevails toward the disabled in this society.

Social Effects of Physical Limitation
Effect of Hospitalization

During the acute care of illness and injury and during hospitalization, the patient is obviously limited in his social contacts and undergos a change in his social status by adopting the "sick role."[8] It is generally accepted that when a person becomes ill he is not required to work and earn a living, but he must make an effort to regain his health so that he can assume his former role.[5]

The patient's acceptance of the sick role *per se* requires only a minor adjustment; however, unavoidably, hospitalization takes him away from his family and usual surroundings. It interferes with his sex life and his customary associations with family and friends. However, it can be compensated for by visits from friends and family, get-well cards, flowers and gifts. It is important, then, that his hospital life permit as much social contact as possible. In certain instances, however, because of the nature of the injury or illness or the nature of his treatment, the patient may suffer social deprivation, the effects of which will be emotional. These effects will be discussed in more detail under Emotional Effects of Disability, p. 50.

Hospitalization also leads to the involuntary association of the disabled patient with hospital staff and fellow patients. This new association may be salutary if the patient has a friendly relationship with the staff and if he encounters a patient with a similar disability who makes him feel less isolated. On the other hand, incompatibility and, worse, hostility towards staff or fellow patients may create emotional problems which delay his recovery.

Whatever the social stresses of hospitalization may be, they are only temporary, and the patient realizes that sooner or later he will return to his own life. On the other hand, some underprivileged patients adjust so well to the hospital society that they fear and resist discharge.

Effects of Permanent Disability

Once the patient's condition has stabilized and he has left the hospital or rehabilitation center, he may still be physically limited by a permanent disability which may affect his social role and status. If he is too disabled to earn a living, his wife may become the supporter of the family. In some instances, he may become a welfare recipient and experience a considerable decline of his social status. The physical disability may also lead to a change in his associations. Not uncommonly, the disability of one partner affects marital or sexual life and leads to divorce.[1] On the other hand, a single disabled person might find it desirable to get married and may choose a partner who fits his needs. Disabled people do not necessarily change their social associations, but it is likely that a former hunter or fisherman may lose contact with his sports associates and, instead, join an indoor sports club or another organization such as the Paraplegic Association. It is certainly not necessary for a disabled person to become socially isolated unless he desires to do so.

Social Effects of Public Attitudes

The public has a generally negative attitude toward the disabled and the elderly.[7] That this is so is indicated immediately by the fact that there has to be protective legislation for both elderly and disabled citizens. If special laws are necessary to protect these people or to assure the employment rights of members of other racial or cultural minorities, there is clear evidence that these groups are being mistreated, abused or discriminated against by the public. The prejudice in the public is most clearly seen with respect to attitudes in employment. The elderly are not only unable to find employment, but their work is often arbitrarily ended when they are retired, frequently at the age of 65 or earlier, regardless of their competence. The employment difficulties encountered by the elderly are similar to those of the minorities, and of the disabled. It seems that close contact with the disabled is most objectionable to the public.

Attitudes of Employers

In general, employment policies are directed toward screening out the disabled and there is no indication that these policies are closely related to the requirements of the job. As a matter of fact, the elimination of the disabled has totally different rules from the placement of individuals according to their physical capacity. The object seems, rather, to avoid the possibility of Workmen's Compensation Insurance or other legal matters having to do with injuries on the job. Aside from this simple background cause, there is a basic mistrust of disabled people, and a prejudice against them. One of the authors was once asked to sit on a Civil Service Review committee preparing to employ someone to fill an administrative position in public health. The brochure indicated that only individuals with all limbs intact and in excellent physical health would be considered for the job. This seemed remarkable in view of the fact that the employing agency was a public health department. When the question was raised, there was considerable shock among the members of the health department staff and a general sense of uneasiness about the requirements. When it was indicated that the examiner would not sit on the committee unless this provision was removed, it was, in fact, modified. There is no information to date that this resulted in any impairment of the quality of the staff member selected. It is hard to see why a man in an administrative position needs two arms, two legs, or even two eyes.

There are many forces at work attempting to improve the attitude toward the employment of the handicapped, including the Vocational Rehabilitation Department and the League for the Handicapped. There are, indeed, employers whose principal objective seems to be the productive use of handicapped workers and places where an impairment may actually be a requirement for a job. For example, according to our information, there are noisy foundries which employ only deaf workers, and Mr. Viscardi's Abilities, Inc. requires that every applicant be 100 per cent disabled. While these examples are special circumstances, they do serve to point out that economically sound enterprises may be built upon handicapped workers.

We are probably a long way from unprejudiced equality in the employment of handicapped and nonhandicapped workers. There is now a great tendency in one direction to specify requirements of health and, in the other, to specify requirements of the job with respect to the abilities of the person. It is hoped that the latter tendency will be the winner in the end.

Attitudes of Family and Close Relatives

These attitudes are extremely variable and their basis is far from clear. In his book, *Physical Disability and Human Behavior,* James W. McDaniel goes into the question of family attitudes in terms of scientific investigations made to date. On the less technical level, it seems that there are differences which are culturally determined, as well as differences which are based mainly on personality. In those cultures where elderly people are revered—such as the oriental cultures, particularly those of Okinawa and China—the attitude toward the disabled family member of advanced years is quite different from that which prevails in this country. Here there is a strong tendency to send disabled, elderly people to institutions where they may be "filed away" and never taken home again. The tendency to improve the quality of these institutions has not succeeded in making them agreeable places.

On the basis of observation of disabled people and their families over many years, it seems to us that there are no cut and dried rules. There is pretty good evidence that a close family which has good supportive features in terms of common experiences, sexuality, etc., is likely to support the disabled person and welcome his homecoming. On the other hand, if there is basic hostility, a sense of threat or any other factor which makes for alienation, the tendency is to have a poor relationship and therefore a poor outcome of rehabilitation with respect to returning home. At any rate, the whole subject is one which requires much more investigation and consideration than can be given here.

Attitudes of Staff and Professionals

In consideration of this phase of individual attitudes toward the disabled, one must differentiate between staff members in rehabilitation oriented facilities and those in the community at large. Every rehabilitation facility, whether it is a center, a ward, a service or just a practicing group of experts in the same environment has, in a sense, a personality of its own. It is usually accepting and supporting of disabled persons, and the team members work together toward the suitable outcome of the rehabilitation program. Occasionally it may be poisoned by one or more individuals whose intent may seem to be good but whose methods are provocative and destructive.

On the other hand, in the community at large we face totally different situations. Many health professionals and, in many instances, the medical establishment have a negative attitude toward the disabled and the elderly. After all, it is the medical community, as well as society at large, which permits the existence of the nursing home-convalescent hospital situation, where people frequently receive inadequate care. These patients are sometimes kept alive even against their will, but they are not given lives to lead. Even in the best of the institutions, little is done in the way of rehabilitation or effort to offer patients a dignified means of existence. Many members of the medical community have little interest in the care or management of the disabled or elderly. They frequently use derogatory terms, such as "old crock," and are in a hurry to transfer them to another ward or institution. The number of physicians who specialize in the care of the disabled and elderly is unusually small, and their prestige in the community is often low. The average physician does not want to learn about the care of the disabled even if such information is offered. He prefers to leave the rehabilitation of these patients in the hands of therapists, social workers, and nurses. Fortunately, most nurses, therapists, and social workers are quite the opposite of physicians and they are very much concerned with the disabled. As a result, they are the principal agents of rehabilitation within institutions and outside of them. Nurses and therapists are often frustrated by the lack of medical direction. A common complaint of nurses in convalescent hospitals is that they cannot obtain physicians' services on the basis of even one visit a month.

At this point, it is appropriate to state our philosophy of care. We believe that each injured or damaged patient is, in fact, an individual. He may or may not be separated from reality by his injury, but until we are positive that this is the case, we prefer to treat him as though he were a dignified, normal, understanding human being.

In that respect, we know that he has reasonable aspirations, that his goal is recovery of function, and our objective is to do him no further injury and to support him in every inch of his way toward improvement.

We believe that each human being has the right to identity. He should have a name and unless he authorizes us otherwise, we should use his surname in addressing him. It is as improper for staff members to address a patient as "Willie," or "Tom," as it is for the patient to address the staff members by their first names. If there is to be a first name basis, it should be by mutual agreement and should be so stated by the staff members individually.

In other respects, the person deserves to have his integrity maintained. He should be allowed to wear everyday clothing and should not be separated from the staff by social distance. He should be as independent as possible and provide all self-care activity of which he is capable. If he is incapable he, of course, needs assistance and this should be proffered without any admonition.

The person being treated should be kept clean, but not to the point of excluding other necessary kinds of care. He should be kept free of contamination by feces or urine, and this should be done by the least damaging method to him.

It should be recognized at once that medication is a useful instrument, but that it is often overused and misused. It is necessary for the treatment of some conditions but, in general, it should be avoided as much as possible. The person who is injured or ill should be allowed to sit as soon as possible, and he should sit in a chair from which he can stand if he is able. If he does not have this ability some gentle restraint may be necessary, but this should be eliminated as soon as possible.

In any institution, those who are confined should have freedom within the limits of the institution. They should be able to dine among a group of their peers and to have their meals in as nearly a normal fashion as possible. They should be kept fully informed about their medical care. They should know what is going on and the reason for every procedure, and they should have a say about how such procedures are carried out. This does not imply that as soon as there is what seems to be an irreconcilable conflict between staff and patient, the patient should be given his walking papers. Many times there are apparent discrepancies and differences, but these are often worked out eventually to the advantage of the patient. It should be borne in mind that though we are dealing with sick people, we must not treat them with a sick attitude.

EMOTIONAL EFFECTS OF DISABILITY

Emotional Reactions to Injury or Illness

Illness is one of the facts of life commonly accepted by society and by the individual. The patient assumes the sick role, does not go to work and allows his family to care for him. If the illness is known to

General Considerations

the patient as a cold or a stomach upset, he adjusts readily to it and considers it only as a minor nuisance. If the diagnosis is not immediately clear to him or to the physician, and if hospitalization is required, he may experience a considerable degree of anxiety. In a known and possibly serious illness, the patient usually assumes that his disease is curable and that within a reasonable time he will return to his former healthy state. If the patient suffers immediately or later from a severe disability, such as paralysis or widespread, painful joint inflammation, his anxiety may be heightened and he will wonder whether he may remain permanently disabled. Thus it is very important to arrive as soon as possible at a diagnosis and prognosis which will make it possible to reassure the patient to some extent. Regardless of the reassurance, however, one must understand that disability produces considerable anxiety, and for this reason the patient's answers to questions and responses to management may sometimes seem erratic and confusing. Unfortunately, the patient is rarely seen by the rehabilitation staff during the acute phase of his illness and little is done to relieve his anxiety.

If the disability is caused by injury, the immediate initial reactions are the same as those of illness. Temporary disability following an injury somehow seems less frightening to a patient than if the disability had occurred in the course of an illness. Somehow, one expects to be temporarily disabled following an injury, and the expectation of complete recovery seems to be greater than in illness. Occasionally, however, patients who have suffered only a minor injury may become severely disabled from a psychological mechanism which is called traumatic neurosis.

Emotional Reactions to Hospitalization
Effects of Social Isolation and Degradation

As pointed out before, hospitalization removes the patient from his customary social world and suddenly forces him into a new system of associations and way of life which deprives him of freedom and civil rights. His own clothes and belongings are removed and he is dressed in institutional garb. He has absolutely no freedom of action and must receive permission for every activity he wishes to carry out; neither is he informed of the purposes of all the activities in which he is asked to engage nor the procedures to which he must submit.

This sudden change will cause definite emotional reaction in all patients. These reactions will, however, vary with personality and prior experience. A former business executive, an independent person, may feel angry and frustrated at the way he is being pushed around while the patient with a dependent personality may be delighted that everything is determined for him by the hospital and its staff. In general, the degrading measures of hospitalization, such as loss of clothes and possessions and the requirement of strict obedience, do cause anger, resentment and sometimes fear. Frequently, patients are so afraid of staff members that they will not report any errors in management, or voice any complaints. After prolonged hospitalization, there may be considerable regression in the patient's initiative as a result of the bureaucratic process in the hospital. This untoward side-effect of hospitalization can, of course, be avoided by allowing patients to wear street clothes, keep their belongings and voice their opinions and vent their feelings in conversations with nurse, social worker, physician or even in public at general patient meetings.

Effects of Motor and Sensory Deprivation

Frequently, the severely disabled patient may have to spend considerable time immobile in one position, often unable to see his environment. Examples of patients who suffer extreme sensory and motor deprivation are the poliomyelitis patient in the iron lung and the spinal cord injury patient on the Stryker frame in a prone or supine position. Even with lesser disabilities, such as a lumbar disc lesion or a heart attack, a patient may be confined for a considerable length of time to one position.

Research studies on this topic have been conducted by subjecting persons to severe sensory and motor restrictions.[2] The subjects reported peculiar bodily sensations and became irritable and suspicious. It has also been reported that sensory restriction leads to immaturity and negative attitudes toward social and occupational opportunities. A good bibliography on the effects of motor and sensory deprivation can be found in the thesis by Lillian Hoyle Parent, OTR, who also points out how sensory deprivation can be minimized by appropriate recreational measures.[4]

Effects of Sexual Deprivation

Medical and nursing literature abound with discussions on the problems of human sexuality. While no definite studies are available on the possible influence of sexual deprivation on the hospitalized patient we should mention it here. It appears to us that in the early phase of disability the patient is so overwhelmed by the many problems and worries that his nonexistent sex life is of little concern to him. In the latter phase of rehabilitation, home visits should give patients an opportunity for sexual activity. It does not seem to us that sexual deprivation has interfered with successful rehabilitation. In fact, the desire to return home to a regular sex life, among other things, may be an important motivating factor for rehabilitation.

Emotional Reactions to Permanent Disability

Adjustment

When severe disability first occurs, it is not always immediately clear to what extent the patient will recover function. During this period of uncertainty, he usually remains rather optimistic of full recovery. This is true, for instance, of a patient with a stroke or a spinal cord injury. This optimism is reinforced when partial recovery occurs during the first few weeks. At some point, however, the patient becomes aware that he will be left with a permanent disability. If the rehabilitation program is carried out appropriately, most patients go through this phase satisfactorily without serious, untoward, emotional reactions.

If the patient shows continuous, progressive improvement in his activities of daily living despite his disability, the emotional impact of permanent disability is somehow lessened. The fact that the patient is doing something constructive about his disability lessens his emotional turmoil.

Depression

A few patients will become depressed when faced with the prospect of permanent disability. This is a state of diminished activity and retreat from social association, in which the patient will have feelings of worthlessness and sometimes suicidal tendencies. Such an emotional state interferes seriously with the course of physical rehabilitation and may lead to secondary disabilities, such as contractures and pressure sores. The degree of depression may depend more upon extraneous factors, such as the ways in which the professional personnel deal with the patient, or the economic realities of his family situation, than on the patient's innate psychological makeup or the psychological effects of injury.

Depression can frequently be avoided by instituting a proper rehabilitation program which affords continuous progress in the activities of living and which provides a good relationship between the patient and the rehabilitation personnel.

From the practical standpoint, the professional person dealing with disabled patients must be guided by a few basic ideas. The first principle is to do no harm. (Primum non nocere.) This adage, meaningful as it is, is easier to state than it is to carry out. A careless lack of concern, a thoughtless word or a shrug of the shoulders may be damaging to an injured person who only appears to be unable to perceive what is going on around him. It is a good principle to assume that the disabled person, no matter what his state of consciousness, understands what is being said. Everything that is done to or for a person must be done with a minimum of unpleasant reaction, and everyone who deals with the disabled must be attentive and careful. It is usually the attentive nurse who perceives the first evidence of communication from the person who seems to be completely "out of it."

As suggested in the section on Social Effects of Disability, the hospital itself is a prime offender in establishing bad attitudes in patients. A good case could be made for the proposition that a hospital is a poor place in which to care for the disabled. Rituals which determine kinds of social reaction and interaction, rules which have no basis in medical necessity, and methods of care which have been established by tradition are frequently harmful. As indicated above, in discussing aspects of care, procedures used in routine nursing are often harmful. To change them requires perseverance and tact almost beyond human ability.

The significance of early rehabilitative care has been stressed already. What is even more important is to emphasize that delay is fatal among the elderly. Our attention to the immediate needs and the mere survival of the patient often militates against adequate care.

A few principles which apply to rehabilitation especially are as follows:

1. No patient should remain in bed when his treatment does not require bedrest. This implies that everyone, except the person on a conservative low-back or disc program, should at least be up in a chair or wheelchair.

2. Whenever it is possible to have a patient participate in a stand-up, walking, or stair-climbing program, this activity must be assured.

3. Patients who do not require hospital gowns should be in civilian clothing.

4. For patients in a wheelchair, position should be changed every 20 minutes, and persons in bed should be turned at least every 2 hours, especially if they have sensory defects.

5. Independent activities of daily living should be promoted among all patients.

6. Deformity must be prevented by footboards, splinting, Dennis-Brown braces or other supports, if it is reasonable or possible to do so.

7. Advantage should be taken of the many beds and devices which provide an opportunity for change of position.

8. Every effort should be made to limit the amount of physical lifting necessary by staff.

Attention to these many details, which help preserve the patient's personal and social abilities and dignity, along with an efficiently operating staff, do much to heighten morale and improve motivation.

Honesty is another principle which is important when dealing with disabled persons. Rehabilitation is one field of medicine in which there is no such thing as a kindly lie. The encouragement of false hopes is an obstacle to recovery. Patients are, at least at the end, invariably grateful to therapeutic personnel who "level with them." It is, of course, the responsibility of the physician to communicate prognosis and to discuss progress with the patient. But all those who deal with him must refrain from such well-intentioned statements as, "Of course, you know it is a matter of time," or "It takes a long time for this paralyzed hand to get better." The role of the nurse, the therapist and the social worker should be to communicate the patient's anxiety to the physician. It is then the responsibility of the physician to use his best judgment in revealing the truth and only the truth when the time is right to do so.

Denial

Denial is a form of psychological defense which interferes with the rehabilitation process. By denying that he is disabled, or by denying that he will remain disabled, the patient boycotts the rehabilitation program and remains entirely dependent. The denial of permanent disability may lead to costly, time-consuming, endless attempts to restore function to paralyzed extremities through exercises, electricity, or other mysterious measures. It is interesting to note that persons who lose a limb completely, by traumatic amputation, for instance, adjust much more readily to their loss than patients with a paralyzed extremity. The fact that the extremity is still there, visible and palpable to the patient, apparently makes it much harder to accept the fact that it does not function. Denial is much more frequent in paralysis than in loss of limb.

MOTIVATION

Definition.   A patient is said to be motivated toward rehabilitation if he shows a strong desire to become independent and faithfully and eagerly follows the rehabilitation program prescribed for him. If he fails to do this, he is said to lack motivation.

The Process of Motivation

The process of motivation can best be understood by considering positive and negative motivational factors.[9] Such factors may be designated as motivating and demotivating factors respectively.

Motivating Factors

The motivating factors are more easily understood. One motivating factor, the desire to be independent, may be inherent in the patient's character. However, this desire is not necessarily present in all people. Another motivating factor is the challenge of achievement. Some patients because they are physically weak and disabled want to show the world and themselves that they have the power to become independent. Finally, some patients just enjoy the exercise and activity that lead to rehabilitation. In these three instances, the motivating factors rest within the patient in the sense that the satisfaction from the rehabilitation is *primary*. Most patients are prompted by these *primary motivating* factors.

Often the patient is motivated by the advantages, pleasures and satisfactions in his life which are possible only with a certain degree of physical ability. For instance, the satisfaction of living at home, being with his wife, driving a car, pursuing a hobby or even returning to vocational usefulness. These are factors outside the patient which may spur his effort at rehabilitation for the sake of the secondary gain resulting from physical ability. These outside motivating factors are numerous; they depend, of course, upon the patient's interests and inclinations. It is certain that for some disabled patients there is a paucity of outside motivating factors, particularly in cases of severe disability and bad social situations. In some instances, even the usually optimistic rehabilitation staff may find no good reason for rehabilitative effort.

Demotivating Factors

The demotivating factors may also be considered in two groups, those inherent in the patient's character, and those outside the patient.

Factors inherent in the patient include depression, anxiety and regressive tendencies. *Depression* is a condition characterized not only by pessimism and despair, but also by a general diminution of all activity. *Anxiety, fears* and *phobias* may prevent the patient from carrying out activities necessary for his rehabilitation. *Regressive tendencies* may be aggravated by prolonged illness and hospitalization and may lead to an inherent motivation for dependency rather than independence.

Demotivating factors outside the patient are more numerous. They can be divided into two groups: those resulting from the patient deriving secondary gains from his disability, and those stemming from unpleasant aspects of the rehabilitation program.

Secondary Gains.   We have seen previously that a patient who can benefit from independence will be motivated to work on his rehabilitation. In some instances, however, where a patient benefits more from disability than independence, a demotivating factor for rehabilitation exists. This is the case with those rare people who receive special cash benefits for their disability which may exceed anything they could earn if they were not disabled at all. Other secondary gains may be emotional and social, as in the case of the patient who gets considerably more attention as a result of being disabled than he would if he were able bodied.

Of course, a reward for disability is not necessarily a demotivating factor for everybody depending upon how important the reward, or secondary gain, is to the patient. Furthermore, the demotivating effect of a reward for disability does not always lead to failure in rehabilitation. This demotivating factor may be outweighed by other motivating factors which will make the patient decide that he would rather be independent. However, an unusually large number of disabled patients fail to recover adequate function because of the secondary gains which may be derived from their disabilities.

Discouraging Rehabilitation Program.   Unpleasant, frustrating or discouraging experiences in the rehabilitation program itself constitute the second group of outside demotivating factors. These factors can also increase and precipitate such inherent demotivating factors as depression, fear, and anxiety. The total management of the patient, and particularly the management of the rehabilitation program can therefore have a great impact upon the patient's motivation.

Evaluation of Motivation

Once it has been clarified that the patient's motivation to be rehabilitated is not a fixed characteristic but the result of multiple motivating and demotivating factors acting upon him, the question arises whether the rehabilitation staff will be able to evaluate the patient's motivation and how they can do so. From a practical standpoint, we can postulate four conditions necessary for motivation.

1. The patient must *desire* to be rehabilitated to a higher degree of independence rather than remaining in his disabled state.

2. He must *believe* that the prescribed rehabilitation program is necessary to restore him to greater independence.

3. He must believe such rehabilitation can be accomplished by the program prescribed for him.

4. He must be willing to pay the price of rehabilitation, that is, to make the effort to improve his physical ability and skill, suffer the pain and discomfort of therapeutic procedures, and overcome the distaste he may have for appliances and the fears of injury or failure in carrying out activities independently.

The first two conditions cannot be influenced by the rehabilitation program and if they are not fulfilled, the prognosis for rehabilitation is poor. The last two conditions, however, can be greatly influenced by a well-managed rehabilitation program. We shall analyze each of these conditions briefly.

The patient has no desire to be rehabilitated. This is usually the case when the patient is actually motivated to remain disabled and dependent. There is very little the rehabilitation staff can do to motivate this patient in the opposite direction. It could be done only by manipulating the circumstances in such a way that the patient would find it more advantageous to be rehabilitated. Failing this, it would be advisable to leave him in his dependent condition. After all, it is not the function of any form of medical care to do things to patients against their will, even if it was possible to do so. One problem the rehabilitation center is faced with, however, is that the patient rarely (practically never) admits that he wishes to remain disabled. The patient often realizes that his behavior is socially unacceptable, and will usually state that he would like to be rehabilitated and would do everything in his power to achieve it. Such patients are very frustrating to the rehabilitation staff, and it is best to recognize their true motivation early and explain to them that further rehabilitation is not possible.

The patient does not believe that the rehabilitation program is necessary. These patients are suffering from a form of denial. They do not accept their disability as permanent and expect that it will disappear completely by itself. To them, the acceptance of braces or other appliances would be an acceptance of the disability. They may be willing to exercise, not for the purpose of improving their ADL ability, but solely in order to restore normal function. Nothing can be done in terms of motivation so long as a person is in the phase of denial.

The patient does not believe that rehabilitation can be accomplished by his present program. This attitude denotes *lack of confidence* in the ability of the rehabilitation center to deliver what has been promised (or what seemed to be promised). Confidence, of course, is a motivating factor which stems from the outside to a considerable extent and can be greatly influenced by rehabilitation management.

The patient is not willing to pay the price. This means that he has been scared or discouraged either by the presentation or by the conduct of the rehabilitation program.

The patients who fail in rehabilitation because they do not fulfill the last two conditions are frequently the victims of an inadequate rehabilitation program.

Principles of a Motivating Rehabilitation Program

The program must be designed in such a way that the patient will believe that rehabilitation helps, that is, he must notice success. In addition the program must be acceptable to the patient so that he is willing to carry it out. This goal can be accomplished by following certain principles.

Principles for Communication

Verbal Understanding. There must be an understanding between staff and patient as to the purpose and results of rehabilitation measures. Most patients do not understand that rehabilitation measures give increased function but do not affect the primary disability (e.g., paraplegia). Many assume that spontaneous recovery from disability is due to exercise. Others fear that activity may aggravate their disability. It is important to make it clear from the outset that three factors influence recovery:

1. Improvement of the primary disability, which is either spontaneous (e.g., in the early phase of neurologic disability) or due to medication (e.g., in arthritis).

2. Prevention of secondary disabilities by the rehabilitation program.

3. Increased function despite permanent disability.

Improved function is achieved through the rehabilitation program. While it is not advisable to inform the patient immediately of the degree of permanent primary disability, if known, it should be made clear to him at the earliest opportunity that rehabilitation cannot influence it. Initially, the purpose of rehabilitation is best presented as a means to prevent secondary disability, so that the patient can most benefit from any spontaneous return of function. Under this pretext, the patient can be given all necessary appliances and training. By the time he accepts his degree of permanent disability, he will be able to function despite it, and not become depressed. Of course, all staff members must follow the same line, and it is important to determine a policy or attitude during the evaluation conference. There should be a feedback on how the patient understands his rehabilitation, and, if necessary, the staff's attitude must be explained repeatedly to him.

Communication by Action. Communication is not only verbal. Every action conveys a message to the patient. If he is provided with a brace, this conveys the message that he will always need a brace. Such an impression can be counteracted by verbal assurances that he may not need the brace in the future. If nurse and therapist continue to hold on to the patient during every move, it may be difficult to convince him verbally that his stability is improving.

Principles of Goal Setting

a. Concentrate on one goal at a time. Success is more likely and the strain is less if only one or two goals are set at a time and others reserved for later on.

b. Set intermediate goals. If the final goal is ambulation (e.g., of a hemiplegic patient), make stand-up ability the first intermediate goal, transfer ability the second, stair-climbing the third and finally, ambulation with a cane.

c. Achieve one goal before the next one is started. Set intermediate goals in such a way that the easier ones come first, and set a difficult goal only when the prerequisites are accomplished. For example, standing up is always the first goal for a hemiplegic patient, and is a prerequisite for transfer. Transfer is a prerequisite for activities of daily living training in use of toilet, bath, etc.

d. Base the immediate goals on abilities the patient has now, and not on abilities he may have later. Initially, all goals must be based upon the patient's uninvolved limbs or functions; e.g., first goals for the hemiplegic, one-legged stand-up; for the paraplegic, chinning; for the aphasic, communication by gestures.

Principles of Exercise

a. Start the program with an activity the patient can do unassisted. Assistance denotes helplessness and causes depression and discouragement; e.g., start the stand-up exercises for the hemiplegic patient from a very high chair (see p. 225).

b. Do not progress until the patient has mastered the first phase of the program.

c. Progress in very small steps so that the exercise remains easy; e.g., lower the stand-up chair 1 inch at a time.

d. Keep an ongoing record and make the patient aware of his progress.

Principles of Bracing

a. Overbrace at first so that the patient gets maximum security; e.g., for paraplegia, start with a pelvic band with hip locks.

b. Brace early. Possible spontaneous recovery should not prevent the early use of braces. They are easy to discard and the patient does not mind. However, if a patient goes without braces and ambulates already, the prescription of braces will seem like a step backward. He will be discouraged and depressed.

c. Do not discontinue bracing unless the gain in function warrants it; otherwise the patient may look better but function worse. If this is the case, regression in function will be demotivating.

Principles of Scheduling

Though the patient's activity tolerance is limited, activity is the key to successful rehabilitation. It is necessary to strike a proper balance between needed exercise and the patient's exercise tolerance.

The patient's daily schedule must include sleep, food intake, elimination and diagnostic and therapeutic measures, in addition to the rehabilitation program. If the patient's schedule is overloaded, he will perform poorly and become depressed. The rehabilitation schedule can be lightened by the following means:

a. Reduce waiting and transportation time to a minimum by performing rehabilitation in or near the patient's room.

b. Combine basic maintenance and rehabilitation; e.g., change of position with exercise; bed bath with either range of motion exercises or with speech stimulation.

c. Ascertain that a given exercise or training is given often enough and long enough to achieve quick results; e.g., stand-up exercises for 10 minutes, once a day, are useless and will only discourage the patient.

Motivating Psychosocial Measures

Short Term Motivation in a Rehabilitation Program

The patient may be motivated to participate in the rehabilitation program, to carry out exercises and to use the necessary appliances without being motivated by the final goal of functional improvement. This is true particularly where the patient is hospitalized. While hospitalized, he is accustomed to follow physicians' orders and to do what the nurses and therapists tell him to do. This assures the feasibility of the initial rehabilitation program and, if well conducted, may motivate the hospitalized patient for the long range goal of functional improvement.

Economic, Social, and Emotional Effects of Disability   61

Besides helping to initiate motivation, short range motivating factors can reinforce the motivation for the long term goal. The immediate rewards may consist of the attention of a sympathetic therapist. At the same time, involvement in a group program provides the patient with an opportunity to exchange thoughts and feelings about his condition with other patients similarly afflicted, which in itself is a reward. Finally, it is possible to organize the rehabilitation program in such a way that there are competitions and special rewards for good rehabilitation performance: medals, certificates, or even tangible rewards such as a party or a special trip to the theatre. Short range motivation is most important with children, because they frequently do not have the necessary intellectual development to conceive of a long range program. But short term measures can also work wonders with adults.

Transition to the Community

One of the fears frequently encountered among disabled persons is the thought that life in the community will be impossible or at least very awkward. To dispel this fear, contact with the outside world is necessary. Visits by motivating visitors such as family members, friends, employees or business associates must be encouraged. Realistic plans for the patient's return to the community must be discussed and developed early. This includes consideration of financial problems, living problems and working problems.

As soon as feasible, the disabled patient should visit his home during the day. Later, trials of home living of 2 to 3 days' duration should be arranged so that problems can be detected and solved. Thus the patient gains confidence in his ability to return home and will be motivated to increase his rehabilitation efforts. Day trips to community events (football or baseball games, and the theatre) are helpful in stimulating a return to normal life.

Pharmacological Methods

Drugs cannot produce motivation. Some inherent demotivating factors, however, such as anxiety and depression, can be successfully treated by pharmacological means.

Drug Treatment of Anxiety

A large number of tranquilizing drugs have a beneficial effect upon anxiety. The phenothiazines, reserpine and its derivatives, meprobamate and diazepam are examples of commonly used tranquilizers. However, two considerations must be kept in mind:

1. Some tranquilizers are more depressing and sleep-inducing than others. The depressing tranquilizers are indicated for a very anxious, agitated patient who has no serious respiratory impairment. Where alertness is required, however, which is most often the case in rehabilitation, one must use nonobtunding drugs, such as Compazine and Stelazine.

2. Patients with brain damage may be very sensitive to cortically acting drugs such as phenobarbital and meprobamate, and become easily disoriented. These patients function better with drugs which act on the midbrain, such as the phenothiazines.

Drug Treatment of Depression

The antidepressant medications are classified as monoamine inhibitors (Parnate), tricyclic drugs (Imipramine) and psychomotor stimulants (Dexedrine, Ritalin). The first two groups are used for long range treatment of severe depressions. Dexedrine has a direct stimulating effect upon the brain, and we have found it most useful in the following circumstances:

1. In the initial management of any severe depression Dexedrine is effective immediately while the major antidepressants may take several weeks before a therapeutic effect is noticeable.

2. In minor depressive states and fatigue states where the stimulating effect of Dexedrine makes it easier to initiate an activity program. Within a few weeks, the patient will become accustomed to the activities, notice progress and the medication can be discontinued.

3. In initiating weight-reducing programs.

REFERENCES

1. Carpenter, J. O.: "Changing Roles and Disagreement in Families with Disabled Husbands." APMR, 55:272, 1974.
2. Heron, M. T.: "The Pathology of Boredom," in Coopersmith, S. (ed.): Frontiers of Psychological Research, Readings from Scientific American. San Francisco: W. H. Freeman, 1966.
3. McDaniel, J. W.: Physical Disability and Human Behavior. Elmsford, N.Y.: Pergamon Press, 1970.
4. Parent, L. H.: "The Effects of Environmental Deprivation on Patient Behavior." Thesis, University of Southern California, 1972.
5. Parsons, T.: "Definitions of Health and Illness in the Light of American Values and Social Structure." Patients, Physicians and Illness, JACO, Ed., 1958.
6. Smolkin, C. and Cohen, B. S.: "Socio-economic Factors Affecting the Vocational Success of Stroke Patients." APMR, 55:269, 1974.

7. Wright, B.: "A Physical Disability: A Psychological Approach." New York: Harper's, 1960.
8. Wu, R.: Behavior and Illness. Englewood Cliffs, N. J.: Prentice-Hall, Inc., 1973.
9. Zane, M. D. and Lowenthal, M.: "Motivation in Rehabilitation of the Physically Handicapped." APMR, 41:400, 1960.

PART TWO

Activities of Daily Living

5

Levels of Independence

Rehabilitation medicine strives to develop whatever potential abilities a person may have, regardless of physical or psychological impairment. Therefore, methods have been developed to appraise and to improve, in the disabled, those activities that are generally carried out by a normal person in his daily routine. In the terminology of rehabilitation these are called Activities of Daily Living or ADL.

The concept of ADL is significant not only medically, but also socially and legally. In medical rehabilitation, the disabled person's ability to care for himself is first appraised and then improved by instruction, exercises or appliances. When maximal improvement has been attained, he may still require varying degrees of assistance that determine his living arrangements. Legally, his eligibility for financial or other assistance from public agencies may be determined by his abilities to perform ADL.

The degree to which a patient can carry out ADL determines his level of independence. To define the degree of independence of a disabled person, we must consider his ADL capabilities if he is (1) bedfast, (2) home-bound or (3) able to move freely within the community.

A patient is completely independent in *bed* if he is able to feed himself, wash himself and use the urinal and the bedpan. However, such a patient is dependent on a person who will serve him food, bring him his wash tray and carry away appliances, such as the bedpan and the urinal.

A patient is completely independent in the *home*, in terms of ADL, if he can go to the bathroom unassisted and can feed, wash and dress himself. If he lives alone he may need a housekeeper to shop, clean house, cook and serve meals. If, in addition to his abilities in ADL, he has the physical capability and the knowledge needed for housekeeping, he may be self-sufficient even if home-bound. Shopping can be accomplished and social contact maintained by telephone.

In order to be independent within the *community*, a patient must be able to get in and out of his house unassisted and to use either public or private transportation. Both the home-bound patient and the completely independent patient need a certain level of communication ability for their independence.

The patient who is not completely independent may need care at one of three levels:

1. *Nursing care* is required for the patient who needs considerable assistance in bathing and elimination or who needs such nursing procedures as wound dressing, irrigation of catheters, intravenous or nasogastric feedings. Usually, the nursing-care patient is a bed patient, although he may be placed in a chair or a tilt table for change of position.

2. *Attendant care* is required for the patient who needs assistance not in the order of specialized nursing. For example, the independent bed patient requires attendant care, since someone has to serve his meals and bring him water for the bath. A disabled patient who is mobile within his home or within the community may still require an attendant to assist him. For example, the quadriplegic patient cannot wash himself entirely and needs help to transfer from bed to wheelchair. Once he is in a wheelchair and fitted with his appliances, he may be entirely independent for prolonged periods of the day. (See Chap. 15.)

3. *Housekeeping service* may be needed by a patient who is capable of all ADL within the home but cannot cook, clean house or order necessary supplies.

From the foregoing it is clear that achieving the ability to carry out ADL is an important goal for every physically disabled patient. To carry out ADL, three functional abilities are required: (1) mobility, (2) self-care and (3) communication. The principles and the methods for restoring these three basic abilities in the disabled patient will be discussed in the following chapters.

CHAPTER
6

Patient Mobility

The achievement of mobility is of considerable importance for the elderly or the disabled patient. Patient mobility serves at least three purposes:

1. A physiologic purpose, namely, to prevent disuse phenomena.

2. A psychological purpose, namely, to stimulate and motivate the patient.

3. A rehabilitative purpose, that is, to enable the patient to carry out the activities of daily living, and those activities required for recreation and for his vocation.

In a disabled patient, usually, mobility progresses through three stages: (1) mobility in bed, (2) mobility within the room (transfer and locomotion) and (3) mobility within the community. The last stage requires the ability to use private and public transportation.

MOBILITY IN BED

Problems of Bed Mobility in the Elderly and Disabled

For a young, able-bodied person, the bed position does not constitute a necessary obstacle to mobility. Such a person can assume face-lying, back-lying and side-lying positions, as well as intermediary positions. He can twist, turn and scoot (i.e., slide up and down or across the bed), sit up and stretch. However, most elderly patients seem to shun certain positions and favor others. This may be partially due to joint stiffness but it may also be due to rigidity of attitude. Usually, the elderly patient is accustomed to one position in bed and finds it most comfortable; therefore, he refuses to change position. Often, it is impossible to persuade elderly persons to assume the flat face-lying position which tends to extend the neck, the trunk and the hips. On the contrary, they have a tendency to assume a flexed position of the neck, the trunk and the limbs when they are in a back-lying or a side-lying position. In back-lying position they frequently request additional pillows under their heads and knees. Once they have developed flexion contractures, change of position becomes extremely difficult.

Disabled patients have specific mobility problems for their particular disability. Patients with quadriplegia (paralysis of all four extremities) or generalized rheumatoid arthritis are frequently helpless and require passive positioning by a nurse or an assistant. Patients with hemiplegia (paralysis of one side of the body) have some potential for mobility, though moving about in bed is very strenuous and requires special instruction and the use of side rails and an overhead trapeze. Usually, paraplegic patients (with paralysis of both legs) are able to sit up with the help of an overhead trapeze and to turn from side to side by using the side rails or the bed frame.

Methods of Promoting Mobility in Bed

There are three ways to promote mobility in bed: training, use of aids and passive positioning.

Training. To train the patient to become mobile in bed requires a bed exercise program, which will vary with the disability. Some bed

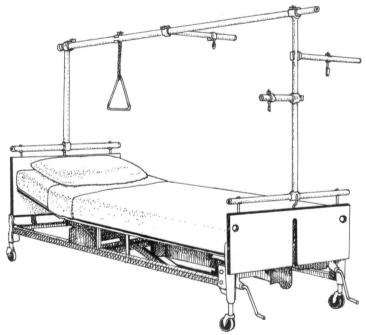

Fig. 6-1. Overhead frame with trapeze. (Orthopedic Equipment Co.)

Activities of Daily Living

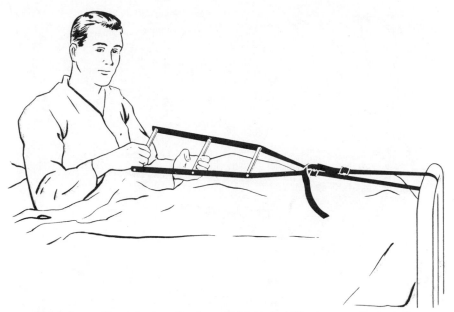

Fig. 6-2. Pull-up device, "Patient Aid." (Rehabilitation Products; J. T. Posey Co.)

exercises can be carried out without special provisions, while others require the use of aids or passive positioning. As a general rule, it is extremely difficult to institute an effective program of bed exercises for elderly disabled patients because these exercises are the most strenuous ones in any rehabilitation program. It is very important to be aware of this fact in the management of the patient, and one must avoid overestimating his strength and endurance and not expect more than he can do.

Aids. A number of appliances are available to assist the patient with mobility in bed. The mattress should be firm so that he does not become stuck in a hollow; the sheets should be smooth so that he can slide back and forth. The cover should be supported over a foot-board or cradle to give his legs room to turn and to prevent him from becoming tangled. Finally, he needs something to hold on to while he turns or slides. The bed frame itself, side rails, an overhead trapeze (Fig. 6-1) or a pull-up device (Fig. 6-2) will serve this purpose.

Positioning. If a patient is unable to turn in bed or sit up by himself, passive change of position will increase his mobility. For instance, a quadriplegic patient in face-lying position can only extend his neck

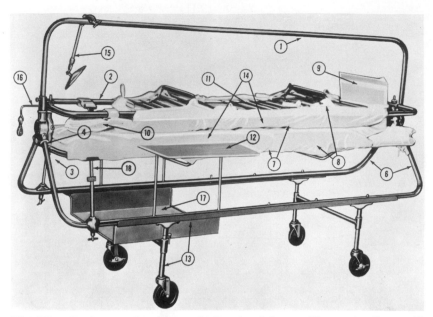

Fig. 6-3. Stryker turning frame. (1) Overhead frame; (2) anterior frame; (3) posterior frame; (4) end turning assembly; (6) support runner; (7) sheet set, anterior and posterior; (8) canvas cover set (anterior, posterior); (9) foot support assembly; (10) forehead bands; (10A) face support assembly (optional for fracture dislocations of the cervical spine); (11) evertaut fasteners complete, rubber bands only, wire hooks only; (12) arm support assemblies; (13) cart assembly; (14) polyfoam mattress set: anterior polyform mattress, posterior polyfoam mattress (end section), posterior polyfoam mattress (center section); (14A) plastic mattress cover set; (15) mirror assembly (optional); (16) head traction attachment; (17) reversible utility tray and bed pan holder; (18) stabilizer arm (optional—recommended for additional stability on 7′ models). *Dimensions:* 6½′ or 7′ inside length. All frames minimum 33″ from floor, adjustable to 38″ in height. Width of frames is 17″ on 6½′ models, 19″ on 7′ models. (Rehabilitation Products; Stryker Orthopedic Frame Co.)

but cannot flex it, while in back-lying position he can flex his neck but cannot extend it. To give him full neck mobility, it is necessary to turn him periodically from face-lying to back-lying position. Similarly, a patient with weak neck muscles may not be able to raise his head at all when lying flat. However, he may be able to do it from a semireclining position. The patient may be brought to various positions by turning or adjusting the backrest of the bed. An electrically powered hospital bed allows the patient to change his position by himself if he is able to push a button. There are also a number of mechanical beds that

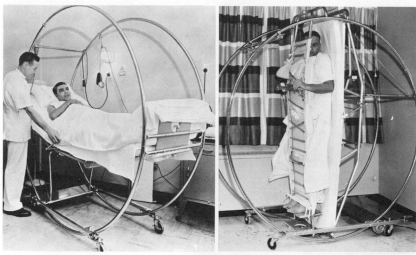

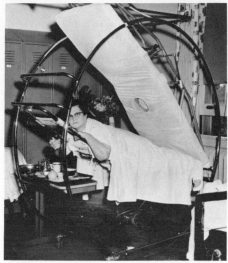

Fig. 6-4. CircOlectric bed.
(Top, left) Patient in back-lying
position. *(Bottom)* Patient in
face-lying position. *(Top, right)*
Upright position. The patient
may stand between the 2 panels
of the bed as shown or may be
supported by belts placed
around his lower extremities and
trunk and the lower bed panel at
appropriate levels. In this way
the bed is used as a tilt table. Precautions to prevent postural
hypotension apply as in the use
of the tilt table. (Rehabilitation
Products; Stryker Orthopedic
Frame Co.)

facilitate change of position. The Stryker frame (Fig. 6-3), essentially
designed for patients with spinal cord injury, permits the patient to be
changed from back-lying to face-lying position by simply pivoting the
bed around a longitudinal axis. The CircOlectric bed can be pivoted
around its transverse axis, thereby putting the patient upright from a
back-lying position and down forward into a face-lying position (Fig.
6-4).

TRANSFERS

A transfer is a single displacement of the patient from one piece of furniture or equipment to another (for instance, from bed to chair or from bed to commode or from bed to wheelchair).

Horizontal Transfers

If the patient transfers in a lying position, for instance, from bed to the stretcher or from a stretcher to the x-ray table, he carries out a horizontal transfer. This may be a necessity if the patient is not allowed or is not able to sit or stand. This would apply to a paraplegic with an ischial pressure sore or a patient with a bilateral hip spica cast. A horizontal transfer can be carried out either by rolling or by sliding. Since it requires above average strength, the patient will frequently need some assistance in such a transfer.

Vertical Transfers

In a vertical transfer the patient transfers from one seat to another. According to his disability, the patient may perform either a weight-bearing transfer, that is, by putting weight on his lower extremities (or one lower extremity) or a non-weight-bearing transfer, that is, without using the lower extremities.

Weight-bearing Transfers. These can be carried out by patients who have at least one stable lower extremity (Fig. 6-5). Hemiplegics, unilateral lower extremity amputees or patients with hip fractures are candidates for one-legged weight-bearing transfer. Even if both legs are available, only one leg is frequently used for weight-bearing trans-

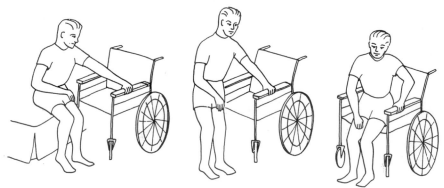

Fig. 6-5. Weight-bearing transfer from bed to chair. The patient stands up, pivots until his back is opposite the new seat and sits down.

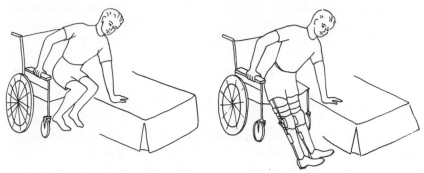

Fig. 6-6. *(Left)* Non-weight-bearing transfer from chair to bed. *(Right)* With legs braced.

fer since it is easier to pivot on one leg than on two. In the weight-bearing transfer the patient first comes from the sitting to a standing position. This can be accomplished by the use of lower extremity muscles alone if they are strong enough or by pulling up with the arms, provided the lower extremities are stiffened by voluntary motion, a brace or a cast. After the patient has come to a standing position he pivots slightly so that his back is opposite the new seat and then sits down either by bending the knees or by letting himself down by the arms with the legs extended. If the weight-bearing transfer is done by an elderly patient with a stiff leg he needs very secure support to pull himself up and let himself down.

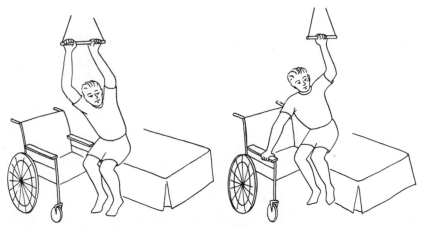

Fig. 6-7. *(Left)* Nonweight-bearing transfer, pull-up method. *(Right)* Nonweight-bearing transfer, combined method.

Non-Weight-Bearing Transfers.   This type of transfer is indicated for the double lower-extremity amputees or for paraplegics who are not braced. There are three methods for performing a non-weight-bearing transfer. The most useful one is the push-up method, in which the patient pushes himself up with his arms as he moves from one seat to the other (Fig. 6-6). The pull-up or chinning method is possible only if the patient has an overhead support (Fig. 6-7, *left*). In the combined method, the patient may push himself up with one arm and pull himself up with the other arm (Fig. 6-7, *right*). This is also useful in moving from bed to wheelchair and back. In some instances, the type of non-weight-bearing transfer is determined by the disability. A patient may have power of arm flexion but not extension and, therefore, may be able to pull himself up but not to push himself. If the patient is weak or unstable, a sliding board may be used to bridge the gap between the two seats. With the sliding board, the patient may still use the push-up, pull-up or mixed method. Usually, the patient requiring a sliding board will also require the assistance of an attendant.

Transfer by Lifting

Lifting is a passive transfer; nevertheless, it helps to increase patient mobility. If a patient is unable to transfer independently or with minor assistance by only one person, usually it is safer to lift him from place to place. It is safer not only for the patient but also for the personnel assisting him. The patient may be lifted manually or by mechanical lifts.

Manual lifting may be done by one attendant if the attendant is strong. It may require two, three or four attendants according to the weight or disability of the patient.

If the patient is too heavy for the number of available attendants, a mechanical hydraulic lift should be used. Several models are available. They all work according to the same principle. The patient sits or lies on a canvas seat and backrest that is raised by the lift (Fig. 6-8). Then the patient is either pivoted around the vertical arm of the lift, or the lift is wheeled on casters until the patient is over the new seat. Then he is lowered into it.

LOCOMOTION

Locomotion is the act of moving from place to place. Two methods of locomotion, ambulation and wheeling, are commonly used by disabled persons. Ambulation or walking is locomotion carried out in the upright position with some degree of weight-bearing on one or both legs (even prosthetic ones or braced legs). In wheeling, the patient

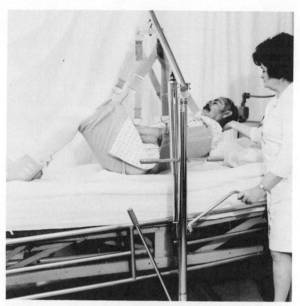

Fig. 6-8. Patient lift.

propels himself or is propelled on wheels or casters in a sitting position. While these two methods are the usual ones, it should be noted that under primitive conditions and in emergencies disabled persons may move from place to place by unorthodox methods, such as hopping on one leg, crawling or performing seated push-ups. In fact, it may be desirable for some patients to learn these methods so that they

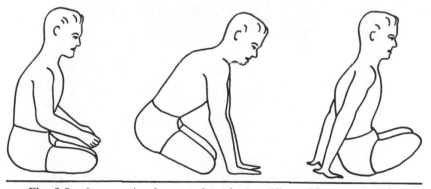

Fig. 6-9. Locomotion by seated push-ups. Bilateral lower extremity amputee.

can help themselves in emergencies. Bilateral amputees frequently move by seated push-ups (Fig. 6-9). A paraplegic sometimes may have to ascend or descend a flight of stairs by a similar method.

Wheelchair Locomotion

Wheelchair locomotion is indicated for those patients who are entirely unable to ambulate. It is indicated also for those patients who have the potential to ambulate but whose ambulation is unsteady, unsafe or too strenuous. Furthermore, a wheelchair may be needed for those patients who can ambulate but are unable to arise unassisted

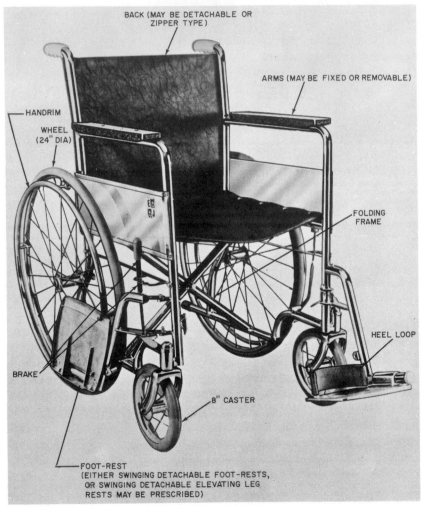

BACK (MAY BE DETACHABLE OR ZIPPER TYPE)

ARMS (MAY BE FIXED OR REMOVABLE)

HANDRIM

WHEEL (24" DIA)

FOLDING FRAME

HEEL LOOP

BRAKE

8" CASTER

FOOT-REST (EITHER SWINGING DETACHABLE FOOT-RESTS, OR SWINGING DETACHABLE ELEVATING LEG RESTS MAY BE PRESCRIBED)

Fig. 6-10. Wheelchair.

Activities of Daily Living

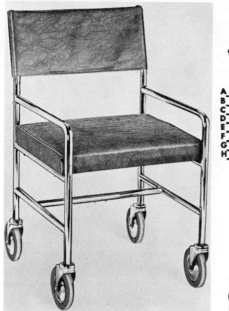

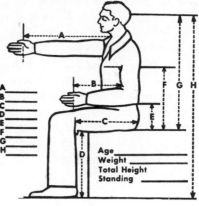

Age _____
Weight _____
Total Height
Standing _____

Fig. 6-11. *(Left)* Glide-about. *(Right)* Wheelchair prescription guide. (Everest and Jennings)

from a sitting to a standing position. A patient who needs crutches to ambulate and has to carry things from one place to another may at times be better off in a wheelchair, since both hands are immobilized by crutches.

Standard Wheelchairs

General Features. The most commonly used type of wheelchair is made of metal and has four wheels (Fig. 6-10). Two of the wheels are large, 24-inch (60.96-cm.) diameter, and have a separate rim that the patient can grasp to propel the chair by turning the large wheels. The two small wheels are casters which pivot freely. They are either 5 or 8 inches (12.7 or 20.32-cm.) in diameter. Three models of standard wheelchairs are commonly used: the Universal model, which has the large wheels in the back and the casters in the front, the Traveler model, which has the casters in the back and large wheels in front, and the Amputee model, which has a longer frame on which the rear wheels are set back to prevent the chair from tipping backward. Names of component parts of a wheelchair are indicated in Figure 6-10. Wheelchairs are available in standard sizes but can be ordered also according to prescribed measurement for height, depth and width. (See Fig. 6-11, *right.*)

Special Parts and Features. The special features of wheelchairs are numerous and can be studied in detail in the catalogues issued by wheelchair manufacturers. The most important additional features are brakes and brake lever extensions, removable sides, reclining backs, folding mechanisms, adjustable footrests, elevating legrests, swing-away footrests and others. The dimensions of the wheelchair as well as the special features should be prescribed for each patient.

Method of Propulsion. The standard procedure by which a patient propels his wheelchair is to turn the large wheel with his hand. He may also push with his feet or use a combination of hand and foot action. The wheelchair can also be pushed by another person or can be powered by an electric motor.

Other Types of Wheeled Chairs

In addition to the standard wheelchairs described above, other types are manufactured. Chairs with four small pivoted casters are called glide-abouts (Fig. 16-11, *left*). They have to be either propelled by use of the legs or pushed by another person. Battery operated electric wheelchairs are useful for patients with upper and lower extremity disabilities.

There are also strollerlike wheelchairs that cannot be propelled by the patient at all and require another person for locomotion.

Prescribing the Wheelchair

The suggested order form, which is explained below, comprises all the specifications which are required to meet individual needs. Each item should be designated when the prescription is submitted to the vendor.*

Type

Large Wheel in Front (Traveler). This chair is more easily self-wheeled by people who lack shoulder motion and have limited elbow motion. However, it is more difficult for another person (attendant) to wheel up curbs or steps, because the larger front wheel does not permit the back-tipping and maneuverability that is provided by front casters.

Large Wheel in Back (Universal). This is the more commonly used chair and with 8-inch (20.32-cm.) casters is more easily maneuvered over rough ground, curbs, etc.

*Literature supplied by the manufacturer will contain important suggestions and will include full directions for the care of the wheelchair. The prescriber and the user should familiarize themselves with this information.

WHEELCHAIR ORDER BLANK

Room _____

Bed _____

Name _____ Address _____ Date _____

TYPE	Large Wheel		Adult	Junior	Child
	Front _____ Back _____		_____	_____	_____
	One-Arm Drive				
	Right _____ Left_____		_____	_____	_____
	Seat-O-Matic: Catch				
	Front _____ Side_____		_____	_____	_____
	Amputee _____				

WHEELS   8″ casters _____ 5″ casters _____ Caster pins_____

             Brakes _____ Rubber tires_____ Squeezer_____

SEAT   Standard _____ Extra wide _____ Slide-eze_____

             Seat board_____ Extra height_____ Extra deep_____

CUSHIONS

         Seat cushion: 3″ foam ____ x ____, 4″ foam ____ x ____,

                   Air ____ x ____

BACK AND   (Back)

HEADREST   Foam_____″   Size_____ x _____

CUSHIONS   (Head)

             Foam_____″   Size_____ x _____

BACKREST   Standard _____ Zipper _____

             Full-reclining _____ Semireclining _____

HEADREST   Channel _____ Hook-on_____

Foam rubber padding, cloth or leatherette covered, is available in 1″ to 4″ thick foam rubber in the dimensions required for back and headrests.

ARMS   Standard _____ Removable _____ Desk Arm _____

ARMRESTS   Upholstered_____ Metal _____ Wooden _____

LEG AND   Standard _____ Heel Straps _____ Calf Straps_____

FOOTRESTS

         Swing-away _____ Elevating _____ Combined _____

         Adjustable panel _____

SLING   Standard   Adjustable

SUPPORTS   supports   supports _____ Slings _____

REMARKS _____

_____

_____

_____

_____

_____ M.D.

One-Arm Drive.　This is propelled by wheeling with the right hand alone or the left hand alone. This chair has two rims on the propelling side, one rim activating each wheel. Used simultaneously, the chair moves in a straight line. Used separately, the chair turns.

Seat-O-Matic (E & J only).　This is a chair with a special seat; loosening a catch will open a part to permit use of the toilet by the occupant of the chair. The seat may be ordered on any type of E & J chair except the one-arm drive. The driving bar on a one-arm chair precludes backing the chair over the toilet.

Amputee.　This type of chair has special balancing to offset the loss of weight caused by leg amputations.

Wheels

Eight-inch (20.32-cm.) Casters.　These permit wheeling over rough ground with less danger of tipping than 5-inch (12.70-cm.) casters.

Rubber Tires.　These appear to be satisfactory for all patients. There are pneumatic tires available that would absorb bumps on rough ground somewhat more and might be more comfortable for a patient with pain, but they would also take more care and maintenance. They are not recommended for most patients.

Caster Pins.　Caster pins lock the casters in place, keeping them in a straight line from front to back of the caster.

Brakes.　All chairs need brakes to stabilize them while the patient is transferring himself or while the attendant is moving the patient into a chair, etc. There are various types of brakes available, all of which stabilize the large wheels.

A Squeezer.　This is a device by which the chair can be narrowed slightly for getting through doorways; the narrowing is done by the same means that the chair is folded, but it is difficult for many patients to handle.

Seat

For some patients the depth or width of the seat needs to be especially measured to fit the patient properly. This also applies to the height of the seat from the floor. These factors depend on the height, weight and general build of the patient. When the patient requires other than a standard dimension chair, it is best to have the vendor do the measurements, although the physical or occupational therapist may also do them (Fig. 6-11, *right*).

Width.　The seat must accommodate the patient's hips comfortably, without crowding. If the patient uses respiratory equipment, such as a chest cuirass, measuring must include additional width for the cuirass.

Depth.   The patient should have support under the thighs to about 2-inches (5.08-cm) above the break of the knee.

Height.   The seat should be high enough from the floor to permit full support of the thighs with the feet on the footrests. By sitting farther forward in the chair, the patient can rest his feet on the floor.

Slide-eze Seat.   This is a seat covered with plastic material, allowing the patient to slide more easily.

Seat Board.   A plywood board is sometimes ordered to give a firmer sitting surface.

Cushions

Seat Cushions.   Seat cushions are available in various dimensions to fit the prescribed seat. Although foam rubber cushions of 2-inch (5.08-cm.), 3-inch (7.62-cm.) and 4-inch (10.16-cm.) thickness are used, the 3-inch (7.62-cm.) and 4-inch (10.16-cm.) foam rubber are more protective. Various types of air-filled cushions are available. These are very satisfactory when individually prescribed.

Cushions for Back and Headrests.   Foam rubber padding is available, as indicated on the order blank.

Backrests

There are various types of backrests available to suit the patient's needs. A *standard* backrest is the most common and is satisfactory for most users. It may also be ordered extra high.

Zipper.   The zipper may be placed on either the right or the left side of the upholstered back according to the convenience of the disabled person. This type of back will allow the patient to slide backward from the chair onto a bed or toilet.

Semireclining.   The chair can be let down to a 45-degree angle, or several positions between 90 degrees and 45 degrees. This is important for some patients with respiratory difficulty who breathe better at such an angle and it also allows some change of position for a patient who must sit for long periods of time.

Full-reclining.   The chair can be let down to a point level with the seat or placed in several positions between that and upright. This allows the patient to rest in a flat, supine position and avoids his having to get back into bed for rest. It is an advantage for many patients with respiratory difficulty. In both the semi-reclining and full-reclining models, the axle for the rear wheels is farther back than in nonreclining chairs, a fact that must be considered if the patient is capable of wheeling himself. Across the backs of both these types of chairs is a collapsible bar that can be dropped down in order to fold the chair, and connected together to hold the back firmly when the chair is opened. The center section of the bar screws in and may be tightened to take up slack in the back as needed.

Headrest

A headrest is necessary if either a semireclining or full-reclining chair is used.

Channel.   This type fits into the hollow, upright tubes holding the back of the chair. The chair may be used with or without the headrest. It is removed when putting the chair into a car, etc.

Hook-on.   This type attaches to the upright tubes by hooking over, not into them. It is removable when desired. This type may become disconnected by the patient's movements, unless it is carefully put on. The advantage is that it can be used on any type of back.

Arms

Standard.   These are permanent, nonremovable arms, of round tubing.

Removable.   Removable arms may be plain round tubing or any of the types described below. A removable arm facilitates many means of transfer from wheelchair to other objects. A front pin helps to lock armrests in place.

Desk Arms.   One portion of the arm is cut about 4-inches (10.16-cm.) lower than the others, making it possible to roll the chair under desks, tables, etc., instead of up to these objects. This arm may be put on with either the high or the low part toward the front, which also facilitates transfer technique with some patients.

Armrests

Wooden.   A flat, polished, wooden piece is bolted to the armrest tubing. The flat surface is more comfortable for resting the arm.

Upholstered.   A padded, leatherette-covered armrest which matches the rest of the chair is attached to the tubing.

Leg- and Footrests

Standard.   Standard leg- and footrests are metal, hinged footrests which may be turned up, out of the way when the patient gets in or out of the chair.

Heel Straps.   These are heavy straps across the back of the footrest to prevent the heels from sliding backward.

Calf Straps.   These are similar straps midway up the footrest bar so that the calf of the leg rests against them.

Swing-away. By releasing a pin lock on the side, this entire footrest assembly may be swung out toward the outside of the chair, along the wheel.

Elevating. The entire legrest assembly may be elevated so that it is horizontal. This is used with full-reclining chairs or when elevation of the leg is essential.

Combined. The legrest will both elevate and swing away.

Adjustable Panel. This long panel supports the calf of the leg. It is used with elevating legrest to support the calf.

Sling Supports

Standard. These sling supports are unbroken rods to hold arm slings, attached to the back of the chair by clamps.

Adjustable. These sling supports are broken rods with ratchet devices to stabilize them in the position needed to hang the slings at the desired angle from a semireclining or reclining wheelchair. (When the chair back goes down, the sling supports must be brought forward to position the slings properly.)

AMBULATION

Indications for Ambulation for the Disabled Patient

Ambulation has been defined as locomotion in an upright position, which includes weight-bearing on the lower extremities. While normal gait is included in this definition, the ambulation of disabled patients may differ considerably in mechanism and appearance from normal walking. Nevertheless, psychologically, the idea of getting around on his own feet gives the patient the feeling of lesser disability than if he is bound to a wheelchair. For this reason alone, a disabled person with limited ambulation potential should be given an opportunity to ambulate occasionally, even if it is done only for short periods and essentially as a recreational exercise.

There are also practical advantages of ambulation over wheelchair locomotion. The ambulatory patient has access to areas that are too narrow or small for a wheelchair, and he may be able to negotiate steep ramps and stairs inaccessible to the wheelchair patient. Very often, personnel concerned with the rehabilitation of the patient take great pride in the patient achieving ambulation, and frequently they urge him to use this method of locomotion exclusively. Such attitudes are as unwise as discouraging all ambulation. The factors that must be considered in advising a patient whether to ambulate and how much to ambulate are: (1) safety of ambulation—he must be sufficiently skilled so he will not fall, (2) effort required for ambulation, (3) possible damage to joints and muscles by ambulation and (4) the efficiency of ambulation, as compared to wheelchair locomotion, in relationship to daily occupation.

Very often, it is advisable for a paraplegic, arthritic or even hemiplegic patient to use wheelchair locomotion for certain activities and ambulation for others. The details of these activities should be prescribed for him by the physician.

The Normal Gait

The normal person walks with a bipedal gait, i.e., on two feet. Each leg goes through two phases: the stance phase, when it stands on the ground, and the swing phase, when it is off the ground and swings forward. The legs alternate so that one leg goes through the swing phase while the opposite leg is in the stance phase. Only for a short time are both legs on the ground. Therefore, normal gait requires the ability to stand on either of the two legs and to lift either of them off the ground and to bring it forward. During each cycle, flexion and extension of all joints of the lower extremities and rotation of the pelvis occur.

Slight disabilities, such as paralysis of one or several muscles and mild joint stiffness, instability or pain, will cause the patient to limp more or less severely. Major disabilities of the lower extremities, such as complete paralysis, amputation, severe joint instability or pain, will make it impossible for the patient to ambulate without special aids.

Special Aids to Ambulation

Special aids are used by the patient who is unable to walk without them. They may also be advisable for the patient who can walk without them, since they may be needed to protect him against musculoskeletal damage and may render his gait more efficient and esthetic. Walking aids for the lower extremities either replace a missing limb (artificial limbs) or stabilize a paralyzed or unstable limb (braces and splints). Walking aids for the upper extremities are used either for weight-bearing or for improving balance and stability (walkers, crutches and canes).

Artificial limbs will be described in the section on amputees (Chap. 16, Sect. D), since their application is limited to that particular disability.

Lower Extremity Aids to Ambulation

Leg Braces. Leg braces (Fig. 6-12) are constructed in many different ways, but the majority follow a standard pattern. Two *lateral bars* or

Activities of Daily Living

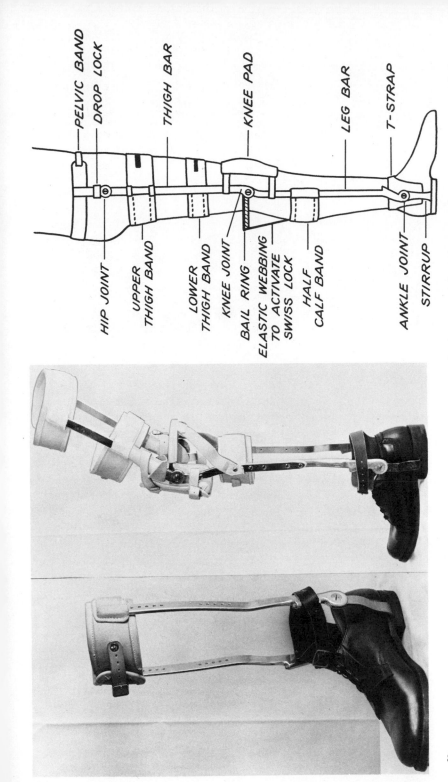

PELVIC BAND

DROP LOCK

THIGH BAR

KNEE PAD

LEG BAR

T-STRAP

HIP JOINT

UPPER THIGH BAND

LOWER THIGH BAND

KNEE JOINT

BAIL RING

ELASTIC WEBBING TO ACTIVATE SWISS LOCK

HALF CALF BAND

ANKLE JOINT

STIRRUP

Fig. 6-12. (*Left*) Short leg brace. (*Center*) Long leg brace. (*Right*) Diagram of parts.

87

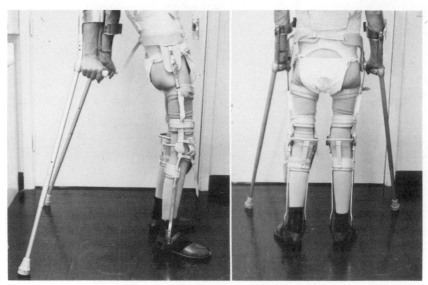

Fig. 6-13.   Long leg braces with pelvic band.

uprights are attached to the shoe or a foot plate. In a *short leg brace* the bars end below the knee in a leather-covered metal cuff, the *calf band*. In a *long leg brace* the bars extend upward to a *thigh band* below the buttock. Usually, there is an upper and a lower thigh band for better stability. The calf band and the thigh bands buckle in front with leather straps. Insead of two thigh bands, a long leg brace may have a laced thigh cuff. A short leg brace has only one joint, at the ankle. The long leg brace has an ankle and a knee joint. The ankle joint may either move freely or have a so-called *posterior stop* at 90 degrees to prevent footdrop. Occasionally, it is provided with anterior and posterior stops to limit mobility in both directions. Complete immobility of the ankle would hamper walking. The knee joint may either move freely or be completely locked. The two kinds of knee lock commonly used are the *drop lock* and the *Swiss (or French) lock*. The latter is preferable since it can be unlocked by pressing the bail ring behind the knee against the edge of a seat. The *drop lock* must be pulled up by hand.

If the patient has poor hip stability, the long leg brace may be extended and attached to a *pelvic band* (Fig. 6-13). A *hip joint* is then needed to permit flexion of the brace when the patient sits. The *hip joint* may be free or have a lock; most commonly, a *drop lock* is used here since it is easily accessible at this high level.

Care of Braces. Every person who wears braces should be instructed in these procedures necessary to keep them in good condition:

1. Clean all the locks every week; use a hairpin or a fine wire to remove the lint that collects in the joints.

2. Place a drop of fine machine oil in each joint every week, and wipe off all excess oil.

3. Keep leather parts in good repair. Have tears repaired at once. Little can be done about perspiration stains on leather parts. Leather should be cleaned with a cloth dampened in lukewarm water and a very mild hand soap. Never saturate leather in water.

4. Keep the heels and the soles of the shoes in good condition so that no part of the brace touches the floor while walking.

5. When the brace has been removed, prop it carefully against the wall or place it on the floor or table in good alignment. Do not bang braces about. Handle them with care.

6. Examine the body nightly for brace pressure marks; no metal should rub on any part of the body.

7. Joints should be checked for correct alignment and wear at least once a year by an orthotist.

8. Before applying, inspect braces for worn parts, loose or missing screws and defective straps and buckles.

9. If possible, have an extra pair of braces.

Splints. Leg splints are cumbersome devices since they do not flex for sitting. However, they have their indications, especially when complete immobilization is desired. They can be made from plaster of Paris, molded leather or plastic materials. In form of a half shell the knee splint is held in place by bandages. The molded leather splint forms a complete sleeve. Two plastic or plaster half shells may be fastened by buckles forming a bivalved cast (Fig. 16-5).

Knee cages and leather anklets have a splintlike effect although they allow some motion (Fig. 16-4).

Foot Appliances. Since the foot plays an essentially passive role in civilized ambulation, very little attention is paid to foot problems in the rehabilitation of the severely disabled patient. However, it is known that foot problems alone can disable an otherwise unaffected person and interfere greatly with his ambulation. For a braced patient with a severely deformed or involved foot, it may be best to attach the brace to a plate that will correct the foot position. In a patient without a brace, foot deformities or foot pain may be managed by the use of arch supports, which are leather or metal inlays placed into the shoe. By means of elevations in some places and cutouts in others, they can improve foot position and eliminate pain.

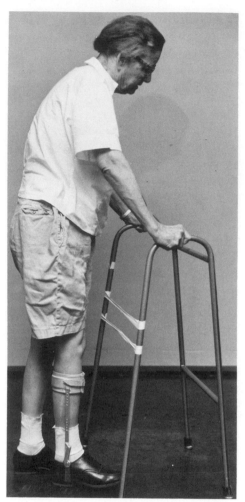

Fig. 6-14. Walkerette without casters.

Upper Extremity Aids to Ambulation

Walkers. Walkers are 4-legged stands that can be displaced by the patient by lifting (Fig. 6-14) or by wheeling on casters (Fig. 6-15). A walker on casters may have a seat that allows the patient to use it like a glide-about. Walkers give maximum stability and permit full weight-bearing on the upper extremities. However, they are bulky and clumsy and therefore are frequently used only temporarily, to be eliminated later on or to be replaced by canes or crutches.

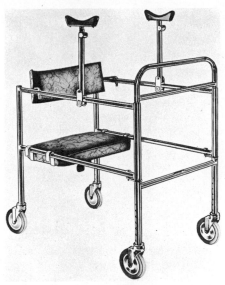

Fig. 6-15. Walker with casters. This type of walker has adjustable underarm supports and a removable seat. (Everest and Jennings)

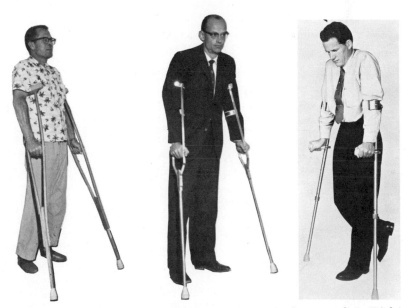

Fig. 6-16. *(Left)* Underarm crutches. *(Center)* Warm Springs crutches. *(Right)* Loftstrand (Canadian) crutches with pivoting forearm cradle grip (Everest and Jennings).

Standard Crutch Gaits

The Point Gaits
1. The 4-point gait (4-point alternate crutch gait):
   Crutch-foot sequence: (1) right crutch, (2) left foot, (3) left crutch, (4) right foot.
2. The 2-point gait (2-point alternate crutch gait):
   Crutch-foot sequence: (1) right crutch and left foot together, (2) left crutch and right foot together.

These 2 gaits can be used only by patients who can move each leg separately and bear a considerable amount of weight on each of them. The term 4-point refers to the number of phases involved in each step cycle. The word alternate refers to alternating movements of the crutches.

The Tripod Crutch Gaits
In these gaits, the patient constantly maintains a tripod position. At the start he has both crutches fairly widespread out front and both feet together in the back.
1. The tripod alternate crutch gait:
   Crutch-foot sequence: (1) right crutch, (2) left crutch, (3) drag body and legs forward.
2. The tripod simultaneous crutch gait:
   Crutch-foot sequence: (1) both crutches, (2) drag body and legs forward.

Both tripod gaits are slow, labored and should be used only as emergency gaits.

The Swinging Crutch Gaits
In the swinging crutch gaits, both legs are lifted off the ground simultaneously and swung forward while the patient pushes up on the crutches.
1. The swing-to gait:
   Crutch-foot sequence: (1) both crutches forward, (2) lift and swing body to crutches, (3) place crutches forward and continue.
2. The swing-through gait:
   Crutch-foot sequence: (1) both crutches forward, (2) lift and swing body beyond crutches, (3) place crutches in front of body and continue.

Crutches.   Crutches are sticks which are stabilized by the upper extremity in at least two places, the lower of which is at hand level (Fig. 6-16). For the underarm crutch, the upper point of stabilization is the axilla. For the Warm Springs crutch it is the upper arm and for the Canadian (Loftstrand) crutch it is the forearm below the elbow. Of these three types of crutches, the underarm crutch gives the greatest stability and the Canadian crutch the least. The elbow crutch, or platform crutch (Fig. 16-17) is designed for patients who either cannot extend their arms or cannot bear weight on the hands or the wrists. The main indications for platform crutches occur in rheumatoid arthritis.

Standard Crutch Gaits.   When walking with crutches, a disabled patient may either take a step with one leg and then the other as in normal walking, or he may move both legs simultaneously. In the former case, the 4-point or 2-point crutch gait is commonly used, while in the latter case the tripod or swinging gaits are used. An explanation of the standard crutch gaits is contained in the box (p. 92).

Canes.   Canes have a function similar to crutches, but lack a second point of impact and, therefore, give much less stability. Usually, a patient uses only one cane for additional weight-bearing or balance on one side.

REFERENCES

1. Fahland, B. and Grendahl, B. C.: Wheelchair Selection: More Than Choosing a Chair with Wheels. Minneapolis: American Rehabilitation Foundation, 1967.
2. Flaherty, P. T. and Jurkovich, S. J.: Transfers for Patients with Acute and Chronic Conditions. Minneapolis: American Rehabilitation Foundation, 1970.
3. Lawton, E. B.: Activities of Daily Living for Physical Rehabilitation. New York: McGraw-Hill, 1963.
4. Licht, S.: Physical Medicine Library, Vol. 9, Orthotics Etcetera. New Haven: Elizabeth Licht, 1966.
5. Perry, J. and Hislop, H. J.: Principles of Lower Extremity Bracing. American Physical Therapy Association, 1972.

CHAPTER
7

Self-Care

TYPES OF SELF-CARE ACTIVITIES

Self-care is the term used in medical rehabilitation for the ability to carry out unassisted the ordinary activities of personal care, such as feeding, dressing and bathing. Of course, the total number and the nature of self-care activities depend on individual and group standards. Eating with specialized tools and using a sanitary toilet for excretion are minimal standards in our culture. Dressing and bathing are also expected of all well-adjusted able-bodied people. However, among the disabled, the home-bound patient frequently passes up daily bathing, while the institutionalized patient often omits dressing.

Self-care may be divided into four categories: (1) eating, (2) dressing, (3) toilet activities and (4) miscellaneous hand activities.

Eating activities include taking meals in bed, in a wheelchair and at a table. While it is desirable to achieve ability to eat with knife, fork and spoon and to drink from cups and glasses, specially adapted tools may sometimes be used.

Toilet activities include washing the whole body, either in bed or in a shower or bathtub, combing hair, brushing teeth, applying make-up, etc. Also included in this group is the use of a bedpan or urinal for the bedfast patient, and the bedside commode or toilet bowl by the mobile patient for purposes of elimination.

Dressing activities include the use of ordinary or special clothing. Certain adjustments and selections of type of clothing must be made according to the disability of the patient. He should not be satisfied to wear night clothes and a bathrobe.

The miscellaneous hand activities include smoking, handling money, operating light switches, opening and closing curtains, doors and windows, writing, page-turning, using the telephone and acts associated with mobility, such as pushing an elevator button and driving a car.

CAUSES OF DEFICIENCY IN SELF-CARE

Disability of any part of the body may impair self-care. For instance, lack of spinal mobility may make it impossible for the patient to reach his feet, creating a problem in putting on socks and lacing shoes. A long leg cast will be an obstacle to the usual way of bathing and dressing.

Since self-care activities are for the most part carried out by the upper extremities, their involvement contributes heavily to limitation in self-care, particularly when both upper extremities are affected. The major disabilities affecting upper extremity function are amputation, paralysis, limitation of range of motion and pain.

Interference with self-care can result from the following:

1. Disabilities of both upper extremities, such as bilateral upper extremity amputation, rheumatoid arthritis involving both upper extremities or paralysis of both upper extremities.

2. Disabilities involving one upper extremity, such as hemiplegia or a unilateral upper extremity amputation.

3. Disabilities interfering with trunk mobility, such as paraplegia, quadriplegia, spinal rigidity due to arthritis, pain or the use of a body cast.

4. Disabilities interfering with lower-extremity mobility, such as paraplegia or arthritis of the lower extremities.

THE EVALUATION OF SELF-CARE ABILITY AND SELF-CARE POTENTIAL

It is important to be able to evaluate the self-care ability and potential of disabled persons, not only in order to assess prognosis for rehabilitation but also to determine eligibility for financial and medical care under the various categories of public welfare programs. Although attention is directed particularly to the medical and rehabilitative aspects of self-care, the legal and administrative issues are important in determining resources for rehabilitation services. Evaluation of self-care involves three steps:

1. Determination of what self-care activities the individual can carry out and what he cannot carry out. This is the diagnostic step.

2. Evaluation of the extent to which self-care ability can be increased, that is, what additional activity the patient may be enabled to carry out by himself as a result of rehabilitation procedures. This is the prognostic phase of evaluation.

3. Determination of the methods by means of which the patient

can achieve his potential self-care ability. This phase of the evaluation leads directly to the management of the self-care problems.

One must always consider not only the potential ability of the individual concerned, but also the cost in strain and effort required in considering whether it is worthwhile to attempt to assign a specific self-care task to the patient. Quite often, a patient with an affliction like multiple sclerosis has the neuromuscular potential to feed himself, but incoordination superimposed upon weakness of the upper extremities transforms his meals into frustrating ordeals. He gets no pleasure out of eating but only struggles to get his food to the proper place. In such instances, enthusiastically imposed self-care training is not a rehabilitative measure but a means of torture. Self-care is of value only if it gives the patient pleasure and dignity and the feeling of achievement. Therefore, it should not be forced. A severely disabled person who has had adequate evaluation and has a full understanding of the problem involved should always be given the choice of being assisted if he is happier that way.

METHODS OF RESTORATION TO SELF-CARE

Problems of self-care are specific for each given disability and will be discussed in detail with these disabilities. However, the general principles may be mentioned here. The following methods are used in rehabilitation or restoration to self-care: (1) physical conditioning techniques to increase strength and range of motion, (2) training or instruction in self-care methods by circumventing disability, (3) use of assistive devices and (4) use of adapted equipment and modifications of clothing and living arrangements.

Physical Conditioning

Improved self-care is achieved by increasing strength, mobility and agility. Therefore, well-directed therapeutic exercises and methods of physical conditioning may be the proper preliminaries to improving self-care. However, the indications for exercises and the exercises prescribed must be specific and consistent with neuromuscular physiology. One must not confuse physical deconditioning that results from disuse with motor loss due to organic neurologic disorder. One should not assume that paralysis can be reversed by exercise in the same way that disuse can be reversed.

It is true that agility and coordination can usually be improved to some extent by practice in both the impaired and the unimpaired extremities. However, there is no reason for prolonged, frustrating exercise for the achievement of negligible gains. It is necessary to weigh potential achievement against the cost in time and effort.

Conditioning of intact muscles is never contraindicated. For example, the muscles of the amputated upper extremity stump should be exercised to improve strength and shoulder range of motion. Both should be brought to optimal levels.

The nonparalyzed side of the hemiplegic should be exercised for strengthening and trained in new activities, especially if the dominant side is paralyzed.

Training in Self-Care Techniques

Specific training in self-care techniques helps restore independence. This involves more than practice to increase strength and agility. To train the disabled person in a specific technique, he must be shown an effective method of dressing or bathing or feeding. It is in the two fields of self-care (dressing and bathing) that training is most helpful. For example, when the hemiplegic patient is told how to place a shirt in front of him, to pass the hemiplegic arm through the sleeve with the aid of the uninvolved arm and then to lift the shirt up over his head and pass the uninvolved arm into the sleeve, he can perform this task at once. If he tries it the opposite way, he will be unable to put on the shirt. Instruction in all acts requiring upper extremity function may involve methods of using the uninvolved upper extremity to overcome the obstacle of the paralyzed, once dominant, hemiplegic hand.

Upper Extremity Appliances and Assistive Devices

A bilateral upper extremity amputee is utterly helpless so far as self-care is concerned. However, if he is provided with bilateral upper extremity prostheses, he will be able to feed, wash, and even dress himself. However, training is needed to develop skill in the use of prostheses. This may be prolonged and difficult.

For paralyzed patients, there are now a great many assistive appliances. One of the most useful is the ball-bearing rocker feeder (Fig. 7-1) which enables a patient with complete upper extremity paralysis, but with some trunk motion, to feed himself.

Adapted Equipment

Although last to be considered, this is probably the most important avenue to restoration of self-care. The use of adapted equipment and modification of the environment to meet the needs of the patient are applicable in nearly every disability. Successful adaptation of the environment illustrates the basic principle of rehabilitation, that is, to

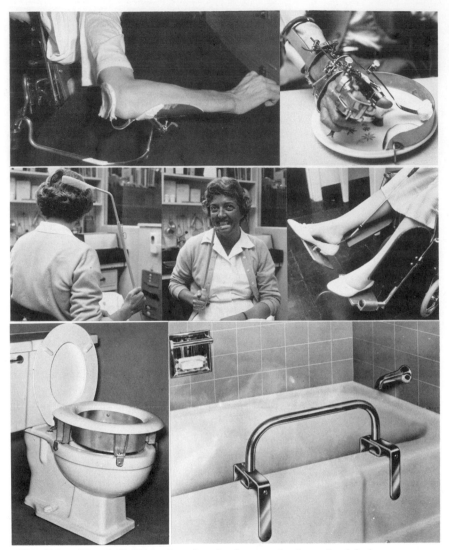

Fig. 7-1. *(Top, left)* Pivoted rocker feeder attached to wheelchair.

Fig. 7-2. *(Top, right)* Plate guard. Permits disabled person to handle food by preventing spillage. This photograph also shows a special hand splint with fork attachment.

Fig. 7-3. Long-handled utensils. *(Center, left)* Comb. *(Center)* Toothbrush. *(Center, right)* shoe horn.

Fig. 7-4. *(Bottom, left)* Portable raised toilet seat with shield.

Fig. 7-5. *(Bottom, right)* Bathtub rail.

enable the patient to live with his disability by using what he has left. Adapted equipment is used in all phases of self-care. For instance, in feeding activities the weak and ataxic patient is helped by a plate guard on a plate (Fig. 7-2). The plate may be fastened to the table by means of a suction cup. To help the patient with an arthritic hand to grasp a utensil, a padded handle is provided. To assist in bringing food to the mouth, special long-handled or curved implements are designed to overcome limitations of motion or weakness.

A long-handled shoehorn, elastic shoelaces, wide sleeves, front fastening brassieres and zippered trouser legs will facilitate dressing for the disabled patient. A long-handled comb or toothbrush may solve problems associated with grooming (Fig. 7-3). A raised toilet seat (Fig. 7-4) may enable the weak person to become independent in elimination since he will be able to get up and down unassisted. A bathtub rail (Fig. 7-5) makes it safer to get in and out of the bath.

Use of adapted equipment and changed environment should not be limited to the phase of rehabilitation. The patient should be given the benefit of this type of self-care assistance from the beginning of disability and continuously thereafter. The bed patient should have access to all the things he needs. Two night tables or a large bedside table with shelves may help him store his personal belongings and equipment. He should have access to the telephone, signal light and a good reading lamp; he should be positioned and supplied with devices to give him the opportunity to feed himself. The rehabilitation center or rehabilitation ward should be arranged in such a way that a patient has access to his clothing, a mirror, lavatory, shower or bathtub and toilet to allow him a maximum of self-care. Before discharge to his own home, the necessary steps should be taken to adapt the home environment to the disabled patient. This should be done before he gets home and should be planned and modified with his assistance, preferably during week-end visits home.

REFERENCES

1. Bumbala, J. A., et al.: "The Self-Help Phenomenon." Amer. J. Nurs., 73:1588, 1973.
2. Hallburg, J. C.: "Teaching Patients Self Care." Nurs. Clin. N. Amer., 5:223, 1970.
3. Lowman, E. W. and Klinger, J.: Aids to Independent Living. New York: McGraw-Hill, 1969.
4. Lowman, E. W. and Rusk, H. A.: Self Help Devices, Rehabilitation Monograph No. XXI. New York: The Institute of Physical Medicine and Rehabilitation, 1962.
5. Robinault, I. P.: Functional Aids for the Multiple Handicapped. New York: Harper and Row, 1973.

CHAPTER

8

Communication
BRUCE E. PORCH

Communication is an act by means of which one human being conveys to another his ideas, thoughts, needs or feelings. It is not only an activity of daily living like mobility or self-care which may need to be restored if impaired, but it is also a necessary tool if those working in rehabilitative medicine are to effect restoration of any functions. Since communication is the means by which the rehabilitation team interacts with the patient from the very beginning of the rehabilitative effort, a means of communication must be found quickly.

The severely impaired patient, the passive patient or the resistive patient can be fed, clothed and transported without his active participation in the process. This is never true of communication. A patient must have the desire to communicate and have some communication channel open to him if he is going to convey ideas to those around him. One of the greatest challenges in rehabilitative medicine is the patient who desires to communicate but is unable to do so because of serious breakdowns in his communication system. In these cases it requires great diligence and creativity to reestablish communication with the patient. For instance, there is the example of the patient who had complete paralysis of all his muscles except for a small group around one eyebrow. By putting an electromyographic electrode on this muscle group and amplifying the sounds of the muscle activity when he moved the muscle we were able to establish quite a rich communication channel. With this device, he was able to answer yes and no questions as well as number questions with considerable facility where he previously had been completely motionless and non-communicative. In other cases we have used microswitches to provide patients with signals, amplifiers to increase the intensity of a nearly inaudible voice and pointing boards for patients who are unable to speak or write.

Communication defects, especially those of speech and hearing, often are difficult to analyze and require highly specialized services. Whenever possible, the patient with communication disorder should be provided with the diagnostic and therapeutic skills of the speech pathologist, the audiologist or other indicated specialist. Many of the suggestions in this chapter are based on the assumption that specialized personnel may be inaccessible or available only for the most severely impaired patients. Emphasis is placed on the ways in which nonspecialized staff may favorably influence the patient who has a communication disability.

THE COMMUNICATION SYSTEM

When considering the communication system it is useful to think of the human being as a brain, isolated in the bony, protective vault of the skull. The rest of the body is designed for nourishing, informing and carrying out the mandates of the brain. Communication involves getting information about the environment to the brain, processing the information and then transmitting the brain's response back to the environment, as shown in the schematic representation in Figure 8-1.

Input: Information to the Brain

Physical stimuli relentlessly bombard the body from every side. Each stimulus is received by one of the five senses or input pathways. Here, it is converted from physical energy to neural energy by receptors, such as the eyes, the ears, the touch receptors, the taste buds and the olfactory hair cells. In truth, the eyes do not see, and the ears do not hear, but each changes only one kind of energy into another so that the energy can be transmitted along nerves. Once generated, the neural message travels to the first junction in the brain where several paths may be open to it. If it is a message of pain or heat, it may be channeled to cause movement away from the harmful stimulus by bringing into play a fast-acting warning or monition system that can bring about change without waiting for the slow-moving conscious pathways to do so. If it is one of many unimportant messages entering at that moment, it may be stopped or "gated" at this point in order that the higher centers of the brain might restrict attention to more important messages entering.

If the message continues on to succeeding neurons, its various characteristics are perceived, and it is differentiated from other messages. The message begins to assume an individual identity that can be associated with other related messages and labeled. When the characteristics of the message are erroneously perceived or if the message contains insufficient or distorted information, the association must await additional messages before being completed.

Therefore, it may be noted that it is possible to perceive something

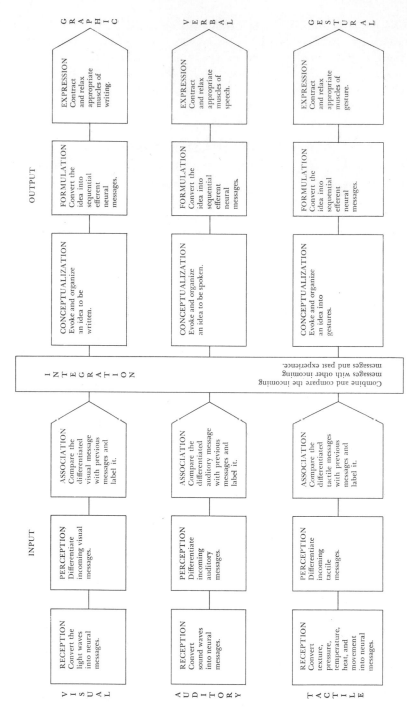

Fig. 8-1. A schematic representation of the communication system.

102

without being able to label or recognize it. For example, as you are confronted with the word (Θx$\pm$) your eyes receive the physical energy of the light waves reflected from the markings on the paper and convert it into a neural message. Your optic nerves transmit the message to the centers for perception where you differentiate one marking from another, but you find yourself unable to associate these symbols with anything in your past experience even though you can duplicate them with paper and pencil. If the symbols (M X Q) are substitued, you can then perceive and associate each symbol, but they remain symbols and take on no combined meaning. When the symbols (C A T) are substituted, reception, perception and association yield a word that can be integrated with other previously processed messages and can generate a wide variety of thoughts about cat.

Output: Messages from the Brain

As the integration of messages takes place, responses to the environment must be generated. Communication must become an outgoing, efferent motor process through one of three primary pathways, i.e., gestural output, speech or verbal output and writing or graphic output. Once the output pathway is chosen, the appropriate idea or concept to be transmitted is selected from the many being integrated at that moment. The component ideas are selected and combined into a concept that must then be formulated into a series of message impulses to be transmitted to the appropriate expressors, such as the lips, the tongue, the larynx, the arm, the hand or the face in exactly the right sequence and duration to produce the movements necessary for speech, writing or gesture.

To return to the example—you have visually received (C A T), perceived the distinctive characteristics of each symbol, associated these symbols with the word cat and have aroused a number of thoughts related to the word. If you want to express one of these ideas, you might choose to use verbal output to say something about the eating habits of small domestic felines. You would select and order a series of message units into the concept, "A cat drinks milk." This conceptualization is then submitted for formulation into the neural patterns that will activate the expressors, which in this case would be the diaphragm, the larynx, the soft palate, the tongue, the lips and the jaw muscles. Each of these expressors must move in exactly the right sequence to contribute to the production of a certain series of sounds and noises that when received by the auditory input pathway of another communication system will be interpreted as the message, "A cat drinks milk."

Your response could have been via graphic output. The idea is then conceptualized into visual symbols and formulated into motor patterns that would contract and relax the muscle groups of the arm and the hand necessary to move a pencil over paper to produce accurate visual symbols imparting the idea. Or, perhaps your response to (C A T) might have employed the most primary and automatic of the three output modalities, gesture, with the conceptualization and formulation activating the muscles of the arm simply to point to a cat sleeping in a chair across the room.

All of the steps outlined above are vital to maintaining contact with one's surroundings. Each step can be affected or eliminated by disease and injury or by various psychological causes. The resulting problems of communication may be temporary or permanent, mild or severe, hardly noticeable or completely disruptive. They may represent the primary goal of rehabilitation or a secondary, complicating factor in disability.

THE EXAMINATION OF COMMUNICATION ABILITY

Although comprehensive examination of communication usually requires the skill of a speech pathologist or speech clinician, everyone taking part in the rehabilitation process can and should have some basic skill in evaluating communication. The information gained may have to serve in lieu of a diagnosis by a speech pathologist since specialized services may not always be readily available. Speech evaluation by other staff members will complement specialist examinations if they are available. Most important, knowledge of his communication problems will lead to a better understanding of the patient and thereby save much time and effort in carrying out effective treatment.

Some of the most important fundamentals of evaluating the communication process are outlined below. Many of the significant symptoms can be obtained through careful observation of the patient during the course of his daily schedule. When it is necessary to evaluate the patient's communication by direct examination, the best results will be achieved by first preparing him for the tests. If the observer is unfamiliar to the patient, he should be informed by whatever means necessary of the identity of the observer and the reason for interest in his communication ability. Once acquainted, one should try to elicit the patient's thoughts about his difficulties by inquiring if he feels that he is having trouble talking, what kind of trouble he is having and if he has tried reading or writing and with what results. The testing can then be introduced by saying, "I'm going to try to help you with the trouble you are having. Before I can do this I must find out what you can do and what you cannot do. I want you to do some things for me. Some of them will be easy, and some will be very hard to do. Try to do as well as you can. Take all the time you need to do them. Are you ready?"

Clear, concise instruction should precede each test. Whenever possible, the patient should be examined in a quiet, well-lit room, free from noise and distraction and preferably without onlookers. The patient should be rested and comfortable, wearing his glasses, hearing aid or dentures if these are customarily used.

Examining the Input Modalities

Visual Input

Visual Reception. Assess visual acuity. Does the patient wear glasses? Perhaps he wore glasses before his present illness, and members of his family can provide them. The physical examination will provide information about cataracts and other peripheral disorders.

A common visual involvement in cases of hemiplegia is hemianopia, the loss of vision in half of the visual field of each eye due to damage to one side of the posterior part of the brain that receives the nerve pathways from the eyes, or due to damage of the pathways. This problem is somewhat similar to trying to see through a pair of glasses that have been painted black on one half of each lens. The patient sees only to the front and to one side but sees nothing to his blind side. Interestingly, the patient is often aware that his vision is changed but does not realize the true nature of the difficulty. He may eat only the foods placed on his sighted side. When given a series of sentences to read, he may read only the last few words in each sentence, those which he can see.

Visual Perception. Determine if the patient can differentiate basic visual characteristics, such as shape, color and size. Place a few objects, pictures, letters or words in front of him; then hand him one item that is identical with one of those in front of him, and ask him through speech and gesture to put the item with the one just like it. Repeat with other items. In most cases, even a patient with no auditory input ability will succeed in this task if his visual reception and perception are intact and if he has enough integrative ability to understand what he is to do.

Visual Association. To determine if the patient is able to associate and categorize visual messages, have him match the printed name with the object or picture or match related items which are dissimilar in structure, such as a knife with a fork, a cigarette with matches, a quarter with a dollar bill and a key with a lock.

Auditory Input

Auditory Reception. Generally, peripheral hearing problems do not result from strokes. However, hearing loss stemming from other causes is always a possibility with any patient and especially in older persons. The case history or the family and friends can supply information about existing hearing deficits, chronic ear pathology and whether the patient uses a hearing aid. Ear canals should be inspected and cleared of cerumen if necessary. The patient's hearing aid should be kept in good working order and should be used whenever verbal communication is necessary. If there is no history available and a hearing loss is suspected, tests of hearing should be carried out.

Auditory Perception. Determine if the patient can differentiate sound by having him imitate single, short, common words. Imitative ability does not imply that the patient understands the meaning of the words. Failure to imitate may also result from impaired verbal output.

Auditory Association. Determine if the patient attaches some meaning to words. Place several common objects or pictures in front of the patient and ask him to point to each as it is named by you. Body parts and objects in the room may also be used.

Tactile Input

Tactile Reception. Peripheral receptors for the sense of touch are not impaired by strokes but may be affected by peripheral nerve and spinal cord injuries accompanying traumatic brain lesions. In these cases, the physical examination will provide information about the patient's ability to feel touch, pressure, pain and temperature.

Tactile Perception. If the patient with hemiplegia begins to get some return of the affected side, his ability to perceive differences between objects through touch should be tested. The procedure is to hold something in front of the patient so that he cannot see objects you will place in his hand. An opened manila folder or a large plain piece of cardboard can serve to obstruct his vision. If he can speak, place a common object, such as a comb, a key, a pencil or a coin in his affected hand and ask him to name it. (Be sure that he has adequate verbal output for this task.) If he cannot speak, hold the obstruction in front of him, allow him to feel the object, take the object and place it with the other objects on the table in front of him, remove the visual obstruction and ask him to point to the object he had been feeling. (It is also common practice to have the patient close his eyes rather than to use an obstruction. However, this is sometimes confusing to the aphasic patient, since he must carry out two tasks, closing his eyes and feeling the object, and often he opens his eyes as soon as his hand is touched, and the test must be repeated.)

Examining the Output Modalities

Verbal Output

Verbal Expression.   Many things can interfere with the patient's peripheral speech mechanism. Paralysis on one side of the face is common, as is unilateral paralysis of the tongue, the palate or the larynx. In general, unilateral involvement of any of these structures does not seriously affect speech but may produce some dysarthria. Bilateral paralysis of the face, the tongue or the palate are not commonly seen. Usually, bilateral paralysis of the pharynx or the larynx is associated with bilateral or multiple cerebral vascular accidents. In these instances, dysarthria is usually more severe.

Weakened facial muscles will sag on the affected side and will not move when the patient smiles or is asked to show his teeth or say "eee." The tongue will deviate toward the weak side when the patient is asked to stick out his tongue. The palate pulls away from the weak side which does not rise when the patient yawns or says "ah." Bilateral pharyngeal weakness results in complaints of food sticking in the throat and usually requires use of a soft or a liquid diet. Bilateral laryngeal weakness results in poor protection of the respiratory tract due to the inefficient valving of the larynx. Liquids, especially water, move rapidly down the pharynx and find their way through the smallest opening in the laryngeal valve. This produces choking and coughing. The liquids should be replaced with soft slippery food (but not ground meat), gelatins and custards. Sometimes, patients find that they can swallow liquids which are hot, cold or sweet since these can be better felt as they move through the pharynx, and the valving of the larynx can be timed more efficiently.

Lack of teeth or poorly fitting dentures can reduce greatly the intelligibility of speech, especially when there is also facial and tongue weakness. Too often, dentures lie in the drawer of the patient's bedstand while the hospital staff struggles to understand what he is trying to say. When the patient has dentures, he should wear them, and they should be checked for fit and comfort.

Verbal Formulation.   The ability to convert a verbal concept into neural messages is tested by having the patient imitate words and short phrases. (This cannot be done if he has lost all auditory input or integrative ability.) After you explain the task to the patient, pause briefly and then say each word clearly with the patient watching your face. If he is having difficulty with verbal formulation, he will appear to understand the task and will make an effort to say the word, but will be unable to speak. He may make several exploratory attempts before approximating the selected word, or after an unsuccessful attempt he may automatically say, "I can't say it!" or swear. This condition is sometimes referred to as oral apraxia.

Verbal Conceptualization.   A patient who has difficulty in conceptualization cannot evoke and organize the components of an idea even though he has integrated the information. The verbal response is on the tip of his tongue, but he cannot elicit it. When asked to name common objects, he might say, "Oh, that's a . . . it's a . . . I know what it is, but I just can't say it . . . it's right on the end of my lip, but I can't do it." He can imitate the word easily and usually can say it if he gets some cues about it. For instance, if you present a pipe for him to name, he is unable to say its name although he may gesturally demonstrate its use; but if you say, "You put tobacco in a . . ." often he will immediately say "pipe." If he is given the first sound of the word, he can frequently complete it. Testing consists of having the patient name objects, colors, letters, pictures, numbers, etc. He should be allowed plenty of time for each response. When he cannot respond, cues should be given to see if the concept can be elicited.

Gestural Output

Gestural Expression.   Gestural ability with the affected side may be reduced or lost depending on the amount of paralysis. Except in cases of bilateral damage, the unaffected side functions adequately and can be efficiently used for communication even if the patient has habitually used the opposite side.

Gestural Formulation.   As with verbal formulation, the ability to convert a gestural concept into neural messages is tested by having the patient imitate simple gestural acts. Gesture is so basic to our communication that this almost automatic skill is rarely lost.

Gestural Conceptualization.   Usually, gesture is the last output modality lost and the first regained after a CVA, and often the patient will rely heavily on it for expressing his needs and thoughts. Ability to evoke and organize gestural concepts can be tested by asking the patient to demonstrate as completely as possible the use of common objects, such as a fork, a cigarette, a key, a spoon, etc. A patient with poor gestural conceptualization who cannot speak will make elaborate gestures in the attempt to convey an idea, but these will be inaccurate and unintelligible.

It is emphasized again that gestural output is very frequently the patient's best means of communicating, if the staff members allow him adequate time and if they make a sincere attempt to decipher his charades.

Graphic Output

Graphic Expression.   Paralysis of the hand and the arm may prevent the patient from holding a pencil and writing as he is accustomed, and he must be taught to use the unaffected hand instead. Sometimes, there is only moderate or mild weakness, and pencils built up in thickness and other devices can be used to good advantage.

Graphic Formulation.   The ability to convert graphic concepts into neural messages is tested by asking the patient to copy simple geometric forms, numbers, letters and words. The patient might be able to tell you what the item is, describe it or spell it, but when he attempts to copy it he cannot make the motions necessary to the act. As one patient stated, "I know what I want, but my hand forgot how!" Treatment for this problem, sometimes called apraxia, is to have the patient use his visual and proprioceptive-kinesthetic input to trace the form with his finger and then try to duplicate the form with pencil and paper.

Graphic Conceptualization.   The ability to evoke and to organize graphic concepts is tested by having the patient write the names, the colors and the functions of objects or pictures presented to him. If he cannot do the more complicated tasks, try saying the word and have him write it. If this fails, spell the word while he writes it.

CAUSES AND MANAGEMENT OF COMMUNICATION DISABILITIES

Although the communication diagram on page 102 and the examination described on pages 104 to 109 may appear complex, there are only four major groups of disabilities from the clinical standpoint. Of the three *receptive input* modalities only *vision* and *hearing* are significant. Tactile input is usually used only to a minor degree in human communication as with a handshake or a slap on the shoulder, for example. However it may serve a major function as a substitute input, as illustrated by the blind patient's use of a cane or braille. The three *expressive output* modalities are disrupted essentially by disturbances in motor function. Disturbances of all higher input and output stages, i.e., perception, association, integration, conceptualization and formulation, are grouped clinically under the term *aphasia*.

We shall discuss briefly causes, diagnosis, prognosis and management of the four major communication disorders: (1) impairment of vision, (2) impairment of hearing, (3) impairment of expression and (4) aphasia.

Impairment of Vision

Visual impairment in the candidate for rehabilitation must be considered under two separate categories. First, there may be preexisting and unrelated visual difficulties, particularly in the elderly, and second, are the visual difficulties induced by the illness or injury which precipitated the difficulty in communication. In the first category we must consider errors of refraction and other kinds of pathology of the eye. The second category involves principally impairments of vision resulting from neurological damage.

Errors of Refraction

Very few human eyes are perfect optical instruments. Most people have ametropia which means that there are minor or severe optical defects interfering with the transmission of parallel rays of light to the retina. The common defects of nearsightedness and farsightedness (myopia and hyperopia) are largely due to congenital disorders. In the myopic eye there is usually prolonged growth of the eyeball so that its anteroposterior diameter is elongated and parallel rays tend to focus in front of the retina. In the hyperopic eye there is generally a failure of normal growth and parallel rays tend to focus behind the retina. In addition, there are characteristic changes in the eye with age, i.e., loss of accommodation and astigmatism.[6] The ability of individuals of varying age to compensate for myopia and hyperopia is lost as the ability of the eye to adjust its focus to objects at different distances diminishes. When the ciliary muscle no longer responds because of normal changes of aging, even the normal eye becomes presbyopic. It is necessary to use a concave lens to correct the defect of myopia and a convex lens to correct hyperopia. The presbyopic eye may have been myopic, hyperopic or astigmatic and corrections will depend upon the visual refractive error. Astigmatism is due to variation in refraction in different meridians of the eye. Such changes are almost invariably due to differences in curvature of the cornea in various meridians. Normally the cornea is spherical but if it is elliptical in any direction the eye will be astigmatic.

The treatment of these eye disorders consists of determining and prescribing suitable lenses. These may be worn in spectacles or they may be applied as contact lenses. In either case, the purpose is to supply externally, a corrective lens which will help focus parallel rays of light on the retina without distortion or blurring.

Defects of the Visual Field

Visual field disturbances not only produce impairment of vision, but often supplement other causes for confusion of the disabled person.[5] The most frequent significant defect encountered in patients suffering from impaired communication is the homonymous hemianopia seen in people who have suffered strokes. The most common area of insufficient blood supply in the brain following a stroke is in the region supplied by the lenticulostriate artery. This lesion often affects that part of the internal capsule along which the fibers of the optic tract pass from the optic area of the occipital lobe toward the lateral geniculate body. The right optic cortex and the right lateral geniculate body innervate the right halves of each retina. A lesion destroying the fiber tracts therefore produces blindness in the left halves of both visual fields, hence homonymous. Since the field defect is usually similar in both eyes, it is also a congruous hemianopia or half blindness. The consequences of this disorder have already been discussed. It is important to realize, however, that the defect is often missed and people who cannot communicate well are particularly prone to be labeled unresponsive or "out of it" because they are approached from the blind side. Following a stroke people with hemianopia often sustain injuries or falls because they fail to recognize obstacles or curbs on the blind side. Eventually, they learn to turn their heads so that they get a reasonable view of the world, but frequently they do not compensate enough for safety. It is especially important, therefore, to guard against injury in the hemianopic person.

Other field defects occur as results of injury, neoplasms, etc., and an essential part of the diagnosis of a difficult neurologic problem is the determination of the visual field by an expert.

Other Forms of Visual Impairment

Aside from errors in refraction and disturbances of visual field, there are numerous other causes of visual disorder in disabled people. In disseminated sclerosis and particularly in the severe form of neuromyelitis optica, progressive impairment of vision occurs. At times this is compounded by nystagmus which leads to visual blurring, but often there is simply progressive damage of the nerve of the eye with pallor of the disc, at first temporal, later generalized.

Older people frequently tend to develop retinal degeneration in the area of the macula where central vision is located, thereby resulting in serious impairment of acuity. Cataracts resulting from thickening or hardening of the capsules of the lens or of the lens itself also lead to progressive impairment of vision. In the elderly person the differential diagnosis between visual loss due to cataract and visual loss due to retinal degeneration is often difficult and requires very special examination techniques.

Other disorders include glaucoma which if undetected leads to destruction of the optic nerve and visual impairment, and injuries to the cornea which often lead to scarring. Both traumatic and spontaneous changes such as retinal detachment, hemorrhage, etc., may occur to complicate the problem of communication. In diabetics particularly the retina is prone to damage from hemorrhage and from accumulations of exudates.

Blindness

Blindness, occurring as the principal defect, is usually treated in special centers for the blind. However, blind people can become otherwise disabled, while blindness occurring with other communication disturbances constitutes a formidable problem.

Causes of blindness are of course legion. In children one encounters congenital amblyopia of variable degree which is untreatable and permanent. Children with crossed eyes almost invariably suppress the vision in one eye, and therefore have what amounts to a partial functional blindness. In the course of life, the eye is subject to injury from direct trauma, from toxic substances, from drugs which may have disastrous effects on vision and from disease.

Whenever blindness occurs in individuals with other motor and communicative disorders it is necessary to find some method of communication through speech and touch which does not involve vision. When both vision and hearing are significantly impaired, it is essential to explore every possibility of remedy. For example, a quadriplegic patient made deaf by antibiotic drugs gradually became blind as a result of progressive cataracts. In this instance the extraction of the cataracts was the only means by which restoration of communication could be accomplished.[13]

Impairment of Hearing

The Hearing Mechanism

The brain is isolated from sound by its protective housing. Before hearing can take place, the sound energy in the air around us must be collected, conducted to the hearing mechanism and then converted to

Activities of Daily Living

neural energy for transmission to the brain. The outer ear collects the sound waves and funnels them into the external auditory canal. As they reach the end of the canal, these waves of energy strike the eardrum and move it in and out slightly. Three small bones in the middle ear form a bridge from the eardrum to a membrane covering the entrance to the inner ear. When the eardrum is moved by sound, the bridge conducts the energy to the inner ear. The sound energy moves through the fluids of the inner ear where it strikes sensitive nerve endings that convert it into neural energy. These neural messages are transmitted to the brain by way of the auditory nerves.

The human ear is a very sensitive mechanism. A young person can hear a range of sounds varying in frequency from 20 to 20,000 cycles per second (Hz). However, the standard tests of hearing with an audiometer sample only the frequencies from 125 Hz to 8000 Hz. The most important frequencies for the discrimination of speech are those between 500 and 2000.

Disease and dysfunction produce two major types of hearing loss. A conductive hearing loss results when any condition prevents the sound from being transported through the outer or the middle ear. A sensorineural hearing loss results when sound energy is not converted and transmitted by the inner ear. Each type has a distinctive set of symptoms and is described briefly here, with particular reference to the hearing of older patients.

Conductive Hearing Loss

Causes. Excessive wax, foreign objects and growths may obstruct the ear canal. Movement of the eardrum and the middle ear bones may be reduced by otosclerosis, middle ear infections and perforations of the eardrum.

Symptoms. Conductive losses are mild or moderate in severity, never severe. All sounds, whether they are of low, medium or high frequency, usually are affected. Only sounds that are loud enough to get through the obstruction or bypass it can be used by the inner ear. Therefore, the patient may have difficulty hearing softly spoken speech but hears and understands louder speech. In noisy places, he does not hear the noise but hears the speech of others well because people with normal hearing automatically talk more loudly when it is noisy.

Some of the clinical symptoms of a conductive hearing loss include:

1. The air-conducted sound from a tuning fork held close to the ear is not easily heard. The bone-conducted sound from the tuning

fork placed on the mastoid bone is easily heard, since the sound traveling through the bone bypasses the defective conductive mechanism and is converted by the intact inner ear.

2. Often, the patient will volunteer a history of middle ear infections, excessive wax, various sensations of fullness, itching or pain in the ears or intermittent hearing difficulty.

3. Frequently, a patient with otosclerosis will report that other members of his family have similar hearing problems and that he has had no ear infections or injury.

Treatment.   An otologist (ear specialist) should examine the ears to determine the cause of the conductive loss and to prescribe treatment. Most conductive losses can be treated effectively by surgery and medication. If there is still a significant residual hearing loss and communication deficit after maximum treatment, the patient will benefit from a hearing aid. Conductive losses respond well to hearing aid amplification since the cochlea (inner ear) is still intact and responds normally once the incoming sound is made loud enough to overcome the conductive "blockage" and stimulates the cochlea.

The first line of defense, however, should be medical management of the conductive loss. The hearing aid should be considered only after maximum improvement has occurred from treatment. Occasionally, a patient will prefer not to have surgical intervention, such as in otosclerosis, and then, of course, the hearing aid becomes the primary "treatment" for the loss.

Sensorineural Hearing Loss

Causes.   1. Generally, in older people, the upper limit of sounds that can be heard gradually descends until the upper speech frequencies are lost and the discrimination of speech is affected. This condition is referred to as presbycusis.

2. Extremely loud noise will damage the inner ear and result in a condition called acoustic trauma or noise-induced loss. Such a loss usually appears first at 4000 Hz and spreads to the other high frequencies if the ear is continuously exposed to noise.

3. Ototoxicity results from the use of large amounts of quinine, aspirin and drugs of the streptomycin family. Characteristically, the hearing loss is seen first at 6000 Hz and may become total.

4. Disease and trauma to the head may damage the inner ear.

Symptoms.   Sensorineural hearing losses may range in severity from a slight loss at one frequency to a profound loss at all frequencies. Typically, the high frequencies are affected more than the lower ones. This means that the patient might hear the voiced sounds of speech but fail to hear the voiceless sounds, such as t, ch, s, f, th, p, k and sh. He hears the speaker but has difficulty understanding what is being said. Noise tends to mask out even more sounds and makes the discrimination of speech difficult.

Treatment.   As in conductive loss, the otologist should examine the ears to rule out any outer or middle ear pathology. The ear specialist will also determine if any conditions exist (Meniere's disease, acoustic neuroma or tumor of the 8th nerve, etc.) which may be treated to possibly lessen the sensorineural loss. Generally, however, most sensorineural losses are untreatable by surgery or medication, but will respond, however imperfectly, to hearing aid amplification.

While the cochlea of the conductively impaired ear responds normally to amplified sounds, the damaged cochlea of most sensorineural losses introduces distortion into the incoming sound, causing imperfect discrimination of speech. Thus, a properly fitted hearing aid will benefit the sensorineural loss by overcoming the associated "loudness loss," but there will usually remain a discrimination or "speech understanding" deficit due to distortion introduced by damage to sensorineural structures. The hearing aid, then, will make sounds easier to hear and thereby improve understanding ability, but even with the hearing aid the person with typical sensorineural hearing loss will have a residual discrimination deficit, i.e., will not understand speech as well as someone with a conductive loss using a hearing aid.

Hearing Aids.   A hearing aid is a device for amplifying sounds in the patient's environment. Just as a magnifying glass makes everything look larger, a hearing aid makes all sounds seem louder. Unfortunately this amplifying is not selective, and background noise is also increased in loudness. It is helpful when talking with a patient wearing a hearing aid to be alert for noise that may mask out your speech. When this occurs, repeat what you said after the noise stops or make sure the patient is watching your face and gestures if the noise is continuous.

Like any device, a hearing aid requires some maintenance. When the patient complains that the aid is not functioning properly, a brief inspection will generally uncover the difficulty. A brief description of maintenance procedures for common hearing aid problems is contained in the box on page 116.

Speech Reading.   If a patient has a marked hearing loss or if there are indications that the hearing loss is getting progressively worse, it is advisable to provide him with guidance and training in speech reading, or "lip reading" as it was formerly called. This type of training teaches the patient to use his visual system to supplement what he is

Hearing Aid Problems

1. Make sure that the aid is turned on. The on-off switch may be a separate switch at the side of the aid or it may be built into the volume control.

2. The battery may be run down or improperly installed. Try a new battery.

3. If the aid is a body type, the plugs on the cord from the aid to the receiver may not be securely in place.

4. The cord may be broken. Check it for damage.

Weak Sound From the Aid

1. The battery may be weak. Try a new one.

2. The ear mold which fits into the ear canal may be plugged with wax. Wash the mold with warm water and then clean the opening with a pipe cleaner.

3. Intermittent crackling noises suggest a damaged cord on a body type aid, or possibly a defective volume control.

A Squealing, Whistling Aid

1. The body-worn aid may be too close to the receiver in the ear. Change the position of the aid to the opposite side of the body.

2. A mold not properly in place or one that does not fit well will cause problems. The fit of the mold is especially important with ear level aids such as eyeglass and behind-the-ear aids. If the mold does not fit snugly into the ear canal, the aid will squeal due to feedback. Inspect the positioning of the mold. If it seems loose it may have to be replaced.

3. Sometimes, a squeal will result if the patient sits too close to a wall. In such cases the squeal will stop when the patient turns his head or moves away from the wall.

hearing. He learns to watch the gestures and the face of the speaker to pick up additional cues about what is being said. Such training is best obtained through a qualified audiologist or aural rehabilitation specialist who can usually be contacted through the local Speech and Hearing Association or Medical Society. Universities, rehabilitation centers and VA Hospitals' Speech Pathology and Audiology Clinics also offer aural rehabilitation courses.

In the event that formal aural rehabilitation training is not available, the patient should be taught to watch the face and gestures of the speaker to assist him in understanding what is being said. Conversely the rehabilitation staff should be advised about the patient's hearing loss and instructed to get the patient's visual attention before giving instructions to him. They should also supplement what they are saying with clear gestures as to the point that they are trying to get across.

Impairment of Expression

Verbal Expression

Verbal expression, the production of speech, is the last step in the process of verbal output. In the adult it seems very simple and automatic, but it is the most complex muscular task the body performs. Each group of muscles of the hundreds employed in speaking must contract and relax with split-second timing to produce intelligible speech. In brief, the process of speech production is as follows:

The power for speech is provided by the respiratory system. The air in the lungs is at a high level of pressure at the completion of inspiration, and so it moves up the trachea as the diaphragm begins to relax. As it reaches the larynx, this moving air vibrates the vocal folds to produce voice. The voice and the air pressure move from the larynx into the pharynx, where some of the sound is absorbed by the soft walls, and the remaining sound takes on its resonance characteristics. Finally, the resonated sound reaches the oral cavity where the movements of the palate, the tongue, the jaw and the lips mold and articulate the sound into intelligible speech.

Disorders of Respiration. When diseases such as poliomyelitis, amyotrophic lateral sclerosis and Guillain-Barré syndrome reduce the patient's vital capacity, the amount of air available for speech is diminished. The patient finds he can say only a few words on a breath. If vital capacity is reduced further, the voice becomes weak. In these cases, usually some form of mechanical respiratory assistance is given, and this imposes an artificial respiratory rhythm on speaking. Communication can be improved greatly if the patient is encouraged to express himself in short ideas that he can articulate in the brief time allowed by his new respiratory cycle.

Another type of respiratory difficulty is due to poor control, as seen in the patient with cerebellar involvement. Instead of producing a steady, controlled air flow, the patient forces air up the trachea in short powerful blasts. Speech is emitted in explosive bursts of one or two words. Frequently, the patient is not aware of the loudness of his voice. With a little gentle assistance he often can learn to monitor his speech and reduce its explosiveness.

Disorders of Phonation.   An increasingly common speech disorder is due to laryngeal cancer. As a growth develops on the vocal fold, movement is impaired, the voice becomes hoarse and eventually cannot be produced. When a laryngectomy is necessary, the removal of the larynx makes normal voice production impossible. The patient must learn to make voice sounds in a new way. He swallows air and then forces the air to vibrate the sphincter at the entrance to the esophagus. This produces a somewhat coarse but usable voice. Information on classes for learning esophageal speech is available at local offices of the American Cancer Society.

A frequent voice disorder, dysphonia, is a change in the voice because of neurological impairment. Sometimes the voice quality is affected as in the case of strokes when the voice becomes strained and hoarse due to the spasticity of the larynx or voice box. Lower motoneuron disorders usually result in poor valving at the laryngeal level which produces a breathy aspirated type voice because of the air leaking through the completely closed vocal folds. Neurological disorders can also result in a reduction in the intensity or loudness of the voice as in Parkinson's disease where the voice might start out at an adequate loudness and gradually become barely audible.

Disorders of Resonation.   Normally, the soft palate acts as a valve to close off the entrance to the nasal passage at the back of the throat. Paralysis of the palate, as seen in bulbar poliomyelitis and amyotrophic lateral sclerosis, results in the voice and air pressure going out through the nose instead of the mouth. The patient's speech, much like that of a child with an unrepaired cleft palate, is emitted nasally. The distortion of articulation and resonation may significantly reduce intelligibility. If the patient's speech is difficult to understand, he should be instructed to try to direct the breath and the voice forward into the mouth, to open his mouth a little more than usual when talking in order to promote the flow of sound through the mouth and to articulate a little more slowly and carefully.

Disorders of Articulation.   Dysarthria, the distortion of articulation due to neurological disorders, is a common clinical finding in the cases of amyotrophic lateral sclerosis, myasthenia gravis, multiple sclerosis, parkinsonism, and cerebral vascular disorders (strokes). Speech may be characterized by only a slight slurring, or in the more involved cases it may be completely unintelligible. The type and severity of the dysarthria are directly related to the site of the lesion in the central nervous system. Cortical lesions due to strokes or trauma usually produce a spastic type of dysarthria in which the voice quality is harsh and strangled and the articulation is imprecise. Lower motoneuron lesions produce weakness and flaccidity which results in poor valving at various points along the speech tract. These patients usually have breathy weak voices and poor palatal action which results in speech being emitted through the nose. Brain damage in the area of the basal ganglia produces hypokinetic dysarthria such as that seen in a person with Parkinson's disease. His articulation is very rapid and imprecise and his speech tends to become poorer the longer he speaks. Damage to the cerebellum produces ataxic dysarthria in which the coordination of the articulatory mechanism is affected and therefore the patient has difficulty controlling the loudness and the smooth flow of his speech.[2,3]

It should not be assumed that unintelligibility is the inevitable outcome of progressive diseases. Frequently, the distortion of speech can be prevented or reduced if the patient is trained to listen to his speech and to compensate for muscle weakness by articulating more carefully and speaking more deliberately, giving the slow-moving muscles time to reach accurate positions of production. Short daily practice sessions during which the patient is asked to articulate slowly and carefully are helpful. These sessions are best if done in the morning, since fatigue tends to reduce the patient's ability to articulate well. This is especially apparent in myasthenia gravis.

Most patients can achieve a reasonable degree of intelligibility once they are aware of the problem and are willing to exert the necessary energy to compensate for the impaired mechanism. When the intelligibility remains poor in spite of training, the patient should be encouraged to use gesture to supplement speech. If speech is unintelligible and the patient cannot write, one or more boards may be made with pictures or names of people, objects, acts or needs that are important to him. Then, he may point to entities to help express ideas.

Graphic and Gestural Expression

The impairment of graphic and gestural output is usually due to an impairment in motor function, the most common of which is paralysis. Very often a disturbance of motor function which impairs gestural and graphic output is also responsible for the impairment of verbal output. A patient who is completely paralyzed may not be able to communicate at all or even respond to simple commands. Thus, it becomes practically impossible to evaluate his input ability. It is usually clear to the rehabilitation staff that the patient is unable to respond because of paralysis and not because he is in coma, mentally disturbed or entirely unable to understand. This is the case, for instance, when the paralysis is due to a peripheral disorder such as Guillain-Barré syndrome. However, when the paralysis and motor impairment are due to a brain injury, it is common for physicians, nurses and therapists to assume that the patient is semicomatose or severely brain damaged and unable to understand what is going on. This can lead to serious mismanagement of a patient, as shown in the following example.

A 26-year-old man was admitted to a Veteran's Hospital following a brain injury suffered in an automobile accident. An examination revealed that he had a complete left hemiplegia and a right hemiathetosis, and his fascies was completely expressionless except for eye movement. For weeks the patient was given basic nursing care. He made no sound, showed no spontaneous motion and, since it was assumed that he was unable to comprehend, the staff did not attempt to communicate with him. However, they did discuss the considerable damage to his brain and his probable prognosis in his presence.

Finally, the patient was visited by an educational therapist with an interest in aphasia. The therapist attempted to establish communications with him, suggesting that he blink his eyes once for yes and twice for no, and within a short time she established that he was able to answer all of her questions intelligently. She then proceeded to use a chart upon which the alphabet was printed, pointing to one letter after another instructing the patient to wink when he wanted a particular letter. By use of this slow method, the patient was finally able to spell out words and sentences and make his wishes and feelings known. The lesson to be learned from this case is that one should never assume that a patient is mentally incompetent so that all attempts at communicating with him are given up.

If a motor disturbance deprives a patient of all expressive ability he should be rechecked from time to time to see if some motor function has returned, making it possible to communicate, such as by blinking the eyes. The most common motor disturbance is paralysis, which may interfere completely with writing and gestures. Other motor disturbances are cerebellar ataxia and abnormal motions, especially athetoid cerebral palsy. It was pointed out above that these patients may have impairments of both verbal and graphic expression.

There are methods to improve the communication ability of patients with severe motor impairment. An athetoid patient, for instance, who cannot use a pen or a pencil may be able to type by using a stick attached to a headband. The use of head motions may also be important in activating an alarm or call light. With modern electronic technology one small switch activated by a finger, a toe or another part of the body may enable the patient to express long and complicated messages.

Aphasia

Perhaps the most dramatic and disruptive of all communicative disabilities is aphasia. As stated previously, the brain carries out all the vital steps of communication between reception and expression. It is easy to understand that even a small injury to the brain might result in a loss or diminution of one or more of the steps. When the brain is unable to fulfill its communicative functions because of damage to its input, integrative or output centers, the patient is called aphasic or is said to have aphasia.

There has been considerable controversy as to whether these centers can be localized to specific areas or if the responsibility for communication is disseminated throughout the brain's many lobes and layers. These academic arguments are not important to this discussion, but a few points dealing with the organizational structure of the brain are of clinical importance.

The brain is divided equally into two parts, the left and the right hemispheres, by a long fissure running from front to back. Each half receives and sends messages to the opposite side of the body because the neural pathways cross over as they reach the lower part of the brain. This curious arrangement explains why a patient with damage to the left side of the brain is unable to move the right side of his body and why brain damage produces weakness or paralysis on one side of the body rather than to one arm and the opposite leg. However, communication does not follow this pattern. Man's communicative processes are controlled in almost all cases by the left side of the brain. Therefore, a patient with right hemiplegia frequently experiences some central communicative disabilities, ranging in severity from a slight difficulty in discriminating the feel of objects with the weakened hand to complete inability to integrate any incoming sensory messages, isolating the patient from his environment.

It is interesting that patients who are partially ambidextrous seem to be less seriously affected communicatively by injury to the left hemisphere than those who do everything with the right hand. Occasionally, a patient with left hemiplegia (right hemisphere damage) and aphasia, after careful examination, shows subtle, right-sided signs of left hemisphere damage or a history of earlier "small strokes."

In the case of left hemiplegia, the patient may have some difficulty with reception or expression, that is, a peripheral problem of hearing, seeing, weakness of the muscles of speech or loss of the use of the left arm for gesture or writing. He rarely has significant difficulty with the central control of communication.

Causes of Aphasia

Traumatic Head Injuries.   The brain is housed in the protective bony casing of the skull for good reason. Unlike many tissues of the body that have the ability to regenerate cells after injury, destroyed brain cells cannot be replaced. The injured brain must operate with a limited number of cells that remain intact after aging and injury take their toll. Once a cell is destroyed, no reserves wait to take its place. It is no wonder nature has provided a hard covering to ward off possible injury.

Even this box of bone cannot protect the cells of the brain from the destructive onslaught of bullets, bludgeonings and expressway collisions. Though often severe, head injuries are usually inflicted on the more active younger members of society who fortunately have great resiliency and are often able to respond to rehabilitation if the injury is not too great.

Obviously, a damaged brain cannot be expected to handle the intricacies of communication as it did before the trauma. Usually, the patient and his family accept these deficits as part of the physical disability. In fact, very often, the communication difficulties are almost disregarded because they are overshadowed by the threat to life and limb. When questions do arise, it is difficult to predict the eventual level of communication that will be reached. It is not uncommon for a patient with severe head injuries to remain semiconscious and uncommunicative for many days or weeks and then have spurts of recovery followed by periods of little change.

Initially, the patient can see and hear but attaches little significance to the messages he receives and does not react to things happening around him. Notable change occurs when perception improves, and he begins to differentiate some sights and sounds. He follows people with his eyes, opens his mouth when food is presented and turns toward sounds. Vocalization, especially in response to pain, begins. In the more severe cases, marked irritability may develop, and the recovery of further communicative ability ceases. If the patient begins to associate incoming messages, he recognizes familiar faces and smiles, becomes more cooperative, responds to tactile and visual stimulation. He may begin to say some words, especially automatic speech, such as "yes," "no," "OK," common social expressions or profanities. Gradually, more understanding develops, limited speech improves and responses become more easily elicited. Finally, as coordination improves, the patient may begin to approach more normal communicative ability if the peripheral and central damage allows. It should be cautioned that throughout the recovery process regardless of outward physical appearances, the patient may understand much of what is done and said around him, and therefore, careless words and acts are always inappropriate in the patient's presence.

The speed with which the patient moves through these recovery stages is highly variable. He may negotiate the complete process in days, remain on a plateau at each stage for weeks or months or permanently stabilize at one stage, depending on the extent of brain involvement.

Cerebral Vascular Accidents. The cells of the brain have an insatiable need for oxygen. This nourishment is supplied in large quantities by an abundant network of blood vessels that make up the brain's vascular system. Conditions involving reduced blood supply to the brain are designated as cerebral vascular accident (CVA). Commonly, the patient is then said to have had a stroke. The nature of the stroke and the course it follows are largely dependent on the location and the extent of brain injury incurred. A gradually diminishing blood supply prodices a slow onset of symptoms, such as weakness, slurred speech, tingling sensations, dizziness and headaches. Intermittent impairment of blood flow may cause transient strokes. Sudden cessation of blood flow may result in immediate collapse, unconsciousness, hemiplegia and aphasia.

Patterns of Recovery

Not all patients with aphasia improve at the same rate. For many years it was thought that "spontaneous recovery" occurred in some degree in all patients but that the amount was variable and unpredictable. More recently our studies of the recovery process in aphasia have shown that there is a definite pattern of recovery which will vary according to the main etiological groups. Before making further comments on the nature of recovery in these groups it is necessary that we discuss the concept of "spontaneous recovery."

It is unfortunate that this term arose in connection with the early months of recovery after brain damage, for it implies that the recovery of communicative ability occurs spontaneously, without any outside intervention. Actually our experience shows that "spontaneous recovery" is in fact a combination of *physiological improvement* and a form of communicative reorganization that arises out of having a fairly *stimulating environment*. If there are no subsequent physical problems and if the environment provides enough stimulation during the first few months of post-onset, the rate of recovery is quite orderly and predictable and it is possible, with a fair degree of accuracy, to predict the eventual level of communicative competency that the patient will reach.

Cerebral Thrombosis or Embolism. The patient who has had a thrombosis or embolus recovers from aphasia most rapidly during the first few months, after which, the rate of improvement greatly decreases until at 6 months after the onset of the illness, it tends to stop. After 6 months there is usually no significant improvement unless the patient is in an active treatment program.

Cerebral Hemorrhage. The patient whose aphasia has resulted from a cerebral hemorrhage will also tend to improve at a fairly steady rate during the first 6 months. After 6 months the recovery rate will stabilize unless there has been a period of unconsciousness for days or weeks after the hemorrhage. In this case, the recovery was delayed because the brain was not stimulated during the period of unconsciousness and the patient will show improvement beyond the 6-month time limit.

Localized Surgical Procedures. A third type of recovery pattern is related to localized surgical procedures such as those used in treating arterial-venous malformations. Post-surgical patients will sometimes show a remarkable recovery during the first month or two after surgery at which time there is a plateauing, with gradual improvements occurring over the next year. The unusual rate of recovery in some of these young patients is probably due to two factors. First, because they are younger their vascular systems have a greater capacity for adjusting to changes in brain structure and therefore the patient has better recuperative powers. Secondly, in cases where there has been longstanding and particularly slow developing pathological states, the brain is able to readjust itself and employ healthy structures nearby which compensate for the "noisy" area. Therefore when the pathological area is removed there is no serious loss in function and the brain is now free to operate without these imperfect areas and it responds with quite a high degree of efficiency.

Massive Trauma. A fourth type of recovery pattern that should be discussed is that of a patient who is recovering from a massive insult to the brain. This category includes both the patient with serious head trauma and the patient who is recovering from extensive brain surgery. Also included in this group are patients who have extensive cerebral edema or those recovering from anoxic states. In all of these cases, the brain seems to react to such widespread insults by closing down some of its systems to preserve the more important vegetative ones. As recovery progresses one system after another is reinitiated as the brain develops the capacity to handle more complexity. The recovery sequence follows a stairstep pattern marked by weeks and sometimes months without significant change, sudden short periods of noticeable improvement, and then another period of little change and so on.

Disuse.   A final type of recovery pattern is that of the aphasic patient who is more than 2 years post-onset. The patient is often admitted to a hospital for some other medical problem but is noted to have "an old CVA with aphasia." Very often it is assumed that the patient is beyond treatment for aphasia and he is not referred for a reevaluation of the communicative problems. However, this assumption should not be made on the basis of a bedside examination or on anecdotal reports of family members who have seen no improvement in communication for months or years. It is not uncommon to see patients who had the potential for significant improvement soon after the onset of aphasia but were unfortunately isolated and deprived of a reasonably stimulating environment. In other cases, the patient makes the expected improvement early in the recovery period but in subsequent years has been without stimulation and has gradually had his communicative ability eroded away by disuse. In either case, the patient's brain has the capacity for much higher levels of communicative ability, but he has not been able to realize this potential because of environmental limitations. His communicative ability suffers from disuse just as a patient's extremities might suffer from disuse if he goes without exercise. It has been clearly demonstrated that a good aggressive treatment program and massive stimulation and encouragement can help produce significant improvement in many chronically aphasic patients. Usually 2 to 4 weeks of intensive treatment and stimulation will indicate whether the patient has potential for further improvement.

In these cases, and in all cases of left hemisphere damage and aphasia, the speech pathologist or clinical aphasiologist can often predict the patient's potential for improvement with a fair degree of accuracy through the use of tests such as the *Porch Index of Communicative Ability*. If such tests are not available, the only way to treat the patient is to provide massive stimulation for as long as it seems to produce noticeable change. If the patient goes for 2 to 4 weeks without demonstrating any changes termination of treatment should be considered.

Management of the Aphasic Patient

The management of the aphasic patient has to be considered from three different aspects, the most important of which is the problem of *communication* for the purpose of medical care, activities of daily living and rehabilitation training. Minimizing the *emotional problems* caused by aphasia and the actual *treatment* of the communication deficit are also important considerations in the management of the aphasic patient.

Communicating with the Aphasic Patient. Though most aphasics, if carefully tested, show disabilities in auditory input as well as verbal output, it is useful to discuss separately the patients who have adequate input ability but who are disabled in output ability. They understand what they hear, see and read in most cases but they may have great difficulty in speaking and writing. In contrast to this group, who have "expressive aphasia," there is a second group of patients with significant input problems, which affect all forms of communication. This condition is often referred to as "receptive aphasia."

The Aphasic Patient with Output Difficulties Only. These patients can understand verbal and written communication but have difficulty in organizing concepts into words or are unable to formulate the words into meaningful expressions. While the degree of disability covers a broad spectrum, only the more severely involved patients present management problems. Patients with formulation problems are sometimes described as having severe oral and verbal apraxia. They are able to make only minimal and usually unintelligible repetitive utterances such as, "wonna wonna" or "all right."

Occasionally patients with severe output problems have some automatic speech such as counting or saying the days of the week, but they are not able to use these words functionally. Another type of frequently occurring automatic speech is swearing. Profanity can be included in a person's verbalization regardless of his previous history of swearing. If the patient or his family become disturbed about the swearing, it should be explained that this is one of the symptoms of aphasia which will usually subside as the patient achieves a broader vocabulary of words.

Communication with patients who have severe output problems is facilitated by use of a few simple methods.

1. The yes-no method. The most common method of communicating with a patient with severely limited output is to ask questions to which he responds by saying or nodding yes or no. As mentioned earlier, patients with severe muscular or neuromuscular prob-

lems can be taught to respond by moving a single muscle, raising a finger, or blinking the eyes for affirmative responses.

2. The pointing method. If the patient cannot talk or write he can frequently use gestural language for communicating. Whenever possible he should be encouraged to point as a means of communicating his needs. Communicating by pointing can be greatly facilitated with a book of pictures, words and numbers. A patient can quickly learn to find the concepts he wishes to communicate, particularly if the book is arranged with topics such as foods, clothes, people and the letters of the alphabet. Some patients are able to point to letters of the alphabet and spell out their ideas quite readily but this is rarely the case with the patient with aphasia. Spelling is one of the more difficult coding activities the brain must do and it is usually impaired in all brain damaged patients.

3. Other methods. Writing can be a supplemental communication channel when speech is grossly impaired. By anticipating what the patient might want to know the staff can reduce the amount of communication he is required to carry out and relieve his anxieties about his general status.

The Aphasic Patient with Output and Input Disabilities. Patients with "receptive aphasia" present special problems to the rehabilitation staff. Imagine awakening some morning to find yourself in a country in which everyone speaks a language you do not understand. Speech and writing would be useless for communication and you would find that gestural and visual systems would become the primary methods of communication. Patients with "receptive aphasia" find themselves in this very situation.

It is not uncommon for the aphasic patient to use his visual input to such great advantage that those unfamiliar with aphasia are deceived and believe that the patient really understands what is being said to him.

In contrast to the patient with expressive aphasia who has halting, distorted and grammatically incomplete speech, the patient with receptive aphasia has speech which is normal in rhythm and melody. However, because he has difficulty understanding his own speech as well as the speech of others he has poor monitoring of what he is saying and therefore can produce quite bizarre utterances. The severely involved patient often talks in rambling and unintelligible jargon. Other patients use a mixture of real words and neologisms or nonmeaningful words.

Communication with a patient with input problems must obviously be founded upon a thorough understanding of the patient's deficits. In cases of severe impairment, staff members and the patient's family should continue to talk to the patient but recognize that most of the communication is being transmitted through visual-gestural systems. The moderately involved patient understands some things but uses the visual-gestural cues to help him organize the auditory signals he is receiving.

A final way of helping the receptively impaired patient is to adhere to a fixed schedule. Since he cannot read and understands very little of what is being said to him, the receptively impaired patient has a great deal of difficulty making sense out of an ever-changing routine. If his schedule is fixed he can begin to regulate his life and learn to anticipate what is expected of him in different situations and what is being said to him from time to time. It is for this reason that many aphasic patients become quite disturbed when their schedules are changed or when something they are anticipating does not happen. Therefore, it is *important to keep the daily schedule as constant as possible and advise the patient well in advance when changes may occur*.

Management of Emotional Problems. Even fully functioning people when they are under stress may experience both input and output difficulties. We sometimes actually block input and do not hear what is said to us when our anxiety level is high. Under stress, we may be unable to find the right word, we may lose an idea or even be unable to express a coherent thought. When the stress diminishes, we find that words and ideas come more easily. Illness itself produces stress. If input information is absent or unreliable, as it often is with brain injuries, stress increases because of anxiety.

The worst frustration is experienced by patients with expressive aphasia because they are aware of their own inability to express themselves correctly. It is more frustrating to be unable to answer a question one understands than it is to not understand a question. As a result, the person with expressive aphasia often becomes irritable, angry and sometimes depressed.

When the patient cannot communicate in a normal manner, he is often treated as a half-functioning human being and the staff assumes that his needs are reduced, when they are actually intensified and must be met in other than traditional ways. The staff must use all available means of communication to repeatedly (because of memory loss) reassure the patient of his location and his illness. They must also attempt to anticipate his needs and to make him as comfortable as possible. Comfort is sometimes withheld from the patient because "he can't understand, anyway," and sometimes, unfortunately, because he is unable to complain.

The patient requires sensory stimulation and isolating him will only deprive him further. Lack of sensory input, compounded by anxiety, fear and frustration will severely limit the patient's ability to cope with his illness and may cause him to withdraw and become apathetic and depressed.

Constant, repeated reassurance and references to concrete demonstrations of progress are necessary. Phrases, such as "don't worry," "you'll be alright" or "I'll take care of you," without explanation only tell the patient that he is, indeed, hopeless. Talking in front of a patient as if he had no faculties is denigrating and certainly works against establishing self-confidence. The patient must be given every opportunity to make choices and decisions to give him the feeling of regaining control. Patients who are able to verbalize in jargon, with automatic responses, or with only some loss are often more frustrated simply because they constantly try but cannot control output. The staff can help the patient to find the right word, deal with profanity and jargon uncritically, help with nonverbal means for identification, anticipate needs and find ways to spend time with him in nonverbal activities. If speech therapy sessions leave the patient exhausted and frustrated, the methods should be evaluated and the format changed. Finally, the family must be informed as to the nature of the disability, and shown ways to help develop two-way communication, rather than encouraged to overprotect the patient and deepen dependency.

Treating Aphasia

During the past 10 years, significant additions have been made to our knowledge of aphasia. The aphasiologists or speech pathologists specializing in the treatment of aphasia now have at their disposal a variety of tools and procedures which were previously not available. Methods developed by linguists and psychologists have been modified for the treatment of the aphasic patient and have done much to organize and structure the rehabilitation of the patient's communication. One of the most productive developments recently has been the devising and standardizing of psychometric methods for assessing the nature and extent of aphasia in the patient. Tests such as the *Porch Index of Communicative Ability* not only help by localizing the site and extent of the brain damage but such tests also quantify the exact extent of communicative deficit, predict with a fairly high degree of accuracy to what extent the patient will recover his communication and indicate specific areas that need to be worked on in the treatment sessions.*

*The reader who is interested in a more indepth consideration of current trends in aphasiology is referred to the works of H. Schuell and of R. H. Brookshire which are listed in the references at the end of this chapter.

The decision as to when and how to treat the patient's aphasia is usually made by the speech pathologist on the basis of test results. However, it is always important to give the patient a lot of communication stimulation from the beginning of his recovery period. This reduces the shock of the patient's first confrontation with his communication problems and it prevents him from developing improper compensatory approaches to communication such as withdrawing or developing the habit of saying "I can't talk" without really trying to do so. We have seen a number of patients who were not treated in the first few months post-onset and they fell far short of what was predicted. It is often possible to recover this lost ground but not without an extended period of time of working to undo the bad habits the patient has developed. This ultimately becomes a very expensive process and wastes months of time.

Ideally, the treatment of aphasia should be done once or twice a day for the first few months of his recovery. However, fewer formal treatment sessions can be productive if they are supplemented with informal sessions carried out by the family or friends under the guidance of the speech pathologist.

Hospital Treatment of the Aphasic Patient. Everyone who has contact with the patient affects the recovery process. Poor handling of attempts to communicate can significantly retard improvement and interfere with the tasks that the patient is asked to carry out, whether the tasks be those of speech, daily living, physical therapy or those related to medical and nursing care. Appropriate treatment based on a thorough understanding of aphasia can facilitate recovery and resolve many of the problems of patient care which result from communication involvement.

The principles outlined below are offered as general guides for increasing communication between staff and patient and for helping the patient to recover functional input and output ability. While these suggestions are particularly important during the early stages of the illness when there is moderate or severe communication disturbance, they are, with some modifications, applicable to any patient with a history of brain injury.

Treat the Patient, Not the Disability. Communication disorders can have quite an impact on the patient. He may try to withdraw from attempts to make him communicate or he may become frustrated when he tries unsuccessfully to speak or write. How he reacts to you and the help you offer depends on the kind of rapport you establish in your first few contacts with him.

1. A positive approach will yield the best results. Demonstrate your interest in the patient and his attempts at communication. Try to appear friendly and accepting but avoid artificial praise.

2. When indicated, simplify your speech and supplement it with gestures. Do not markedly change your usual speaking habits. An unnecessary rise in the pitch and the loudness of your voice does not improve communication and often makes the patient feel uneasy.

3. Remember that the basic intelligence and the personality of the patient are not affected, but his ability to communicate what he is thinking and feeling has been disrupted.

4. Minimize correction and criticism. You are trying to encourage communication, not discourage it.

5. Remember that many things may influence the patient's responses.

    a. Try to eliminate any anxiety and tension related to communication attempts. The patient's apprehensions will subside if you appear relaxed and unhurried.

    b. Give the patient plenty of time to respond. He needs time to sort out the incoming messages, to organize an impaired integrative system and to select and formulate a response. Under time pressure he cannot do this. Instructions or requests given suddenly or rapidly tend to make him feel rushed and should be avoided.

    c. Be consistent. If the patient gets to know you and what you expect of him, he can often follow your instructions even if he understands little of what you are saying. Use the same wording each time you give instructions or ask questions. Keep his daily schedule free of unnecessary changes that may be confusing. When such changes are necessary, inform the patient as soon as possible.

    d. Make a definite transition between tasks. Often, the patient has trouble shifting from one task to another and may continue to give a previous response to new instructions. Tell him you are changing tasks, give the new instructions, then ask him for the new response.

    e. Reduce or eliminate distractions when communication is important. Damaged input pathways cannot keep out many of the distracting stimuli in the patient's environment. These distractions conflict with the important messages and interfere with integration. Small movements and sounds that are unnoticed by you can preoccupy the patient. Develop an awareness of distracting factors and their effect on the patient.

Know Your Patient. Reassess his communication ability often, and gear your actions to his abilities.

1. If you are too simple or too complex with the patient, he may question his abilities, become frustrated and reject further help.

2. Periodic reevaluations will demonstrate to you and to the patient the extent and the nature of improvement taking place. Subjective impressions about change or the lack of it are inaccurate and unreliable. By having the patient perform some standard tasks of speech, writing or gesture periodically, you gain objective information about how his performance compares with earlier samples.

3. Having accurate knowledge of the patient's input and output ability will prevent you from treating him inappropriately. Unless you are fully aware of how he is functioning, you may easily make common errors that accompany unfounded assumptions. For instance, it is often assumed that the patient is understanding what is said to him because he smiles, nods his head and even answers "yes" and "no" to questions. In reality, he does not understand speech but does understand the speaker's gestures, expressions and head nodding. In other cases, a patient with no output ability gives no apparent responses, and so the speaker assumes that the patient does not understand. Consequently, inappropriate comments are made in the patient's presence. A little testing can prevent a lot of mistakes.

The Goal of Treatment. Remember, the goal of treatment is to stimulate attempts at communication.

1. During the first 2 or 3 months after onset of aphasia, the patient's desire to communicate must be kept at a high level.

2. General communication gives the patient a chance to use his intact abilities but minimizes the effect of failure.

3. Do not use repetitious drills. Relate communication attempts to the patient and his needs. When you are with the patient, talk about what you are doing and name the acts and the items of the daily routine as they are carried out.

4. The patient will try to talk or gesture if he feels that the listener is accepting and relaxed. It is not necessary to badger him into talking.

5. At times, you may not be able to understand what he is trying to say. He may talk a great deal, but his speech may be unintelligible. You should not appear anxious about this breakdown in communication. Continue to appear interested in what he is saying and watch his gestures closely for clues about the topic under discussion. Periodically, nod and make neutral statements. At the appropriate moment, shift the conversation to a topic of your choice so that you will have some frame of reference.

Generally, most of the patient's important needs are provided for, and the thing he is trying to tell you is not critical, so he will readily change to another point of interest. If he persists along the same line and seems very intent on getting the idea across to you, explore the various possibilities until you understand his message. Very often, the other patients on the ward will know what he is trying to say or can offer some suggestions.

Home Treatment of the Aphasic Patient. Before the aphasic patient leaves the hospital, many of the problems that may arise later can be anticipated and prevented or minimized by adequate counseling of the family. If the family members can witness and learn to understand the difficulties the patient has with understanding and producing speech, writing and gestures, they can make adjustments in their expectations and plan toward continuing treatment. Without this counseling, the family may impede unwittingly the patient's recovery of communicative ability.

For example, while in the hospital the patient with impaired auditory input frequently appears to understand much more than he is actually capable of understanding. In a consistent, planned program he has learned to associate people and events in his schedule with certain expected responses. When the family members have visited with him, they have seen him apparently responding to verbal instructions, and they are unaware that he is relying almost exclusively on his visual input. Even though he understands very little of what is said to him, he knows that people expect a response when they talk to him, and so he watches closely for visual clues that indicate what is expected of him. He smiles, nods and attempts to speak at appropriate times. His reaction to his environment is not unlike that of anyone who finds himself in a situation where those around him are speaking a foreign language. He attempts to appear as rational as possible, and often he is very successful in his subterfuge.

When the patient is taken home, most of the clues to expected responses are lost. The consistent schedule that he had memorized is replaced by an unstructured situation. The uniforms and the faces that visually suggested certain required responses are gone. The patient in his confusion and doubt suddenly appears much more impaired than he had been previously, much to the consternation of his family. However, this change need not cause undue worry or anxiety. An informed family will be ready for it and will provide a new schedule of activities that the patient can learn. Consistent verbal instructions accompanied by appropriate gestures will be understood by the patient in a relatively short time, and soon he will regain his ability to cope successfully with his environment in spite of input disability.

A second example of the effects of counseling or the lack of it is seen in common family reactions to the patient who cannot speak. Shortly after the patient returns home, well-meaning relatives realize that speaking is now very difficult for him. They begin to anticipate his needs so he will not be required to speak. They speak to him less often so he will not feel that he must respond (and so they will not be embarrassed by not understanding him) and speak for him when visitors come to the house. All these things deprive the patient of opportunities to test his speaking ability, to experiment with his verbal output by making errors and correcting them and gradually to increase his proficiency and confidence. He begins to feel inadequate and loses his motivation to work for improvement. Why should he talk when apparently no one wants him to try? The usual outcome of such treatment is a rather discouraged patient who has a vocabulary limited to phrases such as, "I can't say it" and "I don't know."

In contrast with the family that restricts the patient's opportunities to speak, some families, because of their misunderstanding and misdirected interest in helping the patient, barrage him with speaking tasks. Throughout the day he is asked to say words, name things, imitate sounds and attempt a large number of unrelated tasks, many of which bear little relation to the patient's ability or needs. If the patient understands what is being said, he knows why this attention is being directed at him and will attempt to carry out the many instructions until he tires of the constant pressure or withdraws from requests which are much too difficult or too childish. If he cannot understand speech, he nevertheless can see and feel a certain urgency for his speech attempt (though his speech cannot improve until his auditory input improves) and so he struggles dutifully to imitate the sounds he thinks he hears. In a short time, the high level of frustration he develops begins to interfere with all communication attempts, and finally, improvement stops or greatly slows.

Fortunately, these problems are preventable if the family is motivated to help in the recovery process and if they are provided with adequate information and assistance through effective counseling. Listed below are some of the major points to be covered in discussions with the family after they have some basic understanding of the nature of aphasia and of the extent of the patient's communication disabilities. Shortly before the patient goes home, a brief interview with interested relatives should review the situation, anticipate the problems which may develop, suggest possible solutions and provide sources for securing further information and patient treatment.

Suggestions to the Family. Communication rehabilitation thrives on a consistent environment including considerate, understanding people.

When the patient returns home he should be incorporated into the family schedule as soon as possible. Since he is essentially the same individual psychologically that he was before his illness, he will usually want to assume his previous role in the family constellation, and very often his communication disabilities will not prevent him from undertaking and enjoying a large number of activities. Hopefully, an informed family will allow and encourage him to attempt these things unless they are obviously dangerous to the patient or very disruptive to the family routine.

Above all, the family should understand that reduced communication ability does not necessarily imply reduced intelligence or reduced awareness of feelings and attitudes. Over-reaction to communication disability is quickly sensed by the patient and serves only to remind him of his inadequacies. He does not want overprotection on the one hand or badgering and constant pressure to improve on the other. He wants, as nearly as possible, to live in a normal environment, to be included in conversations, to have people interested in his ideas and his activities and, with a few necessary exceptions, to be treated much the same as he was before his illness.

Whenever possible, it is advisable to continue the treatment of aphasia through the cooperative efforts of the speech therapist and the family. In any case, the treatment should be planned carefully and have a definite direction and purpose at each step. It should avoid random, disjointed efforts which may confuse instead of help the patient. The primary goal is to stimulate improvement in the most natural way. The family members should include the patient in their conversations, encourage attempts at communication but not demand them, give the patient plenty of time to respond and, if necessary, speak in shorter ideas that are accompanied by gestures if the patient has impaired auditory input. Beyond these things, the most important service the family can render is to guard against overprotecting the patient, anticipating his ideas, excluding him from family activities and conversations and generally reducing his opportunities for listening and talking.

If a member of the family has the time and the patience to do more specific speech stimulation, a part of each day's schedule should be set aside for work on speech, writing, reading and listening. During the rest of the day, the patient should be allowed to relax and not be forced to apply the principles of the day's lesson to daily communication attempts. One or two short productive sessions a day will accomplish much more and produce less anxiety and frustration than constant correcting and badgering.

If the patient is agreeable to working on his communication problems, and the sessions are begun, the following points will be found helpful:

1. Do not expect dramatic changes. Improvement may be quite noticeable in the first 2 or 3 months of the illness and then will be less obvious later. Notes on assignments and samples of the work done should be saved so that the patient and the family can compare earlier work with recent samples and observe change.

2. Use a consistent format for these sessions.

   a. Always begin the session with a fairly easy task at which the patient can succeed.

   b. After the beginning tasks, review material previously covered.

   c. Use interesting material that relates to the patient's needs and interests. Be sure the concepts or tasks are not too difficult or too easy.

   d. If the patient handles the review satisfactorily, go on to something new, being careful not to move ahead too rapidly. The patient should master each step before going on to the next.

   e. Maintain a relaxed, friendly atmosphere. If tension develops, stop working for a moment or change to a different task. Humor and laughter are valuable tools in therapy and can do much to relieve tension.

   f. Call attention to the patient's successful experiences with the lesson. Minimize correcting the patient and breaking down his confidence.

   g. Terminate the session before the patient becomes overly tired. Always finish the session with a successful experience and by telling him a tentative time for the next session. In this way, he will develop a positive attitude about the work and will look forward to succeeding sessions.

Bilateral Brain Damage with Aphasia

The patient who has had several small strokes involving both sides of the brain must be viewed differently from the aphasic patient with damage to only the left hemisphere. The bilaterally involved patient presents different symptoms, has different problems and, in general, has a poorer prognosis for improvement.

The classic signs of bilateral brain damage are readily apparent if one looks for them in the patient's medical records or observes him carefully. He usually has a history of small strokes or at least will have had previous dizzy spells, transient weakness of the hand or leg, or temporary slurring of speech. The neurological examination often shows positive findings such as increased tendon reflexes on both sides, although it is possible for the patient who has had a recent stroke to present symptoms on only one side or predominantly on one side when in fact both sides of the brain are damaged.

The clinical signs most frequently seen and associated with bilateral damage are swallowing problems and incontinence. The swallowing difficulty, especially choking from attempts to drink liquids, arises from the fact that the muscles used in swallowing can function adequately only if weakness is limited to one side. When both sides move poorly, the valving necessary to keep food out of the respiratory system cannot be carried out and choking occurs since choking and coughing are natural defenses against aspiration of food into the lungs. Liquids, particularly water, cause more choking than solid food because they move down the throat more rapidly and will enter even the smallest opening in the slow moving, inefficient valve that protects the lungs.

The incontinence of bowel or bladder, to a degree, is a problem of attention or awareness on the part of the patient rather than a disorder of the muscles of elimination. It is uncommon for the aphasic patient even with severe communication breakdown to have confirmed or consistent "accidents." In contrast, the bilaterally involved patient may have little difficulty with communication but will be incontinent repeatedly.

The communicative processes in the patient with multiple strokes are quite different from those of the aphasic patient. As pointed out earlier, the aphasic patient is usually most impaired in the modalities of speech and auditory understanding. He often has difficulty in talking and understanding and relies heavily on gestures for communicating and vision for understanding. For instance, he may not understand a request that he get dressed and then go to the dining room, but he does so readily if he is handed his clothes and then shown through gesture that it is time to eat. The bilateral patient, in contrast, may seem to understand speech and be able to talk quite well but uses vision and gesture poorly. In the same dressing-eating situation he may respond to a request to dress and eat by saying "OK, I'll be right there." But several minutes later he will be found still sitting in his bed, undressed.

Because much of the rehabilitation process is visual-gestural where the patient is shown what to do and then must do it himself, the bilateral patient is very difficult to train and consequently has a poorer prognosis for functional improvement. In addition, because the medical prognosis is poor since it is based on a history of recurring strokes, it is generally ill advised for those responsible for the care of the bilateral patient to embark on a long-term or costly program of treatment such as speech therapy for the patient's slurred speech. However, if the patient has returned to his home and is using his speech, a short period of intensive treatment aimed at improving intelligibility may be in order.

In contrast to the multiple stroke patient whose prognosis must be considered as guarded, there are some patients with bilateral symptoms whose prognosis is much better, such as patients who have increased intracranial pressure due to edema, hydrocephalus or primary lesions in the left hemisphere that are exerting indirect pressure on the right hemisphere. In these cases, the patient does in fact present bilateral symptoms but these are transitory and once the intracranial pressure is reduced, the symptoms change to that of the type associated with the unilateral lesion.

Another type of patient who has bilateral damage with a more favorable prognosis is the patient with head trauma, especially the young patient. Unlike the multiple stroke patient who is a poor treatment risk because another in the series of strokes may wipe out any gains recently achieved with treatment, the trauma patient has a single incident of damage and further extension of the pathology is not expected. Therefore gains made with an aggressive treatment program are cumulative and therapy results in fairly permanent improvement.

REFERENCES

The following sources will provide more detailed information about many of the points discussed in this chapter. These references do not require the reader to have extensive technical training. Additional information and assistance may be obtained at the Speech Pathology and Audiology Departments of local universities or medical centers or by writing to the American Speech and Hearing Association, 903 Old Georgetown Road, Washington, D.C., 20014. Specific questions regarding the content of this chapter should be addressed to Dr. Bruce Porch, Pathology and Audiology Service, Veterans Administration Hospital, 2100 Ridgecrest Drive, S.E., Albuquerque, New Mexico, 87108.

1. Brookshire, R. H.: An Introduction to Aphasia. Minneapolis: BRK Publishers, 1973. An excellent, up-to-date, general consideration of aphasia.
2. Darley, F. L., Aronson, A. E. and Brown, J. R.: "Differential Diagnostic Patterns of Dysarthria." J. Speech Hearing Res., 12:246, 1969.

3. Darley, F. L., Aronson, A. E. and Brown, J. R.: "Clusters of Deviant Speech Dimensions in the Dysarthrias." J. Speech Hearing Res., 12:462, 1969. Both articles by these authors contain excellent discussions of dysarthrias.

4. Davis, H. and Silverman, S. R.: Hearing and Deafness, 3rd ed. New York: Holt, Rinehart and Winston, 1970. This is another text on audiology which explains the various pathologies connected with the ears as well as methods of testing.

5. Harrington, D. O.: The Visual Fields: A Textbook and Atlas of Clinical Perimetry, 3rd Ed. St. Louis: The C. V. Mosby Co., 1971. This is a standard textbook on the subject of visual fields.

6. Hirsch, M. J. and Wick, R. E. (eds.): Vision of the Aging Patient, an Optometric Symposium. Philadelphia: Chilton Book Co., 1965.

7. Longerich, M. C.: Manual for the Aphasic Patient. New York: Macmillan Company, 1958. These are some actual work materials that the author suggests are useful in helping to treat the aphasic patient.

8. McBride, C.: Silent Victory. Chicago: Nelson-Hall. A wife's account of her husband's battle against aphasia.

9. Moss, C. S.: Recovery with Aphasia. Urbana: University of Illinois Press, 1972. This is another self account of a clinical psychologist who had a stroke and recorded all of his observations and feelings during his recovery.

10. Newby, H. A.: Audiology, Principles and Practice, 3rd Ed. New York: Appleton-Century-Crofts, 1972. This is a basic text on hearing and hearing problems and methods of testing hearing.

11. Porch, B. E.: The Porch Index of Communicative Ability. Palo Alto, Calif.: Consulting Psychologists Press, 1967. The most widely used standardized test for aphasia. Volume II of the manual offers a comprehensive psychometric view of aphasia.

12. Sarno, J. E. and Sarno, M. T.: Stroke: The Condition and the Patient. New York: McGraw-Hill Book Company, 1969. This book looks at the problem of stroke both from the standpoint of the physician who specializes in the rehabilitation of stroke patients and from the perspective of the speech pathologist.

13. Schie, H. G. and Albert, D. M.: Adler's Textbook of Ophthalmology, 8th Ed. Philadelphia: W. B. Saunders Co., 1969. This is a standard textbook of the subject.

14. Schuell, H., Jenkins, J. and Jimenez-Pabon, E.: Aphasia in Adults: Diagnosis, Prognosis and Treatment. New York: Harper and Row, 1964. A classic text on aphasia with good description of different types of aphasia and principles of treatment.

15. Taylor, L.: Understanding Aphasia: A Guide for Family and Friends. New York: The Institute of Physical Medicine and Rehabilitation, New York University-Bellevue Medical Center, 1958. This small booklet is made up of questions and answers regarding the problem of aphasia and is written in clear non-technical language.

PART THREE

Organization
of
Rehabilitation

Levels and Places of Rehabilitation

GENERAL CONSIDERATIONS

Rehabilitation can be carried out anywhere, provided an adequate number of knowledgeable personnel are available. Much depends on the patient's condition and his rehabilitation requirements.

If the patient's condition is critical, such as that resulting from a severe brain involvement or respiratory impairment, the patient must be hospitalized. He is admitted to the intensive care unit or to a unit for acute surgical or medical management where the principal objective is preservation of life or body integrity. In advanced medical centers, planning for rehabilitation is started at once. Surgeons and internists are becoming fully cognizant of the measures that must be applied to prevent disuse phenomena, and often, nurses in intensive care units are well trained in the essential techniques. At times, there is early consultation with specialists concerning the eventual rather than the immediate results of injury.

If the patient's condition is not critical, as, for instance, a patient with mild hemiplegia, the advantages of hospitalization must be weighed against the advantages of home treatment. Since it is common practice to perform lumbar punctures on patients with hemiplegia, and in cases where a cerebral angiography and brain scan are recommended it is obviously advisable to hospitalize all hemiplegic patients at least initially. During the diagnostic phase, secondary disabilities must be prevented and, in most cases, active rehabilitation can be started.

Once the patient is over the critical phase and diagnostic study is completed, rehabilitation can be started. At this point, there are four alternative places to carry out the program. Rehabilitation may be started on the *medical or surgical ward* and continued in a *convalescent hospital,* or the patient may be transferred to a *rehabilitation ward* or he may be sent home. The decision must be made in collaboration with the family and the patient and should be based on the following considerations: (1) Are the specialized facilities of a hospital or a re-habilitation center required to accomplish speedy rehabilitation? (2) Is there need for frequent medical observation and close supervision of conditions other than the primary disability, such as hypertension, urinary tract infection or other concomitant disorder? (3) Is it feasible to carry out the program at home? (4) Are there resources, such as a do-it-yourself handyman at home who can construct blocks for eleva-tion of the chair, handrails on stairways, and other simple devices for assistance and protection of the patient? (5) Are there financial cir-cumstances or questions concerning the adequacy of insurance cover-age that must be weighed?

After the patient has recovered his optimum physical ability, he may still require attendant or maintenance care. This can be provided at home or in a long-term care institution.

LEVELS OF REHABILITATION

As shown above, applicable rehabilitation services may vary in nature and intensity according to the degree of disabilty and the general condition of the patient. We shall describe several levels of rehabilitation care though it should be understood that intermediate stages exist.

Preventive Rehabilitation Measures for Acute Medical and Surgical Patients

This is the minimal program required for the prevention of sec-ondary disabilities in patients who are bedridden and immobilized either by their primary disability or its management. This level of rehabilitation is applicable to disabled patients in the ICU and on acute medical and surgical wards.

Short-term ADL Training

Patients with limited disabilities who have completed their acute care on a medical or surgical ward may need short-term instruction and training in crutch walking, wheelchair activities, feeding, and dressing prior to their discharge from the hospital. These are usually patients with fractures who have their limbs in casts and must undergo a period of convalescence with limited activities. The ADL (activities of daily living) training is needed to enable them to function with little assistance and to avoid further disuse. Training in ADL should not take more than 2 or 3 days and is usually carried out on the acute medical or surgical ward.

Rehabilitation of Patients with Limited Disabilities

This group includes patients who are able or nearly able to carry out the activities of daily living but are afflicted with a disability which requires rehabilitation measures. Examples are the blind and the deaf, patients with disability of one or several joints or weakness of one or several muscles. The rehabilitation program required for these patients can usually be carried out on an outpatient basis.

Intensive Inpatient Rehabilitation

Intensive inpatient rehabilitation is necessary for patients who are so severely disabled that it may take several weeks or months of intensive rehabilitation to enable them to become independent or to be prepared for attendant care outside the hospital. To this group belong patients with brain injuries, spinal cord injuries, strokes, and severe widespread rheumatoid arthritis. Usually these patients are transferred to a rehabilitation service after the acute medical and surgical care is completed or after diagnostic measures have been carried to a reasonable conclusion. Intensive inpatient rehabilitation is also needed for those patients who have been disabled for a long time and have never received rehabilitative care and therefore have not achieved their maximum potential. Finally, intensive inpatient rehabilitation is needed for severely disabled patients who were once rehabilitated but have regressed or suffered a complication due to disuse, misuse or additional disease or injury.

Maintenance Care

As the name implies, maintenance care is designed to maintain the patient's optimum level of function already achieved by rehabilitation. This covers a wide spectrum. Many patients are so grossly damaged and so far beyond medical assistance that they are not capable of any function. Organic brain damage, in particular, often presents an insurmountable obstacle to rehabilitation. In this case it may be necessary to limit the therapeutic efforts to humane care which will at least delay deterioration and prevent unnecessary disability and suffering. It may involve little more than periodic turning in bed to prevent effects of disuse; it may require special methods of feeding and even life-long artificial respiration. Regardless of the nature or severity of the disability there is always something that can be done to make life more tolerable, if not for the patient, at least for his family.

The patient who is mentally alert and has some functional ability despite a severe disability may require considerably more intensive and time-consuming maintenance care. He must be given the opportunity to use his available function in activities of daily living to prevent disuse and to maintain the dignity of human existence. He must also be given the stimulation of social life and the opportunity to be creative and useful. This type of maintenance care is best carried out at home and within the family. Unfortunately, few people are willing to take care of their disabled close relatives and the majority of bed patients on maintenance care are housed in nursing homes.

For the mobile patient, maintenance care can be carried out at home and on an outpatient basis. Regular follow-up visits for patients with spinal cord injuries and strokes are very important for the maintenance of their functions. Problems may arise in the health and physical ability of the patient as well as with the condition of his equipment, such as the wheelchair, respirator or artificial limbs. Another reason for closely following such patients is the fact that their maintenance actually depends upon excercise. Unfortunately, exercise is very much like dieting; it takes a good deal of discipline and it needs to be stimulated frequently.

Vocational Rehabilitation

While vocational rehabilitation is not indicated in the elderly or in patients with organic brain damage, it is a very important phase of rehabilitation in many patients regardless of the severity of their disability. In fact, vocational rehabilitation may be considered the highest level of rehabilitation care because it eventually enables the disabled person to be independent not only physically but also economically. Vocational rehabilitation in the form of counselling and instruction can be initiated during the phase of intensive inpatient rehabilitation and may be continued during maintenance care. The disabled person with good vocational potential can usually attend regular classes and receive his training together with able-bodied students. For patients who are not able to achieve competitive skills, sheltered workshops are available to give them the opportunity to improve their work tolerance, to be productive, creative, and earn a small income.

FACILITIES FOR THE CARE OF THE DISABLED

Home Care

One objective of rehabilitation is independent living, and this can be carried out best at home. Sometimes, a home program is feasible immediately after evaluation in a hospital or a center. At home, the rate at which rehabilitation proceeds can be very flexible, since cost is a minor consideration and psychological adjustment is more important than time. The simple equipment for rehabilitation of common disabilities can be acquired inexpensively and often can be constructed by family members. During the course of treatment, simple modifications and additions (banisters, rails, etc.) can be made to make the home more secure.

The virtues of a home are the assurance of privacy and relative independence of action, the comfort of living among familiar people and things and the continuity of normal living which tends to maintain morale. Priority should be given to a good home environment. This is defined as a home in which the handicapped or the disabled person is accepted without hostility or resentment and is assured of affection and adequate attention. It should also have space and facilities which are physically capable of adaptation to the exercise and restorative programs needed. If it is determined by interview with the family and by a home visit that the patient is likely to be confronted by either hostility or overattentiveness, the home may be disqualified as a suitable place for rehabilitation. The primary consideration is the psychological atmosphere of the environment, and this can be measured in terms of manifest affection and interest on the part of relatives or friends. When compared with the psychological environment, the physical accoutrements of the home are secondary considerations.

With the exception of disabled patients who are acutely ill and have to be hospitalized either on an intensive care unit or in isolation, any disabled person can be rehabilitated at home provided adequate personnel are available. Frequently only family members are needed. The patient who has been discharged from the hospital after a brief period of ADL training following a fracture or an acute illness can easily convalesce at home since practically no care is required. The patient with a limited disability usually lives at home and has his rehabilitation supplemented by outpatient care. But even the person with a stroke or spinal cord injury or the amputee who requires intensive inpatient rehabilitation can be handled in the home if members of the health team are willing to make the necessary home visits and if the family is available to maintain a full day's rehabilitation program.

In the past we have successfully rehabilitated hemiplegic patients in their homes with the assistance of family members. We had to give it up for three reasons: (1) It is less and less common to find family members who have the time and desire to take care of the patient. (2) Health insurance will pay for care in the hospital but not for rehabilitation at home. (3) In the time it takes the physician to make a home visit to see one hemiplegic patient, for instance, he or she can easily see 10 to 15 hemiplegic patients in the hospital. Other health team members are also more efficient in an institutional setting. However, there is no question that the patient is vastly better off at home and rehabilitation is less unpleasant and less strenuous and usually proceeds faster with fewer undesirable incidents.

Rehabilitation Centers

Inpatient Rehabilitation Service

An inpatient rehabilitation service is defined as a separate unit specifically dedicated and designed for the rehabilitation of severely disabled patients. The service or center is directed by a physician and staffed by additional physicians, nurses, therapists and social workers. A rehabilitation center may be a service within a general hospital or it may exist as a separate facility. In this case, it is usually affiliated with a hospital for specific diagnostic and therapeutic services. Rehabilitation centers may treat all or various types of disabilities or they may be specialized for children or for patients with specific disabilities such as spinal cord injuries, amputations, etc.

For all practical purposes a rehabilitation center is the only place that provides intensive inservice rehabilitation as defined above. Most inpatient rehabilitation centers also provide outpatient care or at least follow-up care for the patients they have rehabilitated.

Selection of a Rehabilitation Center

When a person has suffered a seriously disabling injury or illness and requires specialized rehabilitation care, selection of a suitable institution is in order. The place selected will depend primarily upon the facilities available in any given community. If there is a choice, the following criteria, listed according to priority, should be considered:

1. The experience and the qualifications of a professional staff.
2. The attitude of the institutional staff and the administration toward the personal rights and privileges of the patient.
3. The physical facilities for treatment.
4. Opportunities for group activities and stimulation through group effort.
5. The physical plan of the institution, with special consideration of opportunities for self-care, for dining in company, for recreation and unrestricted visiting.

Rational selection based upon meaningful criteria may be impossible because of financial considerations.

Nursing Homes

A nursing home is an institution which furnishes essentially nursing and attendant care for the sick and disabled. It is usually licensed by the state health agency. It differs from a hospital in that it does not possess the facilities for diagnosis or for acute or emergency medical care, such as x-ray, laboratory or surgical units. There is no close medical supervision, and physicians are not readily available on a daily basis. It differs from a rehabilitation center in that it has no permanent therapist or psychosocial staff, and the number of nurses is usually inadequate for rehabilitation nursing.

Nursing homes are sometimes called convalescent hospitals, rehabilitation hospitals, or other misleading terms. The physical plant of a nursing home lends itself to the use as a rehabilitation center, provided some space is set aside for exercise, activities of daily living and recreation. But the staff would have to be considerably enlarged and placed under medical directions with daily supervision. As far as rehabilitation is concerned, the nursing home at present serves two distinct functions: short-term rehabilitation and long-term care.

Short-term Rehabilitation

Rehabilitation in this sense is concerned with limited disabilities such as fractures where a patient is mobile but is not capable of all activities of daily living and needs some assistance. This process could well be called convalescence since the patient is only institutionalized until the fractures have healed. After this he is discharged either to his home or to a rehabilitation center for further rehabilitation.

Long-term Care

The nursing home is also (and probably predominantly) used as a lifetime residence and frequently as a storage depot for the permanently disabled. Permanent nursing home patients fall into several categories. Some may have been rehabilitated to their maximum potential and are now in need of maintenance care. Others have never been evaluated for their rehabilitation potential and are simply "stored away" in nursing homes because they have exhausted their acute hospital insurance benefits and either the funds for rehabilitation are not available, or the family and physician are not aware of the fact that rehabilitation is possible. There are probably also a number of elderly people who, while not particularly sick or disabled, are in nursing homes because they cannot quite manage to live alone and it is too troublesome for their family to keep them in their homes.

The maintenance care in nursing homes usually leaves much to be desired. In fact, the conditions prevailing in most nursing homes have become a national scandal. The remedies which have been suggested include: public pressure by more intensive inspection of nursing homes, upgrading of nursing home personnel and evaluation by professional standards review organizations. In our opinion these measures are entirely useless to improve the nursing homes. In order to remedy a situation one has to understand its causes, and the primary cause for the inhumane warehousing of elderly and disabled people in nursing homes is the attitude of the public (see Chapter 4). Public attitudes are difficult to change, but without change it may be difficult to eliminate the other causes of the nursing home scandal.

The second cause for the deplorable conditions in nursing homes in our opinion is the lack of proper segregation of patients. While there are special nursing homes for mental patients, there is apparently no rule to exclude the confused and mentally disturbed from institutions for the purely physically disabled. If confused and incontinent patients are dispersed throughout the nursing home, the mentally alert patients cannot possibly feel comfortable. Even gourmet food would lose its flavor in the squalor of the surroundings. In order to create a proper climate for a maintenance program for these patients, it is necessary that those with socially acceptable behavior be separated from those with socially unacceptable behavior.

The third cause is a complete lack of concern for human values. As pointed out above in discussing the maintenance program, it is not only physical maintenance that is involved, but also social and psychological maintenance. This means there must be space, time, and opportunity for the disabled patient to remain mobile, to socialize, and to carry on creative activities. Obviously, there must be funds to carry out such programs.

Here are a few suggestions for nursing home reform:

1. Patients who do not require nursing care but are admitted to convalescent hospitals or nursing homes because they have no other place to go should be transferred to board-and-care homes.
2. Patients who have not achieved their optimum rehabilitation potential should be evaluated or re-evaluated in a rehabilitation center. If further functional improvement is possible, they should be treated and then sent either to their own homes or to board-and-care-homes.
3. Patients should be separated into the following groups:
    a. Psychiatric patients without physical disability.
    b. Psychiatric patients with physical disability.
    c. Physically disabled patients without psychiatric problems.

These three groups of individuals require entirely different environments and different staffing and therefore should be segregated into different institutions or parts of institutions. Whether the physically handicapped should be separated into categories is another question. Certainly it is discouraging to the young patient with fractures or arthritis to be in a room with a very old person or a person with brain damage.

Convalescent hospitals which give lifetime care to disabled patients should be established primarily as lifetime *homes for human beings*. Secondarily, necessary attention should be paid to their disabilities. Since human beings have different interests, there should be nursing homes available which satisfy different interests. Here are a few examples:

1. For patients interested in learning, reading, and discussion, the institution should offer courses for various interests, should have group discussions, a good library and an efficient library loan service.
2. For patients interested in games, there should be a nursing home where bridge, canasta, pinochle, bingo and various party games are played.
3. For patients interested in crafts, there should be an institution with a workshop for all types of arts and crafts.

A large nursing home may, of course, offer several of these possible activities. Each nursing home should have facilities for physical exercise for the disabled. This should include a gym with mats, therapeutic stairs, stall bars, and opportunities for shuffle board, table tennis, etc. Patients should be able to choose nursing homes according to their spheres of interest and should be allowed to change nursing homes from time to time as their interests change or if they are not satisfied with them.

Some segregation according to age is certainly also desirable. Large metropolitan areas should have a place for disabled children comparable to the Stanford Convalescent Hospital (near Palo Alto, California) where children receive rehabilitative and long-term care. Disabled young people, such as patients with cerebral palsy or head injuries or rheumatoid arthritis, will be much happier in the company of other young people than in a nursing home where everybody else is over 70.

Humane measures are also needed for confused or psychotic patients. This, of course, is an area of considerable uncertainty at present. State hospitals have been closed and communities have been expected to take on their psychiatric clientele, but they have been ill-prepared and ill-supported for this purpose. Nevertheless, halfway houses, long-term facilities and similar programs are being developed to care for these people.

Outpatient Rehabilitation Facilities

Outpatient rehabilitation for patients with limited disabilities allows patients to live at home or in a facility nearby and be transported to the outpatient facility for rehabilitation care. Some inpatient rehabilitation centers also furnish rehabilitation on an outpatient basis. Many hospitals which have no inpatient rehabilitation service still furnish outpatient rehabilitation through their physical or occupational therapy departments and social services. Finally there are independent outpatient rehabilitation centers in many communities. Most of them furnish general rehabilitation services such as strengthening and training in activities of daily living for all types of disabilities. Some outpatient rehabilitation facilities are specialized such as schools for the deaf and schools for the blind. Centers devoted to the rehabilitation of cerebral palsy are also frequently associated with schools. Another outpatient rehabilitation facility is a sheltered workshop, where disabled patients have the opportunity to do assembly or factory work for several hours of the day according to their ability. They are paid a salary for their work.

Living Facilities for the Disabled and Elderly
Board and Care Homes

A boarding home is an institution which provides room and board. In cases of boarding homes for the disabled, special safety features are required by the government, although certain facilities adapted to the disabled may or may not be present. Such a facility differs from a nursing home in that the patients do not get any assistance with activities of daily living. However, it would be desirable to have boarding homes with a certain amount of attendant care. The cost could be substantially less than a nursing home and it would offer a further opportunity to segregate the less severely disabled from the more severely disabled thus giving them a chance to live a more active and complete life.

Housing for the Disabled

Another form of living arrangement is special housing for the disabled who are nearly independent. In some locations, efforts are being made—mostly by the disabled themselves—to establish community housing facilities in which it is possible for them to share expenses and attendant care. The conception of such sharing is as old as the welfare programs. However, the realization of this concept has been relatively recent. Take, for example, Alpha Place, a project founded by an enterprising paraplegic in San Jose, California. Alpha Place is a part of a housing project, containing a series of quadriplex units. Selected ground floor apartments are rented to the disabled. Two adjacent ground floor apartments are usually fitted with ramps to provide easy access, and each person has his own quarters which are provided with any necessary apparatus. Attendant care services, paid for by the welfare department, are shared. One of the most successful aspects of Alpha Place is the air of freedom which prevails. No one is pressured into doing anything. Those who are depressed can have their depressions quietly. Those who want to socialize may socialize. No lines are drawn on ordinary behavior and no censorship prevails with respect to sexuality.

The interesting thing about this project is that it is run by a disabled person and includes all types of personalities who are apparently able to get along well. There are two vans which belong to the enterprise. One is used to transport members to schools and to special appointments, such as vocational rehabilitation counselling. The other van is used to carry food and to serve other purposes related to the unit.

Housing for the Elderly

The project of special housing for the elderly has been approached from many different points of view. There are private institutions where elderly people maintain apartments and have the opportunity either to provide their own meals or to share the meals of the institution in a common dining room. There are also various projects for the elderly where they maintain their own independent lives. In this country, while we have been concerned over the possibility of segregating the elderly away from the other age groups, there have been projects designed to allow for a certain percentage of elderly people to live among younger associates, hopefully to provide contact for the different age groups. In addition, of course, there are middle class developments where individuals can find reasonable comfort, protection, and activities within the grounds of large developments.

Providing adequate housing for our increasing population of senior citizens is a great problem. This country is behind Great Britain, the Scandinavian countries and other Western cultures, where housing for the elderly has been a public concern for years. For example, there is a residence in Amsterdam, Holland, where elderly people have had housing provided for them for many years. In addition, many of the Scandinavian countries have well-developed housing projects for the elderly.

CONTINUITY OF CARE

Rehabilitation has been designated the third phase of medical care, the first two being prevention and definitive medical or surgical treatment. This concept is unfortunate, because it implies a time relationship, with rehabilitation taking up where definitive treatment leaves off. If rehabilitation is understood to encompass prevention of disuse and misuse (see Chap. 3) as well as maintenance of maximal physical function and emotional balance during the course of definitive treatment, it is obvious that rehabilitation must begin in parallel with rather than in series with definitive medical care.

The person who requires rehabilitation services must maintain a relationship with general medical services, whether provided by the private practitioner, the clinic or the medical group. Whenever possible, rehabilitation should be carried out as a continuing program with general medical care. In each instance, a decision must be made whether to treat the patient in a hospital, in a rehabilitation center, as an outpatient or at home. Regardless of the location selected, there should be good liaison and communication between those directing rehabilitation and the family physician, the clinic or other responsible medical personnel.

Basically, the candidate for rehabilitation needs both special medical and psychosocial services. The two aspects of rehabilitation, namely, physical re-education or strengthening and psychosocial adjustment, must go hand in hand. If the combination of skillful health professionals with their essential aides and a skillful social worker with her access to community resources can form a working partnership for the patient's benefit, a framework for a very satisfactory rehabilitation team is established immediately.

If one assumes that a major disability is handled best in a well-staffed rehabilitation center, the course of events should be somewhat as follows: (1) diagnositic evaluative study that analyzes the problem and provides a basis for program planning and a preliminary prognosis; (2) a therapeutic program scheduled according to priorities of goals and consistent with the patient's interests and capabilities; (3) concurrent psychosocial service aimed at utilizing family or community relationships, securing economic resources and exploiting interests and aptitudes that can lead the disabled person back into the normal stream of activity; (4) planning for discharge, a joint enterprise of the medical and the psychosocial staff, preferably initiated early and developed in close cooperation with the patient, and (5) follow-up observation.

Whether postdischarge follow-up is delegated to the family physician or is carried on by the center staff depends in part on the nature of the disability and the need for continued specialist services. However, even when the follow-up is done by the family physician, continued contact with the center is desirable.

REFERENCES

1. Elements of Progressive Patient Care. Washington, D.C.: U.S. Dept. of HEW, Public Health Service Publication, No. 930-C-1, 1962.
2. Fogel, C. D.: "Survey of Disabled Persons Reveals Housing Choices." J. Rehabilitation, 37:26, 1971.
3. Green, R. F., Silber, M. and Hinterbuchner, C.: "Housing for the Disabled: A Follow-Up Study." APMR, 55:447, 1974.
4. "Housing for the Disabled: II. Characteristics of Those Willing to Move to Specially Designed Facilities." Percept. Mat. Skills, 32:212, 1971.
5. Housing for the Physically Impaired: A Guide for Planning and Design. Washington, D.C.: U.S. Dept. of Housing and Urban Development, U.S. Govt. Printing Office, 1968.

10

The Physical Plant

DESIGN OF REHABILITATION FACILITIES

Both rehabilitation and long-term nursing care are now carried out in patients' homes, in so-called rest or boarding homes, in nursing homes or other convalescent institutions, in chronic illness hospitals and in rehabilitation centers or rehabilitation units of general hospitals. Manifestly, it would be impossible to propose any broad pattern for the architectural design of this variety of institutions, even if the authors had professional competence to do so. The function of the architect in designing a new facility is to express in physical structure the most satisfying and efficient integration of a large number of statutory, professional, individual and esthetic requirements. Laws concerned with fire safety and structural quality influence greatly the gross character of the facility. Space needed and interrelationships of treatment, domiciliary, dining and recreational facilities present a major challenge to the architect. In addition, his own ideas must be resolved in the light of consultants, boards of directors, administrators and professional staff who may be concerned with design.

Medical personnel with experience in rehabilitation are qualified to offer suggestions to the architect. Among these are the following:

General Design. A rehabilitation facility must be accessible to the disabled and provide easy means for egress, ingress and mobility within the premises. Accordingly, entrances must be level or adequately ramped or provided with platforms that allow easy transfer from ambulances, invalid buses and other vehicles. Hallways and doorways and particularly entrances to dining, bathing and treatment facilities must be wide enough to permit the easy movement of wheelchairs and such equipment as tilt tables, beds and other apparatus which may have to be moved from place to place.

Unit Size. Variety of size of units is highly desirable. For some types of disability there is great advantage in grouping together compatible people for socialization, mutual stimulation and group treatment. It seems to be economical and satisfactory to group six people together in a living space for rehabilitation. However, there should be private quarters for those who are temporarily ill, who may require relative isolation because of psychological problems or who need a period of quietude before attempting group living. Some persons are particularly unsuited for sharing of space and cannot be rehabilitated in a general ward.

After the rehabilitation program is well under way, sometimes it is desirable to establish people in independent quarters where they may exercise self-care prior to discharge. Small apartmentlike units are highly advantageous for this purpose. Separating living quarters from the treatment area may be economical as well as beneficial in promoting independent living.[2]

Beds. Once, a patient with robust wit, when told by his physician to go to bed for the treatment of a respiratory infection, replied, "Bed! Why that's where people die." However, the bed is a therapeutic modality in rehabilitation. Rest, and especially prescribed rest, is an important part of any medical program. Unfortunately, in many institutions and particularly in modern efficient hospitals, the bed has taken on a role quite independent of prescription and serves as a convenient place to render treatments. Within the past three decades the bed has begun to lose some of its ritualistic appeal, particularly in surgical wards where early ambulation has become routine. On medical wards, and especially in institutions for the treatment of the elderly, the bed is still a dangerous instrument. It has more serious side-effects than the most potent medications, yet it is prescribed and used most casually.

Most of the severely disabling secondary consequences of primary disability are the results of improperly used bed rest. Asher's indictment of the bed should be inscribed on the walls of the staff rooms and the nursing stations of every medical institution:

> Rest in bed is anatomically, physically and psychologically unsound. Look at a patient lying long in bed. What a pathetic picture he makes! The blood clotting in his veins, the lime draining from his bones, the scybala stacking up in his colon, the flesh rotting from his seat, the urine leaking from his distended bladder, and the spirit evaporating from his soul.[1]

From the standpoint of architecture and hospital organization, every effort should be made to de-emphasize the bed. It is suggested that hospitals no longer be measured in terms of bed capacity and that institutions for medical treatment be humanized by substituting such terms as patient units or persons or individuals for the usual unit designation, bed. In an effort to de-emphasize the bed, attempts should be made to detach patient activity from bed spaces. This can be done by designing rooms in such a way as to make the bed less physically evident during the day, by lining beds up against the wall or by having recesses into which they may be moved when not in use. No one has yet developed a satisfactory disappearing bed, but new designs that tend to make the bed a flexible unit may serve to diminish its potential harmfulness. If the bed cannot be de-emphasized physically, an alternative approach is the removal of the patient from the bed area for much of the day. This can be accomplished by locating activity and exercise rooms in close proximity to ward spaces and by adequate provision of multipurpose and recreational rooms to encourage patients to spend much of their time elsewhere than in dormitory areas.

Chairs and Other Furniture.   The type of chair suitable for rehabilitation should be firm, straight and comfortable. The most satisfactory type is a well-designed captain's chair with firm arms and a somewhat contoured seat. Its height should be adjustable by elevation on blocks or a platform or by the addition of risers, firm cushions, or other means of elevating the seat (Fig. 14-4). Training the patient to rise from chairs of graded height is intended to develop enough strength to allow a person to stand up from an ordinary chair. However, some people are too weak or too deformed to achieve this goal. Eventually, they should be provided with higher chairs to use at home. In addition to suitable chairs, work tables and work areas also are necessary as are storage spaces, closets and rooms for items of personal interest. The wards or adjacent treatment areas should be large enough to accommodate tilt tables, wheelchairs, walkers and other necessary devices.

In addition to these basic items, the space designed for patient care should provide a handy location for clothing and accessories that allow the patient to develop independence in dressing. He should be able to reach his clothes from bed or chair and not have to wait for an attendant to bring clothing from a locker placed across the room. Finally, he should have space available where his private belongings may be within reach and within his field of vision. By this means, some of the attributes of home may be transferred to the institution and may serve as a link between the past and the future.

Toilets and Lavatories.   The particular type of receptacle for bladder and bowel hygiene depends on the disability and the stage of recovery. Use of the bedpan should be discontinued as soon as possible. The bedside commode or an adjacent toilet to which the patient may be wheeled on a chair with casters (glider) or a wheelchair best serve the needs in rehabilitation. Western man is accustomed to elimination in private, and this cultural pattern should be maintained if possible. A lavatory should be close at hand and at a level that will permit self-bathing as soon as possible.

In the institution there should be toilet seats of various heights in order to permit the weak and the otherwise incapacitated to learn to use ordinary toilet facilities as soon as possible. Toilets can either be permanently installed at different heights in a toilet area or various devices can be used to raise the seats to appropriate levels. In general, the elderly and the disabled do better with a relatively high toilet, and it might be advisable, especially where space is limited, to install all seats 2 to 4 inches (5 to 10 cm.) higher than the standard toilet. Whichever plan is decided on, either the permanent installation of seats of varying height or of somewhat higher than average height or the provision of special devices to raise the seat temporarily, some provision must be made that will encourage use of the ordinary toilet.

Lavatories also should be of varying height to accommodate patients when they stand or sit and those who may become mobile by lying prone on litters. Since lavatory bowls must be installed permanently, the height must be based on the nature of the disabilities to be treated in any given facility. Near the lavatory basins there should be ample room for toilet articles and cosmetics and for the attachment of special assistive devices which may stimulate or facilitate self-care.

Treatment Areas. The relationship between the medical specialty of rehabilitation and the therapeutic specialties of physical, occupational, speech and recreational therapy is not clear-cut. The evolution of these interrelated fields of medicine has brought about an unjustifiable amount of ritualization. When a hospital administration or a community organization begins to develop plans for a rehabilitation unit, recourse is made usually to documents available from well-established centers or from federal agencies or health organizations that have prepared model plans. The planners and the architect almost invariably lay out well-defined separate units for physical and occupational therapy. If economic support is assured, one may anticipate design of a luxurious therapeutic pool. Though a therapeutic pool is not essential, if there is one in a rehabilitation facility, its use may be helpful for early weight-bearing. Space is allocated for a variety of specialties, and usually the planners proceed to install highly specialized and expensive equipment, much of it designed for mechanization of exercise or manipulative stretching and other physical procedures. Usually, such planning is done without the guidance of a physiatrist or other qualified medical consultant. It is not unusual to find a rehabilitation center fully equipped and even almost thoroughly staffed before the medical director is employed. Often, design and construction are carried out without consideration of the population to be served and without clear understanding of the modalities of therapy that may be necessary.

Since there are already numerous examples of the complex, highly equipped rehabilitation facilities designed for the treatment of every conceivable disability, attention is here focused on the simple necessities for the rehabilitation of common disabilities.

Beyond these essentials, the institution must provide those facilities that are needed in rehabilitation. If the disability is such as to require only the simplest measures, such as standing and stair-climbing activities, usually these are best carried out in the room or ward or in an adjacent space. If very special therapeutic exercises are needed, the equipment must be centralized in a therapy department where prescribed procedures may be carried out. It is important to note that a medical decision must be made concerning the best place to carry out exercises or other treatments in each case. The tendency to develop a routine method of treatment should be strongly resisted.

It should be emphasized that no attempt is being made to offer an either-or alternative of complex versus simple establishment. It may be necessary to have a battery of therapeutic devices for specialized exercises and training. Often, it is highly advantageous to have a closely affiliated speech and hearing unit. Recreational or vocational services may be needed, and these may include training in weaving, ceramics, painting, sculpture, mosaic and many other fields. In preliminary design, the most essential feature is space that will permit the growth of special services as these prove to be necessary. *Whatever may be planned for special therapy units should not prevent the development of exercise areas in close proximity to dormitory space.*

Decor. In addition to the basic requirements of the environment, the therapeutic atmosphere may be heightened in a number of ways. In a rehabilitation setting, it is no longer necessary to maintain the sterile and cold atmosphere of the communicable disease ward. We decorate our homes with paintings, prints, rugs and ceramics because it is more pleasant to live in an esthetically pleasing environment. If we derive psychological and emotional support from agreeable surroundings under ordinary circumstances, is it not probable that we can also benefit from them under trying and difficult circumstances? Should not the environment of the therapeutic institution be developed in such a way as to contribute to therapy? Color, design and opportunity to view the outside world are among the considerations that should be regarded as essentials rather than frills.

Recreation.   With respect to recreation, the taste of the individual should be considered, and the influence on others of his particular interests should also be weighed. It is unlikely that four or six occupants of a ward will all want to hear the same type of music or view the same television program at the same time. Modern electronic engineering makes it possible for individualization of program and for protection of privacy. Group recreational activity is most desirable, but it is almost always unsuccessful unless it is developed and coordinated by an expert in group work. Often, the entertainment that is imposed upon the institutionally confined is more gratifying to the volunteers who provide it than to the recipients.

REFERENCES

1. Asher, R. A.: "The Dangers of Going to Bed." Brit. M. J., 967, Dec. 13, 1947.
2. Mackie, W.: "Planning the Hospitals of the Future." The Lancet, 211, Jan. 26, 1963.

11

The Rehabilitation Process

Since the development of formal medical rehabilitation about 30 years ago, the rehabilitation process has remained virtually unchanged. It starts with an *evaluation* or an assessment of the patient's medical status, disabilities, assets and psychosocial circumstances. This is followed by the application of an appropriate *rehabilitation program,* to bring the patient to his optimal functional ability. Next comes *follow-up care* which is necessary to ascertain that the patient maintains this ability and to assist him with physical and psychosocial problems. Sometimes a *maintenance program* is indicated. Finally, if in the course of rehabilitation the patient is transferred from one institution to another, or to his home, very careful *discharge planning* is necessary.

Basically, the rehabilitation process remains the same wherever rehabilitation is carried out. We shall describe the process as carried out in a rehabilitation center, since this covers all possible phases of the process.

EVALUATION

The term "evaluation" was introduced early in the history of rehabilitation medicine. The traditional medical assessment of the patient resulting in diagnosis, prognosis, and treatment recommendations did not take into consideration the patient's disability and rehabilitation. It dealt only with the pathology, not with the person. In order to assess the patient's rehabilitation potential, it is not sufficient to know the diagnosis. A detailed evaluation of his disability, his economic situation, and his attitudes is necessary for a complete assessment.

It is sometimes possible to evaluate a patient's rehabilitation potential in a single examination. For the severely disabled hospitalized patient, however, it is usually necessary to observe him for 1 or 2 weeks, carry out various diagnostic and functional tests, and interview the patient and his family. Physicians, nurses, therapists, and social workers participate in evaluating the patient and then report their findings during an evaluation conference. The total patient evaluation consists of three parts: (1) the medical evaluation, (2) the disability evaluation and (3) the psychosocial evaluation.

Medical Evaluation

The medical evaluation is generally carried out by the physician. It is frequently supplemented by data furnished by nurses, therapists, and social workers. The data obtained in the medical evaluation include past illnesses and injuries, history of the disease or the injury leading to the present disability and the patient's current medical condition expressed in terms of definite diagnoses. Not infrequently, one cannot be immediately certain of all diagnoses. In this case, a presentation of the possible diagnoses is helpful. Whenever a definite diagnosis is made, prognosis and treatment of this condition should be determined. By knowing the diagnosis of the disease leading to the present disability, it is frequently possible to say whether the disability will progress, improve or remain stationary. This is very helpful in the rehabilitation plan.

Disability Evaluation

The term "disability" has been defined previously (see p. 6). The disability evaluation consists of four phases: (1) evaluation of the physical disability or impairment, (2) assessment of physical assets, (3) evaluation of ADL capabilities, and (4) evaluation of the vocational handicap.

Evaluation of the Physical Disability or Impairment

Frequently, the severely disabled patient is suffering from a number of physical disabilities, which can be classified as primary, secondary and pre-existing.

Primary Disabilities.   Those disabilities which are caused by the presenting illness or injury are called primary disabilities. A patient who has suffered a stroke may present several primary disabilities resulting from the stroke, for instance, hemiplegia, aphasia, and hemianopsia.

Secondary Disabilities.   Secondary disabilities are those which have resulted from inadequate management of the patient since the onset of the primary disability. The secondary disabilities are usually caused by disuse or misuse (see p. 27).

Pre-existing Disabilities.   These disabilities are not related to the present illness but may assume an important role in planning the rehabilitation. Common pre-existing disabilities in the elderly are impairment of sight and hearing, joint pain, limitation of range of motion and cardiovascular disorders.

Besides recognizing the existence of all physical disabilities, it is important to evaluate their extent and nature. If the disability is hemiplegia, it is important to know whether the paralyzed extremities are spastic or flaccid. It is also important to know how complete the paralysis is and which portions of the extremities are involved. In case of a contracture, the physical impairment should be expressed by the number of degrees in range of motion loss.

Assessment of Physical Assets

A second factor in the disability evaluation is an assessment of the patient's physical assets. Let us demonstrate this by the example of two paraplegics. Although their physical disabilities may be identical, one may have very weak upper extremities and be unable to perform a push-up or a chinning exercise; the other patient may have the arms of an athlete and without any training may transfer easily from bed to chair and chair to floor, etc. It is obvious that the prognosis for self-cure for these two patients is quite different and that they also require different rehabilitation programs. The arms of the paraplegic, the remaining leg of the lower extremity amputee and the uninvolved side of the hemiplegic are the keys to their rehabilitation. Unfortunately, a proper evaluation of the physical assets is frequently forgotten.

ADL Evaluation

The third phase of the disability evaluation is the study of the patient's ability to perform the activities of daily living. We have divided the activities of daily living into three goups: mobility, self-care, and communication. The severely disabled patient has many deficits in these areas, which should be recorded and evaluated as to their prognosis and management. For the majority of elderly disabled patients, restoration of activities of daily living is usually the only rehabilitation goal, i.e., vocational rehabilitation is not expected.

Evaluation of the Vocational Handicap

In the younger person of working age, it is important to determine whether the existing disability will interfere with his previous occupation. If that is the case, one has to establish which possible jobs the patient can carry out despite his physical disability. This will require special arrangements for pre-vocational testing.

The detection and evaluation of the physical disabilities is mainly the responsibility of the physician. He may be assisted in grading the disabilities by the observations of nurses and therapists. The ADL evaluation is essentially the function of nurses and therapists.

Psychosocial Evaluation

The psychosocial evaluation is usually carried out by the social worker. It is frequently supplemented by observations of nurses and therapists. This evaluation should include:

1. The educational and social history of the patient.
2. His present social and economic status.
3. His present emotional state including his reaction to the disability and his expectations.
4. His opinion and feelings about his present medical, nursing, and rehabilitation care.

With all the above-mentioned data available, the team involved in the evaluation conference must formulate a *rehabilitation goal and a rehabilitation plan.*

Rehabilitation Goal and Prognosis

The formulation of the rehabilitation goal occurs in two steps. The first step is to determine the physical rehabilitation potential of the patient. This means that one must determine what improvement in his ADL status can be achieved, which requires medical knowledge and thorough knowledge of rehabilitation. It is based upon the diagnoses, the prognosis and the expected permanent disability.

The prognosis for spontaneous recovery from physical disability varies with the disease. In Guillain-Barré syndrome, the patient may be completely paralyzed at the time of evaluation, but spontaneous recovery is usually good and in 3 months minimal permanent disability may exist. In hemiplegia, very few patients recover full muscle strength. If a hemiplegic has not recovered function in 3 weeks, he will remain hemiplegic. His rehabilitation is based on his physical assets and the use of leg braces. The hemiplegic should become ambulatory and self-caring but usually does not regain the use of the hemiplegic arm. Sometimes no spontaneous recovery can be expected. A patient with complete transection of the spinal cord immediately has permanent paraplegia. His ADL prognosis depends upon the level of the lesion. A paraplegic with a spinal level at L-1 with otherwise good physical assets can walk with braces and crutches, but a paraplegic with a spinal level of D-4, even with strong arms, could not comfortably get around all day without a wheelchair.

When the disease is progressive and physical disability is likely to increase in the near future, it is wise to set the ADL goal lower than the maximal level. To have a patient achieve ambulation with great effort, only to have his disability force him back into a wheelchair within 2 months may satisfy professional vanity but does not render a service to the patient.

While *physical* rehabilitation potential can be determined more or less on a scientific basis, the *true* rehabilitation potential depends a great deal upon the patient's motivation and social circumstances. The paraplegic who has a job and family and has adjusted to his situation may function perfectly well for the rest of his life without considerable illness. On the other hand, the paraplegic who does not have the mental or vocational skills to work from the wheelchair and has no family may be unable to maintain his health and may spend most of the rest of his life in a hospital with urinary tract infection, pressure sores, and other complications.

There are, of course, cases where the diagnosis and prognosis cannot be made with certainty, nor is it always possible to assess the patient's motivation initially. In this instance, one must set an *intermediate or temporary goal* and determine the final goal in a later *re-evaluation.* In an elderly, confused, above-the-knee amputee, the first intermediate goal would be healing of the stump and wheelchair mobility. If the confusion improves, the next intermediate goal may be ambulation with a pylon. If the patient accomplishes this, the final goal of ambulation with a prosthesis may be set.

Rehabilitation Plan

Once the goal has been established and discussed with the patient and his family and has been generally accepted, a plan must be set up to carry out the goal. This will include the immediate plan in the hospital as well as a plan for discharge and follow-up when the patient returns home. It will include determining the type of wheelchair and other appliances required, devising an exercise and training program to make the patient self-sufficient, and planning for the immediate economic support of the family, and vocational training, if feasible, for the future.

Re-evaluations

In some instances it is possible to carry out the rehabilitation plan exactly as outlined in the original evaluation. More often, however, it is necessary to make minor or major adjustments. The following reasons account for re-evaluation:

1. The diagnosis and/or the prognosis for spontaneous recovery could not be made at once or were erroneous, and the patient recovers more or less function than expected.
2. The patient suffered additional illness or disability, delaying the rehabilitation program or modifying the expectation of permanent disability.
3. In the course of rehabilitation, a pre-existing disability was discovered which was not apparent in the initial evaluation.

THE REHABILITATION PROGRAM

The rehabilitation program must be designed to carry out several tasks simultaneously. Each task requires different techniques for its accomplishment. We shall first briefly describe the various tasks and the techniques involved and then describe the practical methods of setting up and carrying out the rehabilitation program.

Tasks and Techniques
Maintenance of Vital Functions
In order to achieve rehabilitation, it is of course necessary to keep the patient alive and healthy. Severely disabled patients may have respiratory impairment, inability to swallow or to feed themselves, and bladder and bowel paralysis. Respiratory impairment may require respiratory equipment or respiratory assistance, tracheostomy care and many other important measures (see Chapter 17 on respiratory disability). Nutrition may have to be maintained by intravenous fluids, nasogastric tube or gastrostomy feedings (see section on nutrition in Chapter 2). If the patient is able to swallow, he may still require specially prepared food or may need to be fed or assisted with feeding. Nearly all severely disabled patients have to be on a bladder and bowel program (see section on elimination in Chapter 2). All patients have to be maintained in a certain state of cleanliness and given the necessary medical care to restore or maintain their health.

While this task is not specific for the rehabilitation program and the same techniques are also carried out in an intensive care unit and on medical and surgical wards, it must be pointed out that it takes time and energy. Sufficient time must be left for the four other tasks which have to be carried out simultaneously.

Prevention of Secondary Disabilities
This second task is more specifically a rehabilitation function. It is designed to prevent disability. As pointed out in Chapter 3, a patient who is physically disabled by a primary disability is very vulnerable to the development of secondary disabilities, mainly due to disuse. The

techniques used in the prevention of secondary disabilities are passive and active motion and proper positioning, including frequent changes of position (see Chapter 3).

The first two tasks prevent further deterioration of the patient's condition, but have no restorative function. In some instances, a restorative rehabilitation program cannot be started for days, weeks, or even months because the patient is in coma, is confused, acutely ill or is in severe pain. Until some medical recovery has occurred, maintenance of vital functions and prevention of secondary disability are the only measures to be taken. These patients should preferably be kept in the intensive care unit or on an acute ward until they are capable of participating in restorative measures.

Improvement in Physical Fitness

The purpose of this third task is to restore maximum function to the parts of the patient which are not disabled. It is often said that rehabilitation is achieved with what the patient has left. The techniques used in this task are active exercises and development of sitting and standing balance. Changing to different positions for these exercises is important. Exercises to improve swallowing ability and breathing ability also belong to this group. Improvement in physical fitness is further enhanced by having the patient carry out those activities of daily living which he is able to do.

Training in Activities of Daily Living

This task approaches squarely the very purpose of rehabilitation and must be handled with a great deal of discretion. The ADL evaluation has shown the patient's deficiencies. An inventory of the physical assets may give some clue on how one might proceed to enable the patient to perform certain activities of daily living. It is important that the method used to restore an ADL activity be based upon the patient's present strength and ability; if strength and ability improve, another method can be used. Substitution is the most important technique of ADL training. The right-handed patient who has lost the use of his right arm should be trained to use his left hand for self-care. The aphasic patient who can write should be given the means to communicate in writing. The lower extremity amputee is trained to transfer to one leg, while the paraplegic is trained to transfer by chinning or push-ups.

A second technique for ADL training is the use of special devices and appliances: a long-handled comb, a long-handled toothbrush and a long-handled shoe horn are useful for patients with limited range of motion. Mobility for the paralyzed patient is provided by a wheelchair or through braces and crutches.

Psychological Support and Counseling

This task is accomplished in part by talking to the patient, explaining the purposes of his program and listening to his fears, complaints and worries. A great part of psychological support is provided by the patient's confidence in the staff and the rehabilitation program, and by the fact that he can see that he is progressing satisfactorily.

The Daily Schedule

It is obvious that an attempt to carry out all five tasks simultaneously can easily lead to problems with time and may exhaust the patient's strength. Yet, for successful rehabilitation it is necessary to carry out all five tasks simultaneously. Fortunately, it is possible, and even desirable, to integrate them as much as possible. For example, while the patient is being fed (Task #1), he may be placed into a sitting position (Task #2), and have a short period of training in left-handed eating (Task #4). This activity leads to the strengthening of his trunk and left upper extremity (Task #3). Or, while the patient is given a sponge bath (Task #1), the shoulder may be moved passively through the existing range of motion (Task #2), after which the patient may be asked to move his arm actively through the range of motion (Task #3). Finally, the patient may be given a face cloth and asked to wash his face (Task #4). The bath also offers a good opportunity to talk with the patient (Task #5).

However, certain rehabilitative measures must be carried out in a special place, with special apparatus, or in a group or individual teaching session and cannot be combined with other tasks. It is desirable, therefore, to establish a daily schedule for each patient. This will have as its basic skeleton the time reserved for maintenance of vital functions, such as toilet training, bath, and meals which can and should be integrated with some rehabilitative measures. The schedule should then be filled with special exercise and training sessions. For example, stand-up exercises for the hemiplegic, parallel bar exercises for the paraplegic, gait training for the amputee, etc. The patient should be given enough time for rest, a period of recreation and one of absolute freedom. As he improves and progresses, less and less time will be required for the maintenance of vital functions and the prevention of secondary disabilities, and he can then spend more time on exercise and ADL training. The daily schedule may be readjusted weekly according to the patient's needs.

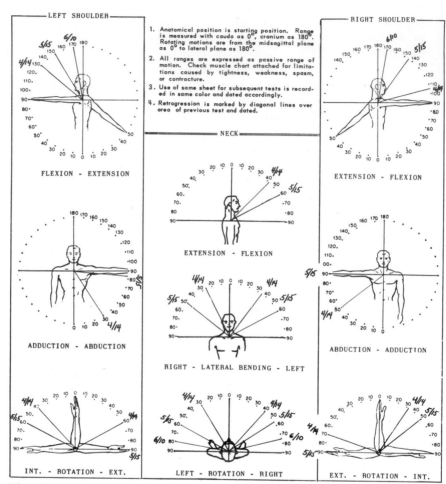

Fig. 11-1a. Neck and shoulder range of motion measurements showing recovery from a whiplash injury.

GERALD G. HIRSCHBERG, M.D.
2435 WEBSTER STREET
BERKELEY, CALIFORNIA 94705

RANGE OF MOTION TEST

Date: *4-11-75*

Patient's Name *Doe, John*   Date of Birth: *6-9-1904*

Diagnosis: *Fracture of Left Hip, Nailed*   Date of Onset: *11-3-74*

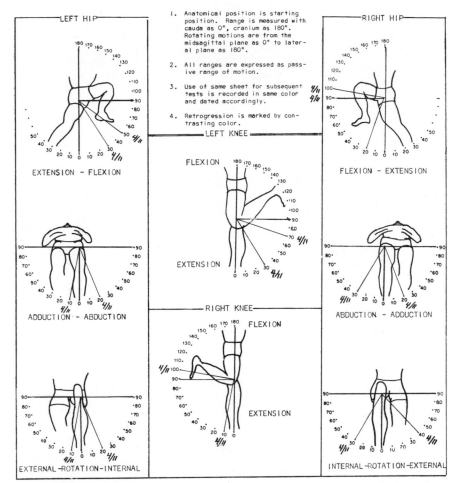

1. Anatomical position is starting position. Range is measured with cauda as 0°, cranium as 180°. Rotating motions are from the midsagittal plane as 0° to lateral plane as 180°.

2. All ranges are expressed as passive range of motion.

3. Use of same sheet for subsequent tests is recorded in same color and dated accordingly.

4. Retrogression is marked by contrasting color.

Fig. 11-1b. Hip and knee range of motion measurements of an elderly patient 5 months after the nailing of a fractured left hip show a marked limitation of range of motion in the left hip and knee, and some limitation in the right.

171

GERALD G. HIRSCHBERG, M.D.
2435 WEBSTER STREET
BERKELEY, CALIFORNIA 94705

RANGE OF MOTION TEST

PHYSICAL MEDICINE
REHABILITATION

Date: 7-16-75

Patient's Name _Doe, John_

Date of Birth: 7-13-10

Diagnosis: _Hemiplegic, Left_

Date of Onset: 6-15-75

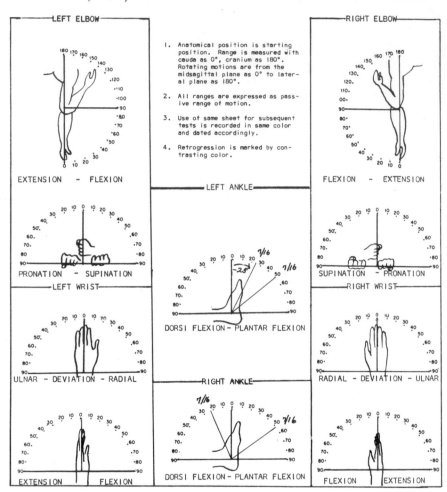

1. Anatomical position is starting position. Range is measured with cauda as 0°, cranium as 180°. Rotating motions are from the midsagittal plane as 0° to lateral plane as 180°.

2. All ranges are expressed as passive range of motion.

3. Use of same sheet for subsequent tests is recorded in same color and dated accordingly.

4. Retrogression is marked by contrasting color.

LEFT ELBOW — EXTENSION – FLEXION

RIGHT ELBOW — FLEXION – EXTENSION

PRONATION – SUPINATION

LEFT ANKLE — DORSI FLEXION – PLANTAR FLEXION

SUPINATION – PRONATION

LEFT WRIST — ULNAR – DEVIATION – RADIAL

RIGHT WRIST — RADIAL – DEVIATION – ULNAR

EXTENSION | FLEXION

RIGHT ANKLE — DORSI FLEXION – PLANTAR FLEXION

FLEXION | EXTENSION

Fig. 11-1c. Range of motion measurements which show a marked limitation of dorsiflexion on the hemiplegic side.

Record Keeping

Since the rehabilitation program must be adjusted and advanced according to the response and progress of the patient, it is imperative to record the date and the patient's status in order to evaluate progress. Frequently, the daily notes of nurses and therapists contain empty phrases, such as "patient doing well," or "patient improved," or "patient had his treatment," or "patient was up in chair." Such entries do not provide useful information. A record of the happenings of the day (nurse's notes) is useful only for a specific incident such as the occurrence of an injury or a turn for the worse. For all other information—treatment, activity, medication record and tests—a table or graphic chart in function of time is much more useful. Several subjects can be listed on the same sheet, for instance: temperature, pulse, respiration and weight may be kept on the graphic chart, a procedure usually done routinely for the charting of vital functions. Charts for the recording of physical fitness may vary according to the part of the body treated and the secondary disability involved. In cases of contractures, repetitive range of motion measurements should be charted at given intervals, as should specific strength measurements in the case of disuse weakness, and weight in cases of obesity.

While the range of motion can be reported in degrees and the strength in pounds or number of repetitions of an exercise, achievement in ADL activities cannot be well measured numerically. It is sufficient to chart on a given date that the patient has become able to feed himself or to wash himself or to dress himself or to wheel his chair. The records mentioned so far are the graphic chart with vital functions, a range of motion test chart (Fig. 11-1) a chart for repetitive strength measurement (Fig. 11-2) and an ADL achievement chart (Fig. 11-3). A fourth record which is very important is a treatment record (Fig. 11-4).

If a patient does not make the predicted progress, an error may have been made in evaluating his potential. Most commonly, however, we have found that such lack of progress is due to the fact that the patient failed to get his treatment. Providing the patient with his proper treatment regularly is one of the most serious problems in the organization of a rehabilitation program. Missed treatments do not seem to result from a single cause. A variety of circumstances, however unconnected, may still have the effect of rendering the rehabilitation program useless. Some of the reasons for missed treatment include: (1) therapist failure, (2) equipment failure and (3) patient failure.

Muscle Examination

Patient's Name **Doe, John** Chart No.

Date of Birth **3-12-50**

Name of Institution

Date of Onset **6-15-70** Attending Physician **M. D.**

Diagnosis: **Guillain - Barré Syndrome**

LEFT **1970** RIGHT

Region	10-20	10-5	7-2	Examiner's Initials / Date	7-2	10-5	10-20		Region
NECK	G	G	T	Flexors	T	G	G		NECK
	G	G	O	Extensors	O	G	G-		
TRUNK	F+	F+	T	Flexor	T	F+	F+		TRUNK
	G	G	O	Extensors — thoracic	O	G	G		
	G	G	O	Extensors — lumbar	O	G	G-		
	G	G	O	R. ext. obl. / L. int. obl. } Rotators { L. ext. obl. / R. int. obl.	O	G	G		
	G	G-	T+	Elevation of pelvis	T	G-	G		
HIP	F-	P+	O	Flexors	O	P+	F-		HIP
	F-	P+	T	Extensors	T	P+	F-		
	F+	P+	O	Abductor	O	P+	F		
	F-	P	T	Adductors	T	P	F-		
	F+	P	O	External Rotators	O	F	F+		
	F	P	O	Internal Rotators	O	P	F		
	P+	P+	O	Sartorius	O	P+	P+		
	F+	P	O	Tensor fasciae latae	O	P	F		
KNEE	P	T	O	Flexor — outer hamstring	O	T	P+		KNEE
	P	T	O	Flexors — inner hamstrings	O	T	P+		
	F-	T+	T	Extensors	T	T+	F-		
ANKLE	O	O	O	Plantar-flexors — Gastroc. & Soleus	O	O	O		ANKLE
	O	O	O	Plantar-flexor — Soleus	O	O	O		
FOOT	O	O	O	Invertor — Anterior tibial	O	O	O		FOOT
	O	O	O	Invertor — Posterior tibial	O	O	O		
	O	O	O	Evertor — Peroneus brevis	O	O	O		
	O	O	O	Evertor — Peroneus longus	O	O	O		
TOES (4 lateral)	O	O	O	Flexors — metatarsophalangeal	O	O	O		TOES (4 lateral)
	O	O	O	Extensors — metatarsophalangeal	O	O	O		
	O	O	O	Flexor — proximal interphalangeal	O	O	O		
	O	O	O	Flexor — distal interphalangeal	O	O	O		
	O	O	O	Abductors	O	O	O		
	O	O	O	Adductors	O	O	O		
HALLUX	O	O	O	Flexor — metatarsophalangeal	O	O	O		HALLUX
	O	O	O	Flexor — interphalangeal	O	O	O		
	O	O	O	Extensor — interphalangeal	O	O	O		

Additional Data:

Face

Speech

Swallowing

Diaphragm

Intercostals

KEY

100%	5	N	Normal — Complete range of motion against gravity with full resistance.
75%	4	G	Good* — Complete range of motion against gravity with some resistance.
50%	3	F	Fair* — Complete range of motion against gravity.
25%	2	P	Poor* — Complete range of motion with gravity eliminated.
10%	1	T	Trace — Evidence of slight contractility. No joint motion.
0	0	0	Zero — No evidence of contractility.
	S or SS	Spasm	Spasm or severe spasm.
	C or CC	Contracture	Contracture or severe contracture.

*Muscle Spasm or contracture may limit range of motion. A question mark should be placed after the grading of a movement that is incomplete from this cause.

Fig. 11-2a, b. Manual Muscle Test. Repetitive tests showing the gradual improvement of muscle strength in a patient with Guillain-Barré syndrome.

174

Region	10-20	10-5	7-2	Examiner's Initials / Date	7-2	10-5	10-20	Region
				Examiner's Initials				
	10-20	10-5	7-2	Date	7-2	10-5	10-20	
SCAPULA	G	G	T	Abductor — Serratus anterior	T	G	G	SCAPULA
	F+	F	O	Adductor — middle trapezius	O	F	F+	
	F+	F	O	Adductors — Rhomboids	O	F	F+	
	G	G	T	Elevators	T	G	G	
	F+	F	O	Depressor	O	F	F+	
SHOULDER	F+	F	T+	Flexors	T+	F-	F+	SHOULDER
	F+	F+	O	Extensors	O	F	F+	
	F+	F	T+	Abductors	T+	F	F+	
	P+	P+	T+	Horizontal Abductor	T+	P+	P+	
	G	G	P-	Horizontal Adductor	P-	G	G	
	F+	F-	T	External rotators	T	F	F+	
	F	F-	T	Internal rotators	T	F-	F-	
ELBOW	F+	F	O	Flexors	O	F	F+	ELBOW
	F+	F+	O	Extensors	O	F-	F	
FOREARM	F+	F-	O	Supinators	O	F-	F+	FOREARM
	G-	F+	O	Pronators	O	F+	G-	
WRIST	F	F-	O	Flexor — radial deviation	O	F-	F	WRIST
	F	F-	O	Flexor — ulnar deviation	O	F-	F	
	F	F-	T	Extensors — radial deviation	T	F-	F	
	F	F-	T	Extensor — ulnar deviation	T	F-	F	
FINGERS	F-	P	O	Flexors — metacarpophalangeal	O	P	F	FINGERS
	P+	P+	O	Extensors — metacarpophalangeal	O	P+	P+	
	P+	P+	T	Flexor — proximal interphalangeal	T	P+	P+	
	P+	P+	O	Flexor — distal interphalangeal	O	P+	P+	
	T	T	O	Abductors	O	T	T	
	T	T	O	Adductors	O	T	T	
	T	T	O	Opponens — 5th finger	O	T	T	
THUMB	F+	F	T	Opponens	T	F	F+	THUMB
	F+	F	T	Flexor — metacarpophalangeal	T	F	F+	
	P	P	O	Extensor — metacarpophalangeal	O	P	P	
	F+	P	O	Flexor — interphalangeal	O	F	F+	
	F+	F	O	Extensor — interphalangeal	O	F	F+	
	F	P	O	Abductors	O	P	F	
	F	P	O	Adductor	O	P	F	
				MEASUREMENTS				
CHEST				Inspiration				CHEST
				Expiration				
ABDOMEN				Umbilicus to Ant. Sup. Spine				ABDOMEN
LOWER EXTREMITY				Circumference — mid calf				LOWER EXTREMITY
				Circumference — mid thigh				
				Ant. Sup. spine to int. malleolus				
				Umbilicus to internal malleolus				

Cannot walk   Date_____   Walks with crutches   Date_____
Stands   Date_____   Walks with canes   Date_____
Walks with braces   Date_____   Walks unaided   Date_____
Walks with corset   Date_____   Climbs stairs   Date_____
Other Apparatus_____

Scoliosis and other deformities_____

Supplied by The National Foundation for Infantile Paralysis, 120 Broadway, N. Y. 5, N. Y., Publication PE 3.

161   Reprinted November 1950

CONTRA COSTA COUNTY MEDICAL SERVICES
THERAPY DEPARTMENT

ACTIVITIES OF DAILY LIVING EVALUATION

Diagnosis:

Examiner's Initials					
Date					
Behavior Effecting ADL Status:					
confusion/disorientation					
poor motivation					
apprehension					
apraxia					
body image distortion					
lack of strength/ROM					
pain					
poor balance					
sensory loss					
Wheelchair and Transfer Activities:					
come to sitting position					
change position in bed					
wheel wheelchair 50 yards					
bed to chair					
chair to bed					
onto toilet					
from toilet					
into bathtub/shower					
from bathtub/shower					
into car					
from car					
Hygiene—Grooming:					
comb and brush hair					
shave and put on makeup					
wash hands and face					
brush teeth					
denture care					
manipulate bedpan/urinal					
use toilet paper					

Fig. 11-3a, b. ADL Evaluation.

Examiner's Initials _____

Date _____

Mealtime Activities:

swallow					
eat with a spoon					
eat with a fork					
cut food					
drink from a glass or cup					

Hand Activities:

Dominence:
Hand Used:

buttons					
zippers					
dial telephone					
handle money					
strike match					
buckle					
snap snappers					

Bathing

Bathtub/Shower   Bed Bath/Sponge Bath

						arms					
						legs					
						body					
						back					
						perineum					

Dressing Activities

On   Off

						bra or T shirt					
						blouse/shirt					
						skirt					
						pants					
						socks					
						elastic hose					
						shoes					
						corset					
						brace					
						sling/splints					

Sensory/Communication

hearing					
vision					
spoken language					
ability to write					
ability to read					

Recommended Aids and Equipment:

Date Provided:

REHABILITATION SERVICES
Patient's Activity Record

Patient's Name: Doe, John   Date of Birth: 4/3/20

Diagnosis: Right hemiplegia with aphasia   Date of Onset: 6/15/75

Start	Activity	Disc.	1	2	3	④	⑤	⑥	⑦	8	9	10	11	⑫	⑬	14	15	16	⑰	18	19	⑳	21	22	23	24	25	26	27	28	29	30	31
6/15	Bed ROM exercise	7/14	X	X	X	X	X	X	X	X	X	X	X	X	X	X	X	X	Disc.															
6/17	Self-care training	7/2²	x	x	T				x	x	T	T	X	x	x	X	X	T	X				X	X	Disc.									
6/17	1st standup period	7/10	x	x	x	x	x	x	x	x	x	x	Disc.																					
6/19	2nd standup period	7/2²	x	x	x	x	x	x	X	P	x	x	x	x	x	X	X	x	x	x	x	x	x	x	Disc.									
7/3	Special training	7/8			T				X	X	X	P	T	x	x	x	x	x	x	x	Disc.													
7/3	3rd stand-up period	7/4		x	T				X	P	X	X	X	x	Disc.																			
7/3	Recreation 2X week	7/2²							X	X	X	X		X	X	X	X	X		X			Disc.											
7/7	4th standup period	7/2²							X	P	P	X	X	X	X	X	X	X	X				X	X	Disc.									
7/10	1st stairclimbing period	7/2²											X	X	X	X	X	X					X	X	Disc.									
7/10	2nd stairclimbing period	7/2²												X	X	X	X	X	E				X	X	Disc.									
7/18	Cane walking	7/2²																X	X				X	X	Disc.									
7/2²	Discharge																																	

MR-49   7/74

178

Therapist Failure

a. No therapist was there, due to sickness, vacations, holidays, important meetings, etc.

b. A substitute therapist was there and did not know the treatment, or did not have an adequate relationship with the patient, or decided to try a different treatment.

c. The patient's therapist was there but has not understood which treatment should be given, or has not recorded which treatment should be given or is unfamiliar with the exact administration of this treatment.

Equipment Failure

The equipment needed for the treatment was used by another patient, was lost or broken, was not ordered or was not delivered.

Patient Failure

Probably the most common cause of missed treatment.

a. The patient is not there. He is having an x-ray, is attending a meeting with the social worker, attending a picnic, or visiting with a member of the family.

b. The patient is there but unable to have the treatment because of severe illness, because he is on the bedpan at that time, because he is not dressed, etc. Finally, the patient is not willing to have the treatment because he doesn't feel well, is too tired, or complains that something hurts, etc.

As one can readily see, lack of treatment is sometimes the result of poor patient motivation, a new incidence of illness or possibly, interference by another treatment or diagnostic procedure. Most often, however, it is caused by a failure of proper organization because of the many demands made upon the patient and staff and because of the complexity of the rehabilitation process. A good treatment record

---

Fig. 11-4. Treatment Record. The prescribed activities, with the dates they are started and discontinued are listed on the left. The days of the month are listed across the top and the weekends are circled, i.e., 12, 13.

An (X) indicates that treatment was given. Self-care and speech training, administered by an occupational therapist, are not given on the weekends. Understaffing is a frequent cause of therapist failure, indicated by a (T).

Stand-up and stair-climbing exercises are administered by nurses. There are only two stand-up periods on Saturdays and none on Sundays. Patient failure (P) is common for the third and fourth stand-up periods.

Equipment failure is indicated by an (E).

may help remedy some of the problems. If the treatment is charted by an "X" as given, or by another letter as not given, the letter could indicate the reason for the missed treatment. For instance T for therapist failure, E for equipment failure, and P for patient failure (Fig. 11-4). If a patient misses too many treatments, it may be possible, by awareness of the fact and its cause, to remedy the situation to the extent that the patient will progress again.

DISCHARGE PLANNING

Discharge planning starts immediately following the evaluation. It is carried on throughout the duration of the rehabilitation program and terminates with the discharge of the patient who has achieved maximum hospital benefit and may then go home or to another facility. Discharge planning may be considered as part of the rehabilitation program and is closely interwoven with psychological support and counseling. It deserves a special section, however, since it focuses entirely on the management of the patient following his discharge, while the rehabilitation program is concerned with the management of the patient prior to his discharge.

The Time of Discharge

At the original evaluation, a determination should be made concerning the approximate length of time it will take to prepare the patient physically for that degree of independence which will enable him to live either at home or in a facility where he will continue his rehabilitation. In general, one might say that the patient is ready for discharge when he needs no assistance in the maintenance of vital functions and has become independent in activities of daily living. If it is possible to achieve these two goals within a reasonable length of time, they are best completed in a rehabilitation center. The time of discharge is then determined by the completion of the rehabilitation goal.

Some disabled patients, however, need permanent assistance in vital functions as well as in activities of daily living and do not become independent. These patients may often need only a short rehabilitation program and may be discharged to a home or a facility where equipment and assistance are available. In this case, the time of discharge is determined by the time necessary to find equipment and services suitable for the patient outside the rehabilitation center.

In a general way the patient is ready for discharge when:

Organization of Rehabilitation

1. Hospitalization in the rehabilitation center is no longer needed.
2. The patient is emotionally ready for a transfer to another place.
3. Such a facility, as well as necessary services, has become available.

For most efficient use of a rehabilitation center, it would be desirable to have all three factors completed and ready at the same time. Unfortunately, it is not always possible, particularly when there are financial problems.

The Place of Discharge

Home

True physical and social rehabilitation is achieved only when the patient can return to his own home. This choice does not depend upon the patient's physical condition but solely upon economic and social factors. If he can live with his family and has the means to pay for an attendant, there is no problem. If he cannot afford such a service but there is a devoted and able member of the family willing to take care of a disabled patient, he can usually be discharged to his home. Welfare and other benefits will cover living expenses for the needy and medical services and further outpatient rehabilitation may be available as well. A patient with no family or no family member able to care for him can go home only if he can arrange for the payment of an attendant's services, which have become quite costly.

Another factor determining the suitability of home discharge is the ability of the patient to handle his own affairs. If he is irresponsible, confused, or otherwise unreliable, he will do better under conditions of supervision. The same consideration also applies if there are children in the home who would be unduly upset by such a patient.

Boarding Home

We shall define a boarding home as an institution in which the patient is given room and board and a certain degree of supervision. To live in a boarding home a patient must be independent in activities of daily living and should not require any nursing care. A wheelchair is not acceptable in most boarding homes.

Nursing Home

We shall define a nursing home or "convalescent hospital"* as an institution in which patients of all levels of independence can be cared for. A nursing home is equipped to help with maintenance of vital functions and prevention of secondary disabilities. It may actually

---

*In California: Extended Care Facility, Skilled Nursing Care Centers, Rehabilitation Hospitals, Intermediate Care Facility, etc.

provide a certain degree of rehabilitation for patients who are not severely disabled. The nursing home is used in various ways. Patients may be discharged from an acute medical or surgical ward to a nursing home for convalescence and minor restorative measures, which is the case in fractures. Disabled patients not capable of participating in an active rehabilitation program may temporarily be "stored" in a nursing home. If a certain degree of recovery occurs, they may well become eligible for transfer to a rehabilitation center. The nursing home also becomes a depository for patients who have achieved their maximum rehabilitation but are unable to live at home because of complex nursing problems or simply lack of friends or relatives willing to take care of them.

Home Evaluation and Adaptation

Evaluation

If the patient is to be discharged to his own home, it is important to evaluate the home in terms of how well suited it is for a person with his disability. This evaluation is done frequently by a public health or community health nurse who has participated in the evaluation conference and is aware of the patient's limitations. She must then be present at the discharge conference and explain the access, layout and any possible hazards in the home. The public health nurse is frequently used because part of her function is to visit homes. It is more efficient for the home evaluation to be done by the person—nurse or therapist—who trains the patient in activities of daily living, because he would be better informed about the patient's limitations.

Special attention must be given to stairs, ramps and stairways inside the house; the width of doorways and accessibility of areas to a wheelchair; and to special adjustments needed for the use of the bed and bathroom.

Adaptation

The need for changes in the home must be discussed with the patient and his family. Some equipment can be purchased and installed easily, such as a bathroom bench and bathtub rail, a raised toilet seat or an overhead trapeze for the bed. Other changes may require the services of a carpenter, such as installing a bannister on a stairway or replacing steps with a ramp. After the adaptation of the home has been completed, it is advisable to make another visit to check that everything is satisfactory. It is very frustrating for the disabled patient to be trapped in his bed or in his bathroom because of inadequate equipment.

Attendant and Nursing Care

If a member of the family takes over the care of the disabled patient, it is important that he be well oriented to the patient's disability and capabilities. He should be instructed to assist the patient when necessary but to permit independent activity when no assistance is needed. He must be trained in the specific techniques of nursing and rehabilitation care required at home, such as changing a dressing or suctioning a tracheostomy tube. If a hired attendant or nurse takes over the patient's care, she must be similarly instructed. This orientation and training should be done at the rehabilitation center and started long before discharge.

Transportation

Some patients, even with fairly severe disabilities, are able to drive their own cars, thanks to adaptations such as hand controls. Other patients are unable to drive or do not own a car and must depend upon friends or community services for transportation. This transportation should be discussed and arranged prior to discharge.

Medical Care and Outpatient Therapy

It is very difficult to assure continuity of care for the disabled. The best continuity is assured if the patient returns to the rehabilitation center for further outpatient rehabilitation therapy and receives his medical care through the same facility. Often this is not feasible because of distance and transportation problems. If the patient is referred to his family physician for further care, this physician should receive a full report of the medical care and rehabilitation plan. He should, preferably, be invited to the discharge conference and become familiar with the appliances used by the patient. The physician should be encouraged to use the rehabilitation center as a consultant facility if he encounters any difficulty with the patient's disabilities.

The Discharge Conference

A discharge conference should be held when all discharge planning has been completed. During the conference, the patient and his family should be present. If everything has been well prepared, it is simply a matter of going down a check list and making sure that nothing has been forgotten. Each member of the team outlines the measures he has taken to assure that the patient can function properly at home and will receive continuity of care. This review gives the physician the material to be incorporated in his discharge summary.

Such a review should not only summarize the course of the patient in the hospital, but should also point out what needs to be done in terms of continuity of care and follow-up.

FOLLOW-UP

The weakest link in most rehabilitation programs is follow-up care after discharge from treatment facilities. Failure in this respect is responsible for much regression and development of preventable disability. Continued use of adaptive appliances, for example, is dependent on maintenance of these devices and encouragement in their use. Frequently, family members, in the interest of speed and apparent efficiency, tend to take over self-care activities that have been learned by patients after much effort, time and expense have been expended. Frequently, patients who have been instructed in crutch ambulation lapse into easier life in a wheelchair and fail even to use their walking ability for maintenance of strength and range of motion.

Therefore, it is essential to continue the rehabilitation process far beyond discharge from a treatment facility. Regularly scheduled outpatient visits, periodic home visits by public or community health nurses or other adequately educated personnel and occasional re-evaluation in institutions are the means to assure maintenance of the level of functional improvement achieved by rehabilitation. In the follow-up process it is well to have records that indicate level of achievement at the time of discharge and allow comparison of function with the passage of time.

In the follow-up, as in discharge planning, psychosocial services play a highly important, often a dominant role. Usually, the danger of psychological regression and the threat of social or economic disorganization are greater than the risk of physical deterioration. The handicapped person is by no means assured a satisfactory adjustment to his family, friends or general environment by reason of his having successfully accomplished a rehabilitation program. The death or illness of a family member, a period of unemployment for a parent or spouse, separation, divorce or other family disruption may precipitate a crisis that can be solved best with the assistance of qualified social workers or other members of the psychosocial team. Such disruptions may necessitate a period of institutional care to provide for the amount of time and intensity of therapy needed to resolve a difficult problem.

In addition to ongoing service and assistance during crises, there is need to keep abreast of changes in benefits under social welfare law and Social Security. The opportunities for vocational training also undergo changes; usually, they tend toward expansion of program, possibly opening new avenues toward self-sufficiency for the disabled.

Since one of the major objectives of psychosocial therapy is the growth of independence and security on the part of the patient, it is desirable to assure him of the availability of a willing ear to listen and a friendly spirit to guide him during his readjustment and survival during the short period of convalescence and the long period of life with an impairment. An adequate rehabilitation service in a community requires the availability, at all times, of psychosocial resources to meet his needs.

The frequency and the extent of re-evaluation necessary at periodic follow-up visits vary according to the disability and are greatly influenced by the personality of the patient. Often, the severely handicapped continue to improve and achieve capacities far beyond the predicted levels. These highly motivated and successful persons require less frequent follow-up and usually make few demands for special services. Usually, they are able to supervise the maintenance of their adaptive equipment, braces, wheelchairs and other devices. They make their own arrangements for repair and maintenance services. They can be relied on to keep appointments for medical follow-up visits. Other people may require more paternalistic relationships between agencies or facilities and have to be prodded to retain the level of independence that has been established. Follow-up plans must take personality differences as well as levels of disability into account. Successful rehabilitation is measured on a time scale as well as a functional scale. It is not sufficient to achieve success in a restorative and treatment program. The ultimate test of a rehabilitation endeavor is the demonstrated ability of the individual to maintain what he has achieved and to use his potential capacities effectively for the duration of his life.

EFFICIENCY AND ECONOMY OF CARE

The initial development of modern rehabilitation and its rapid evolution occurred principally in large rehabilitation centers, many of them supported by public funds and some of them sponsored by voluntary health organizations. In these centers, the concept of the rehabilitation team led to the development of many complex therapeutic programs that, in effect, were dealt with by committees. Often, these committees or teams assumed the responsibility formerly vested in a single physician. Organization and interrelationships of rehabilitation teams vary from place to place, but often leadership is difficult to pin down, and frequently coordination of effort is lost. For example, there is a prevailing idea that rehabilitation cannot be carried out successfully unless the staff includes all the experts who may be required for a wide variety of therapies.

In the course of evaluation, the same patient may be studied by one or several physicians and may be given a muscle check by a physical therapist, a self-care evaluation by an occupational therapist, speech and hearing tests by a speech therapist, psychological evaluation by a clinical psychologist, social evaluation and casework by a social worker and a careful analysis of hobbies and interests by a recreational therapist. Often, the sum total of these diagnostic efforts is presented in a time-consuming conference in which each expert vies for consideration of what he considers to be the all-important phase of care, and eventually the patient may be subjected to complicated but fractionated treatment that delays rehabilitation and becomes extremely expensive.

In the interest of efficiency, it is essential to give priority to certain phases of rehabilitation and to postpone others. For each phase, the simplest possible approach should be used. Nonessential diagnostic procedures should be postponed. While large and well-attended staff conferences may serve educational purposes even when the patient has been treated by relatively few persons, the services of the available specialists should be employed carefully and economically. Emphasis should be placed on the development of relatively standardized technical procedures that will lead to the desired goals. The use of group methods of exercise is desirable because it spares personnel and also adds the element of competition that raises morale.

One of the major obstacles to rehabilitation has been the lack of private or public funds to support the treatment of the disabled. The money available for rehabilitation has been distributed very unevenly.

REFERENCES

1. Daniels, L. and Worthingham, C.: Muscle Testing—Techniques of Manual Examination, 3rd Ed. Philadelphia: W. B. Saunders Co., 1972
2. "Joint Motion—Method of Measuring and Recording." Chicago: Amer. Acad. Orth. Surg., 1965.
3. Packard, T.: Evaluation of Industrial Disability. New York: Oxford University Press, 1960.

12

The Rehabilitation Staff

The single most important factor in successful rehabilitation of the disabled is the rehabilitation staff. At all levels of rehabilitation, the condition of the physical plant and the methods used in the rehabilitation process are of minor importance in comparison to the ability of the staff.

CATEGORIES OF REHABILITATION STAFF

In each institutional rehabilitation setting there is staff needed to direct the institution and to maintain its facilities. We shall call this the *administrative staff*. On the other hand, there are staff members whose main function is the rehabilitation of the individual disabled patient. They constitute the *clinical staff*.

The Administrative Staff

The administrative staff is frequently ignored in books and articles on rehabilitation. However, its importance in the rehabilitation program is considerable. If the direction of the facility by the administrative staff is not geared toward rehabilitation, the clinical staff can be greatly hampered in its efforts. This book is written not only for the clinical staff, but also for the administrative staff since a general knowledge of rehabilitation is necessary to administer a rehabilitation facility.

Many years ago in their initial organization of a county hospital rehabilitation service, two of the authors encountered great resistance from the hospital administration in many aspects of the rehabilitation program. For instance, the administration would not authorize expenditures for assistive devices which a patient needed when he left the hospital. This simply eliminated discharges for paraplegics, double amputees, quadriplegics, etc., and the hospital accumulated a large number of "custodial" patients. Such a restrictive regulation would seem ridiculous today; however, even now administrators can either hamper clinical rehabilitation by bureaucratic regulations or can advance rehabilitation considerably by judicious administrative measures. We shall indicate a few areas in which the administration influences the rehabilitation program.

Fiscal Policies

Today, the financing of rehabilitation is almost entirely in the hands of government. Thus the fiscal policies of government officials in this field can greatly influence the fate of the disabled. Here is an interesting example: Prior to the introduction of Medicare, the decisions of whether or not a patient was eligible to go to a nursing home at the expense of public funds was made at the county level. Contra Costa County in California used a statesman-like procedure. Every applicant for admission to a nursing home was first evaluated for his rehabilitation potential. Over 50 per cent of the disabled patients had rehabilitation potential and were restored to self-sufficiency and could return to their own home. Since the advent of Medicare a disabled patient coming from an acute hospital can go either to a rehabilitation center or to a nursing home. Since most patients do not know the difference between the two types of facilities, fewer disabled people are rehabilitated in Contra Costa County and the nursing homes are overflowing. Thus a liberal fiscal policy apparently ignorant of the importance of rehabilitation leads to unnecessary suffering and considerably higher cost of care.

In a rehabilitation facility itself, the administration has very little choice in fiscal matters since it can accept only patients whose bills will be paid. However, aggressive and alert administrators can assure rehabilitation benefits for a greater number of disabled patients than stoic bureaucratic administrators.

Purchasing

The purchasing department is responsible not only for obtaining the equipment and supplies of the rehabilitation service itself, but also for the appliances and devices needed by individual patients. It is important to develop procedures which enable the patient to obtain his equipment without delay when he needs it. It is very common that a patient has to wait days or weeks for a brace or an artificial limb and sometimes several months for a specially ordered wheelchair. By making contact with cooperative vendors and by accelerating the bureaucratic procedure, the purchasing department can assist clinical rehabilitation.

Engineering, Carpenter Shop, Electrician

Very often a disabled patient needs a device, an appliance or a setup which is not commercially available. A clever and cooperative engineer, carpenter or electrician can do much to assist the clinical staff by manufacturing special equipment for specific patients.

Personnel Management

The administration has the responsibility of providing adequate staffing of the rehabilitation facility. This is not always easy. One has to be aware of the fact that the administrative staff is subject to many outside and political pressures. Fiscal and eligibility policies are laid down by legislation or regulation. Personnel policies are partly determined by pressures of unions and civil service. Certain hospital policies are introduced under pressure from the public. It requires the skill of administrators to work around pressures and regulations and sometimes even to reform the regulations in order to permit optimal and most efficient clinical rehabilitation. It is necessary that the clinical staff constantly inform the administrative staff of its needs, and the administrative staff must assist the clinical staff in carrying out its function.

The Clinical Staff

The clinical staff provides medical care, restoration to activities of daily living and psychosocial services.

Medical Care

Medical care is conducted under the auspices of the physician in conjunction with the activities of nurses and therapists. There are also indirect services by the pharmacist and by the dietitian.

Restoration to Activities of Daily Living

Physical restoration of the disabled has been practiced to some extent for centuries, although it was not considered directly related to medicine and was not practiced in a specific unit in a hospital. In 1949, the first rehabilitation ward in the world was established at Bellevue Hospital at New York University under the direction of Doctor Howard Rusk. It was immediately realized that disabled patients needed more than traditional medical and nursing care. Since no staff specifically trained in physical restoration of disabled persons existed at that time, Doctor Rusk appointed one nurse as "rehabilitation nurse" with the special function of encouraging and training the patients in activities of daily living. In addition, he transferred several therapists from the physical therapy and the occupational therapy departments to the rehabilitation service. While the physical therapists in the physical therapy department continued to give exercise therapy, heat, cold, massage and electrotherapy, the therapists who transferred to the rehabilitation service trained the patients in activities of daily living. Similarly the occupational therapy department continued to do arts and crafts for therapeutic purposes while those transferred to rehabilitation trained the patients in activities of daily living.

Over the years nurses, physical therapists and occupational therapists have to a greater or lesser extent specialized in physical restoration. The number of nurses specializing in rehabilitation nursing is still relatively small though growing. All physical and most occupational therapists (some specialize in psychiatric O.T.) have made physical restoration part of their function.

One of the important activities of daily living is communication through speech and hearing. A special group of therapists was developed for rehabilitation of speech and hearing defects. Instructors for the blind had existed for a long time and now formally joined the ranks of rehabilitation therapists. More recently in the field of respiratory rehabilitation, a new discipline was developed with the name of inhalation therapy (or respiratory therapy). Another special need is fulfilled by orthotists and prosthetists who provide braces and artificial limbs.

Wherever a large number of patients with one type of disability are located in one place, specialization of restorative services is, of course, helpful and practical. However, in areas where general hospitals have small rehabilitation wards with very few patients with respiratory and neurologic disabilities, and only occasional speech, hearing and visual disabilities, it would not be economical or practical to employ a speech therapist or an inhalation therapist. In such areas nurses frequently take care of problems of physical restoration sometimes with the assistance of a therapist specializing in either occupational therapy or physical therapy, and appropriate consultants.

Psychosocial Services

The psychosocial services are carried out by a number of professions. The social worker is usually responsible for the immediate relief of economic and social distress. It is his function to guide the patient toward the proper agencies which will be able to help him. As far as emotional and adjustment problems of the patient are concerned, the

Organization of Rehabilitation

social worker may provide counseling. This could also be done by a psychiatrist or by a psychologist. The choice of the personnel or the discipline must depend on the conditions of the patient and the organization of the particular rehabilitation center. Frequently a recreational therapist contributes to the mental health of the patients.

Vocational counseling and rehabilitation may be directed by a vocational counselor though a social worker could conceivably manage this function. The Veterans Administration has a department of educational therapy and manual arts therapy which have a vocational function.

From the preceding discussion, it becomes clear that a relatively large number of disciplines can be involved in the rehabilitation of the disabled patient. Within the domain of physical restoration and psychosocial services, there is a considerable overlap in the functions which the various disciplines may carry out. This may at times lead to problems and difficulties in the rehabilitation of the individual patient.

FUNCTIONS OF THE CLINICAL STAFF

Direct Care and Consultant Care

We shall define *direct care* as those services provided for the patient throughout the rehabilitation program, such as continuing medical and nursing care, and continuing measures for physical restoration and psychosocial counseling. We shall define *consultant care* as those services which consist of solving a single short-range problem by making a diagnosis, giving an opinion as to future management or even performing a technical procedure. In the medical field the consultant may give his opinion as to the management of an intercurrent infection or a sudden heart condition, or a surgeon may be requested to perform a tracheostomy for a patient in respiratory distress. The continuing care of these patients, however, is carried out by the ward physician who provides direct medical care.

Consultations are not limited to the field of medicine. In our rehabilitation center (Contra Costa County Hospital) we have a consultant speech pathologist who evaluates aphasic patients and outlines programs of management which are carried out by a rehabilitation therapist not formally trained in speech rehabilitation. This rehabilitation therapist is trained in occupational therapy basically and specializes in communication and self-care. She, in turn, becomes a consultant to the nurse by evaluating a patient's self-care problems and developing a program of management. A rehabilitation therapist who is an expert in glossopharyngeal breathing may be a consultant to direct care personnel, initiate the glossopharyngeal breathing program of a patient and then turn it over to direct care personnel. On the other hand, we might decide that in a particularly difficult case, the glossopharyngeal breathing instruction or the speech retraining has to be given by the expert and, in some instances, the consultant may be asked to provide direct care for a certain period of time. The number of direct care personnel for each individual patient should be kept at a minimum to permit continuity. There is no need, however, to limit the number of consultants. The interaction between patient, direct-care personnel and consultant is beneficial to all concerned.

Number of Direct Care Disciplines Required for Rehabilitation

How many disciplines are necessary for direct care in the rehabilitation of a disabled patient? The answer to this question must vary with the disability, state of health and social and economic conditions of the patient. Under some circumstances, the rehabilitation of the disabled patient can be handled by a single discipline. In the case of training a blind person who is otherwise healthy, the specialist may be the only person required for complete rehabilitation of the patient. He is unusually well equipped by his experience to give practical advice as well as psychological support. If a patient suffered a leg fracture a physician may well take on the complete care and rehabilitation of the patient. He sets the fracture, applies a cast, instructs the patient in crutch walking, and later, removes the cast and instructs the patient in exercises.

Rehabilitation by two disciplines is also very common. This applies to the hospitalized patient where only physician and nurse are involved in the care and rehabilitation of the patient, or to the outpatient where rehabilitation is handled by a physician and a physical therapist. In most rehabilitation centers there are at least four disciplines involved in the direct rehabilitation care of the disabled: physicians, nurses, rehabilitation therapists, and social workers.

Function of Direct Care Disciplines in Rehabilitation
Physicians

Rehabilitation personnel should be organized in a team under the leadership of a physician capable of sharing authority while assuming full responsibility for patient care. Teamwork involves much flexibility and integration. Teams function well, not as committees but as complementary groups of individuals capable of carrying out specific tasks while collaborating, under leadership, in achieving a common purpose.

Nurses' Role in Rehabilitation

Nurses may play different roles in different phases of rehabilitation. During the acute phase of the medical or surgical case, the nurse is responsible for preventing secondary disabilities. She is frequently responsible for simple rehabilitative measures such as training the patient to transfer from bed to chair and she also instructs patients with minor disabilities in wheelchair use and crutch walking.

The Public Health Nurse or Community Health Nurse has an important function of helping to evaluate the disabled patients in their home and to evaluate the suitability of their environment for their particular disability. She forms a liaison between the disabled home-bound patient and the rehabilitation center.

Finally the Rehabilitation Nurse will staff the rehabilitation ward or the rehabilitation service. Often a rehabilitation service uses nursing staff only for maintenance of vital functions and for prevention of secondary disabilities. However, nurses do not have to limit themselves to those two tasks. If they have adequate training and, above all, the interest and incentive, they can carry out the complete program of activities of daily living, that is, the restoration to mobility, self-care, and communication. For example, in our center (Contra Costa County Hospital) the nurses are responsible for the restoration of the hemiplegic patients to mobility. They teach the patient how to get out of bed, strengthen him through stand-up exercises, provide him with a temporary short leg brace, help him to progress to stair climbing and follow through until the patient is ambulatory. However, they do not train the hemiplegic in self-care and communication, a function which is left to a rehabilitation therapist. This is, of course, only an example of the possible function of nurses. It could also be the other way around. Nurses could be responsible for self-care and communication and the rehabilitation therapists could train the patient in mobility. In fact, there is nothing that would prevent nurses from performing total rehabilitation of the hemiplegic if there were enough of them. The reason for our arrangement is the fact that we have only a small number of therapists, a relatively small number of nurses, and a rather large number of hemiplegics. There are hospitals which have fewer therapists than we and, if rehabilitation is to be carried out at all, it must be done by the nurses.

Rehabilitation Therapists

We have grouped under this term all those therapists who contribute to the restoration of the patient's ability in activities of daily living. This includes physical therapists and occupational therapists, along with their aides. These two disciplines have the necessary basic training to restore the patient to mobility and self-care. They have a tendency to specialize mainly for the purpose of maintaining their own identity. For instance, it is common that occupational therapists treat the patient above the belt, and physical therapists below the belt. In our opinion, this is a most inefficient arrangement. It is also contrary to the principle of having a minimum of direct-care personnel for an individual patient. A more efficient division of labor could be established, for instance, by assigning the amputees to the nurses, the paraplegics and quadriplegics to the physical therapists and the hemiplegics to the occupational therapists.

PART FOUR

Rehabilitation of Patients with Specific Disabilities

CHAPTER

13

Causes and Types of Neurologic Disabilities

FREQUENCY AND GRAVITY OF NEUROLOGIC DISABILITIES

Statistical data from a variety of studies demonstrate that neurologic disabilities are the most frequent causes of functional impairment. Reports of health surveys of the general population as well as special studies of the patients in county hospitals, nursing homes or other institutions for long-term care indicate that hemiplegia alone accounts for 25 to 30 per cent of all disabled adults. Other neurologic disabilities may account for as much as an additional 50 per cent of the elderly disabled.

An illustration of the causes of neurologic disability among county hospital patients is given in the report of the University of Michigan research and demonstration project on rehabilitation personnel training.* The study population comprised 168 patients in 3 hospitals. Over 60 per cent were seriously disabled, and an additional 16 per cent were moderately disabled. "Disease of the nervous system was the most common cause of disability. Eight out of ten patients had such disease. Cerebral arteriosclerosis was the most important underlying pathological process. This was manifested as a chronic brain syndrome in 42 per cent and as hemiplegia in 33 per cent of the disabled group."

Among children and young adults, the common causes of neurologic disability are congenital disorders of the brain and the spinal cord, muscular dystrophies and myopathies, brain injuries and the aftermaths of central nervous system infections. The latter category, once the chief cause of neurologic disability, has been reduced greatly since the decline of poliomyelitis.

*Rehabilitation Training of County Hospital Personnel, Department of Physical Medicine and Rehabilitation, University of Michigan, August, 1962.

197

UNDERSTANDING NEUROLOGIC IMPAIRMENT

In order to understand the terminology used to record the necessary observations on the patients' conditions and also to comprehend the rationale for the methods of management described later in this chapter, it is important to know the normal function and the varieties of abnormal function of the nervous system. While this may be extremely complex, nevertheless it is possible to present facts relevant to the management of hemiplegia and other common impairments in a fairly logical and simple fashion. From the standpoint of structure and function, the neuromuscular system is more closely related to a machine than any other system of our body; therefore, it can be understood more readily in mechanical terms.

While many diseases and injuries cause neurologic impairment, the impairment itself does not depend on the *nature* of the lesion but only on its *site*. For instance, if a certain area of the brain is damaged, the patient will develop paralysis of the opposite side of the body. His disability and management will be the same regardless of the cause of this damage, which might have been a hemorrhage, a blood clot, a tumor, an abscess or a bullet. To understand neurologic impairment it is necessary, therefore, to know the functions of the nervous system and to know through which structures they are carried out.

Unfortunately, there is little knowledge about the highest function of our nervous system, namely, the thinking process. While it is known that the process of thinking is a function of the brain, its nervous pathways are not defined clearly. Therefore, we understand very poorly in which way damage to the brain impairs thinking and mental processes.

A very important role of the neuromuscular apparatus is motor function. It not only controls mobility and locomotion but it is necessary also in respiration, to activate the pump that gets air in and out of the lungs; in nutrition, to activate the muscles of chewing and swallowing; and in the control of elimination, to activate the muscles of the bladder and the bowel. The heart contraction is also a motor phenomenon, albeit a very special one, influenced but not fully controlled by the nervous system. Motor function in combination with certain intellectual functions is necessary also for the socially important function of communication.

Motor function can be subdivided into two branches. One is the sensory component of motor function. It conducts peripheral impulses to the central nervous system that tell muscles when to move and in which direction to move. The other is the motor component proper that conducts impulses from the central nervous system to muscles. Special structures of the central nervous system serve to coordinate these two components. If muscle power is absent or diminished, we deal with *paralysis*. If movement is erratic and imprecise, we deal with *incoordination*. Excessive activity occurs in *involuntary motions*.

There are other functions of the nervous system that are of lesser importance to rehabilitation and will not be discussed here.

To summarize, neurologic impairment can be:

1. Impairment of thinking or intellectual function (mental retardation, organic mental syndrome, etc.)

2. Impairment of motor function

    a. Loss of motor power or paralysis (hemiplegia, paraplegia, quadriplegia, bladder paralysis, etc.)

    b. Loss of motor coordination (cerebellar ataxia, spinal ataxia)

    c. Involuntary motions (tremor, chorea, athetosis)

3. Sensory impairment (blindness, hearing loss, loss of skin sensation, loss of proprioception).

STRUCTURE AND FUNCTIONS OF THE NERVOUS SYSTEM

Gross Appearance of the Nervous System

The gross conformation of the nervous system is simple and intriguing (Fig. 13-1), consisting of a compact portion that is called the *central nervous system* and a large network of fibers originating from the central nervous system and spreading throughout the organism, the *peripheral nervous system*.

The Peripheral Nervous System

The peripheral nervous system can be subdivided into (1) cranial nerves, (2) spinal nerves, and (3) visceral nerves.

Cranial Nerves. So called because they emerge from the intracranial portion of the central nervous system. Essentially, they serve organs located in the head and the neck.

Spinal Nerves. These nerves emerge by two roots (anterior and posterior) from the spinal portion of the central nervous system and innervate the trunk and the limbs. Fibers of neighboring spinal nerves interchange and form *plexuses* from which the *peripheral nerves* emerge (Fig. 13-1). The peripheral nerves divide into sensory and motor branches and end either in terminal sense organs or skeletal muscles.

Visceral Nerves. The visceral or autonomic nervous system provides sensory and motor innervation to the viscera, the blood vessels and the glands. According to location and function evoked in organs,

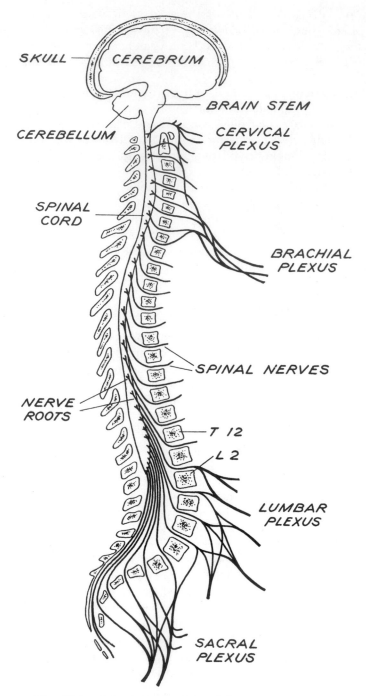

Fig. 13-1. Schematic diagram of the nervous system.

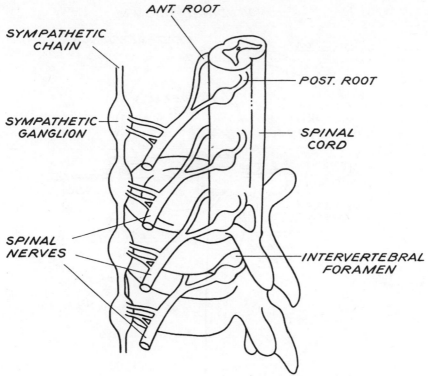

Fig. 13-2. The prevertebral sympathetic chain and its connections with the spinal nerves.

it has been subdivided into *sympathetic* and *parasympathetic* systems. The sympathetic system forms a chain to either side of the vertebrae and sends connecting branches to the spinal nerves (Fig. 13-2). At each of the 12 thoracic segments there is an enlarged portion, the sympathetic *ganglion,* which is a collection of nerve cells. The parasympathetic nerves innervate the cranial, the abdominal and the pelvic organs.

The Central Nervous System

The central nervous system is encased solidly in bone (Fig. 13-3). The portion occupying the skull is called the *brain* and the portion located inside the spinal canal formed by the vertebrae is called the *spinal cord.* The central nervous system is surrounded by membranes, the *meninges,* and is bathed in a clear fluid called *spinal fluid* which

Causes and Types of Neurologic Disabilities   **201**

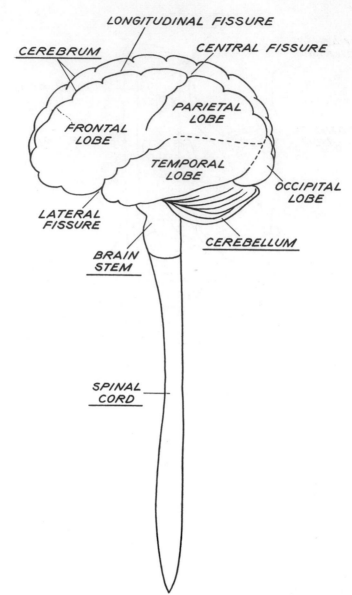

Fig. 13-3. Central nervous system.

flows freely between the meninges and the cavities *(ventricles)* inside the central nervous system.

1. Spinal Cord. The spinal cord extends from the base of the skull to the lower border of the first lumbar vertebra. It is only as thick as a finger but well protected by surrounding fluid, shock-absorbing membranes and the bone of the vertebrae. The spinal cord is the seat of the spinal reflexes. However, its most important function is to conduct impulses to and from the brain. Frequently, an injury to the spinal cord causes a complete transection and interrupts sensory and motor impulses at the level of the injury.

2. Brain. The brain consists of three portions: the *brain stem,* the *cerebellum* and the *cerebral hemispheres,* or cerebrum.

The *brain stem* is a prolongation of the spinal cord. It contains nerve centers controlling respiration and circulation and therefore is a vital part of the nervous system. It is also the area of origin of the cranial nerves.

The *cerebral hemispheres* (cerebrum) form the largest portion of the brain. Their surface is marked by deep fissures dividing them into *lobes* (frontal, parietal, temporal and occipital) and by lesser depressions which divide each lobe into *convolutions.* These are used as landmarks for identification of given areas. The *longitudinal fissure* divides the two hemispheres. The *central fissure* divides the *frontal* from the *parietal lobe.* The *lateral fissure* divides the parietal lobe from the *temporal* lobe. The cerebrum is the seat of sensation, voluntary motion and intellectual function.

The *cerebellum,* which controls coordination and body position, is located posteriorly to the brain stem and below the cerebrum. It is connected to these two structures and to the spinal cord.

A cross section through the brain and the spinal cord shows that they contain cavities that are filled with spinal fluid and that they are composed of gray matter and white matter.

The cavities of the brain (Fig. 13-4) are called *ventricles.* The gray matter forms a thin layer at the surface of the brain called the *cortex* and a number of solid masses at the base called *basal ganglia.* The white matter between the basal ganglia is called the *internal capsule.*

In the spinal cord (Fig. 13-5) the gray matter has roughly the form of an "H" on cross section. The front portions are called the *anterior horns* and the back portions, the *posterior horns.* At each segment strands of nerve tissue emerge from the anterior and posterior horns and from the *anterior* and *posterior roots* of the spinal nerves. The posterior root has a swelling, the *posterior root ganglion.* The white

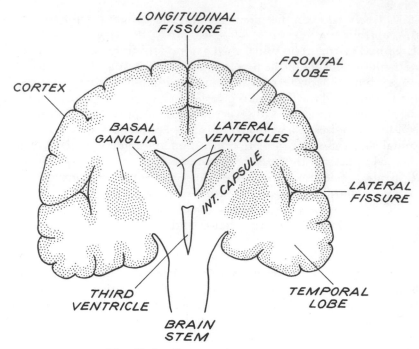

Fig. 13-4. Cross section of the brain.

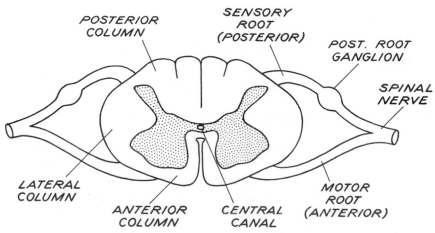

Fig. 13-5. Cross section of the spinal cord.

matter forms an *anterior*, a *lateral* and a *posterior column* on each side. The cavity in the center is the *central canal* which is filled with spinal fluid.

Structure of the Nervous System

The Neuron

When one looks at the nervous system under the microscope with maximum enlargement, one notices that the nervous tissue is composed of two elements, *cells* and *fibers*. Essentially, the gray areas of the central nervous system are composed of cells and the white areas of

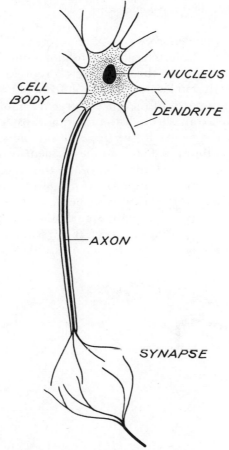

Fig. 13-6. A neuron consisting of a nerve cell and its branches.

nerve fibers. A typical nerve cell has several short branches, or *dendrites,* that connect it with neighboring nerve cells, and one very long branch, or *axon,* that connects it with distant nerve cells and, at the periphery, with sensory end organs and muscle fibers (Fig. 13-6). The axons of the anterior horn cells and the posterior root ganglion cells may be several feet long. They form the motor and the sensory fibers of the peripheral nerves.

A nerve cell and its branches form a functional unit that is called a *neuron.* The nerve fibers cannot live independently, and if separated from the cell body they undergo degeneration and disappear. Nerve impulses are transmitted along the nerve fibers and pass from one neuron to the next through a connecting link between two nerve fiber endings, which is called a *synapse.*

Motor and Sensory Pathways

Voluntary Motion. Voluntary motion originates in the cortex of the frontal lobe. The parts of the body are all represented in a given order in one convolution located directly in front of the central fissure (Fig. 13-7). From this area of the cortex, large triangular motor nerve cells extend their axons through the internal capsule into the brain stem where they cross over to the opposite side and descend in the lateral columns of the spinal cord to the segments which they innervate (Fig. 13-8). At this level, the fibers enter the anterior horn of the gray matter and synapse with motor nerve cells located in this area. The axons of these anterior horn cells emerge from the spinal cord as anterior or motor roots, traverse the spinal canal and finally leave the spinal canal through openings between two vertebrae. The openings are called *intervertebral foramina.* Motor axons, which join sensory and

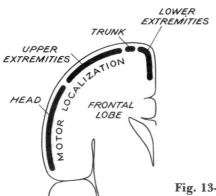

Fig. 13-7. Cortical representation of motor function.

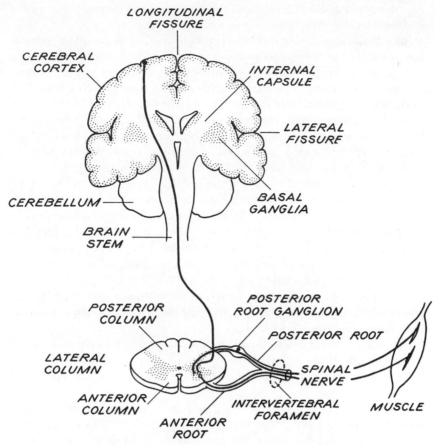

Fig. 13-8. Voluntary and reflex motor pathways.

sympathetic fibers to form a spinal nerve, extend to their peripheral destination in muscle. Before reaching muscle, each axon branches into a great many fibers, each of which leads to a single muscle fiber. The area of union between nerve fiber and muscle fiber is designated as the *motor endplate.*

If a voluntary motion is to be performed, nerve impulses arising in the motor cortex of the frontal lobe are conducted through the first neuron (the *upper motoneuron* of the *corticospinal tract,* so-called because it extends from the cerebral cortex to the spinal cord) to the level of the segment where the motion is performed. Then, they are transmitted by synapse to the anterior horn cell and conducted through a second neuron, the *lower motoneuron* (anterior root and nerve), to the motor endplate. Each impulse is then transmitted through the motor endplate to the muscle fiber, causing a contraction.

Reflex Motion.   Reflex function is involuntary. The simplest reflex is the spinal reflex. It requires a sensory neuron and a motoneuron. The cells of origin of the sensory neuron are located in the posterior root ganglion (Fig. 13-8). The axons bifurcate and one branch goes to the periphery via the mixed nerve. The other branch enters the spinal cord through the posterior root and bifurcates again. The longer branch transmits the impulses to a higher center, while a short branch connects directly with a motor cell at the same level. When a sensory end organ at the periphery in skin or muscle is stimulated, the impulse is carried along the sensory nerve fibers, which follow the mixed nerve, enter the spinal cord through the posterior root and synapse with the anterior horn cells. The nerve impulse is then transmitted by the lower motoneuron to the muscle fiber, as in the voluntary impulse, and causes a muscular contraction. The lower motoneuron serves voluntary as well as reflex motor function and therefore, has been called the *final common path.*

A knowledge of the dual function of motoneurons leads to the understanding of two types of paralysis: lower motoneuron paralysis and upper motoneuron paralysis.

In *lower motoneuron paralysis* the damage occurs in the final common path and leads to impairment of voluntary motion and reflexes. This causes wasting of muscle and flail limbs. It is called *flaccid paralysis.*

In *upper motoneuron paralysis* the damage involves the corticospinal tract, and reflexes are preserved while voluntary motion is impaired. The muscles offer resistance to stretch, and the limbs are stiff. This is called *spastic paralysis.* Despite much research the mechanism of spasticity is not well understood; except for the fact that it is due to hyperactivity of reflexes. Very often spasticity leads to greater disability than paralysis (see p. 286).

Coordination.   The mechanism of coordination is exceedingly complex, and the pathways are only partially known. Coordination is based on a feedback mechanism that informs the central nervous system at each moment of the position of the limbs or the body. This mechanism originates in sensory end organs. Most important for coordination are the sensations that register muscle tension, joint position, etc. They are called *proprioceptive* sensations because they register stimuli from the body itself. These proprioceptive impulses originate at the periphery and travel along sensory nerve fibers that ascend in the posterior columns of the spinal cord after giving off short branches for the spinal reflex, as described above. These proprioceptive impulses are led through synapses to the cerebral cortex for perception and to the cerebellum for coordination. The cerebellum has connections with all portions of the central nervous system and performs the miraculous function of coordinating muscular activity and controlling body position. In addition to the proprioceptive sensations, the cerebellum uses stimuli from special senses, such as vision and equilibrium, for effective coordination.

If a patient's gait has become incoordinated by damage to proprioceptive fibers in the posterior column (spinal ataxia) or peripheral nerve (ataxic form of neuropathy), the use of vision, i.e., looking where one steps, can improve the gait. But if incoordination is due to a lesion of the cerebellum itself or of its pathways (cerebellar ataxia), no such substitution is possible.

Sensory Perception. We have seen that proprioceptive sensory pathways play a role in reflex motion and in coordination. Another important function of the sensory pathways is to make the person aware of a stimulus. This is called perception and occurs in the cerebral cortex. In addition to proprioception (stretch on a muscle, portion of a limb) we can perceive hot and cold, pain and touch which is important for our protection. Sensations perceived through the special senses are also important for communication.

Recognition of perceived stimuli occurs through association pathways which connect cortical areas. Some types of brain damage may interfere with recognition. The patient then suffers from *agnosia* which is very disabling.

PRINCIPAL CAUSES OF NEUROLOGIC IMPAIRMENT

Some degenerative, toxic or infectious diseases affect selectively specific structures of the nervous system (Fig. 13-9). For instance, epidemic encephalitis frequently causes permanent damage to the basal ganglia only and eventually may lead to postencephalitic parkinsonism. Acute anterior poliomyelitis attacks selectively anterior horn cells, leading to lower motoneuron paralysis. Some diseases may attack two structures selectively. For instance, the deficiency disease that causes pernicious anemia may cause, simultaneously, degeneration of the corticospinal tract and the proprioceptive fibers of the posterior columns of the spinal cord (combined system disease).

Multiple sclerosis (disseminated sclerosis) attacks only one type of tissue: namely, the myelinated nerve fibers of the central nervous system. Since many functions of the central nervous system are

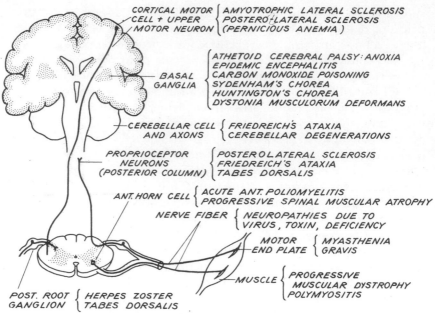

CORTICAL MOTOR { AMYOTROPHIC LATERAL SCLEROSIS
CELL + UPPER { POSTERO-LATERAL SCLEROSIS
MOTOR NEURON ((PERNICIOUS ANEMIA)

BASAL
GANGLIA
{ ATHETOID CEREBRAL PALSY: ANOXIA
EPIDEMIC ENCEPHALITIS
CARBON MONOXIDE POISONING
SYDENHAM'S CHOREA
HUNTINGTON'S CHOREA
DYSTONIA MUSCULORUM DEFORMANS

CEREBELLAR CELL { FRIEDREICH'S ATAXIA
AND AXONS { CEREBELLAR DEGENERATIONS

PROPRIOCEPTOR { POSTEROLATERAL SCLEROSIS
NEURONS { FRIEDREICH'S ATAXIA
(POSTERIOR COLUMN) { TABES DORSALIS

ANT. HORN CELL { ACUTE ANT. POLIOMYELITIS
{ PROGRESSIVE SPINAL MUSCULAR ATROPHY

NERVE FIBER { NEUROPATHIES DUE TO
{ VIRUS, TOXIN, DEFICIENCY

MOTOR { MYASTHENIA
END PLATE { GRAVIS

MUSCLE { PROGRESSIVE
{ MUSCULAR DYSTROPHY
{ POLYMYOSITIS

POST. ROOT { HERPES ZOSTER
GANGLION { TABES DORSALIS

Fig. 13-9. Diseases of specific structures of the nervous system.

mediated through myelinated fibers and since multiple sclerosis may involve any of them in more or less widely scattered small patches, the disabilities which can be caused by this disease are numerous. Attacks of multiple sclerosis may result in complete remissions or may leave some residual disability. With repeated attacks the patient becomes more and more disabled over the years and eventually may die of complications of the disability. However, many patients with multiple sclerosis live remarkably long lives and are able to function for many years.

The disabilities most commonly seen in multiple sclerosis are upper motoneuron paralysis and cerebellar ataxia. They may occur alone or in combination and may be accompanied by blindness, organic mental syndrome, or respiratory paralysis. Multiple sclerosis does not involve the peripheral nervous system. The etiology of this disease is presently unknown.

Some pathologic processes in the nervous system are not delimited by tracts or other structures—for example, transection of the spinal cord by injury or invasion of the cord or brain by tumor results in multiple neurologic impairments, since all structures at the site of the lesions are damaged or destroyed.

Causes of Upper Motoneuron Paralysis

The most common neurologic impairment is paralysis. In upper motoneuron paralysis, three types of paralytic involvement are seen: hemiplegia, paraplegia and quadriplegia (Fig. 13-10). The site of the lesion determines the type of paralysis.

A lesion of one cerebral hemisphere will cause paralysis of the opposite side of the body, that is, *hemiplegia* (Fig. 13-11). A lesion of the spinal cord may cause a hemiplegia if it involves half of the cervical cord. However, most of the time it will involve both sides of the body, since the diameter of the spinal cord is very small and spinal cord lesions are most often more or less complete transverse lesions (Fig. 13-12). If the transverse lesion of the spinal cord is in the cervical spine, the patient will have involvement of all four extremities, that is *quadriplegia*. If the transverse lesion of the spinal cord is in the thoracic and lumbar area, he will be *paraplegic,* and the upper extremities will be spared. The trunk musculature will be involved as high up as the level of the lesion. Therefore, a patient with a transverse lesion in a lumbar segment of the spinal cord will have use of

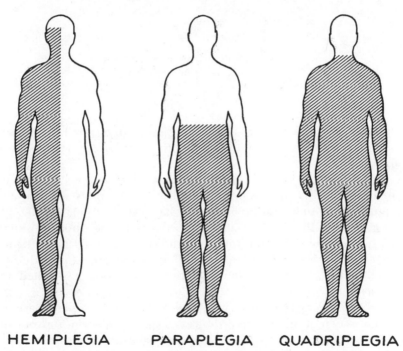

HEMIPLEGIA   PARAPLEGIA   QUADRIPLEGIA

Fig. 13-10. Types of upper motoneuron paralysis. This localization of paralysis also occurs in lower motoneuron disease.

Causes and Types of Neurologic Disabilities   **211**

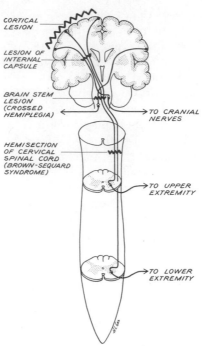

CORTICAL LESION

LESION OF INTERNAL CAPSULE

BRAIN STEM LESION (CROSSED HEMIPLEGIA)

→ TO CRANIAL NERVES

HEMISECTION OF CERVICAL SPINAL CORD (BROWN-SEQUARD SYNDROME)

→ TO UPPER EXTREMITY

→ TO LOWER EXTREMITY

Fig. 13-11. Upper motoneuron lesions causing hemiplegia.

most of his trunk muscles, while a patient with a spinal cord lesion in an upper dorsal segment will have most of his trunk muscles paralyzed.

If a lesion is located within the brain stem, it may create bilateral involvement but since the brain stem is considerably wider than the spinal cord, unilateral involvement may also occur. Since the upper motoneuron for the cranial nerves crosses to the opposite side at a higher level of the brain stem than the corticospinal tract, frequently there is involvement of the cranial nerves at the same side of the cerebral lesion and of the limbs on the opposite side, a so-called *crossed hemiplegia.*

The principal causes of upper motoneuron hemiplegia are: cerebral vascular accident, tumor abscess, injury and surgical procedures. The term *cerebral vascular accident* usually applies to vascular occlusion or rupture of a blood vessel followed by hemorrhage. Occlusion is produced by a blood clot that either forms in the artery supply-

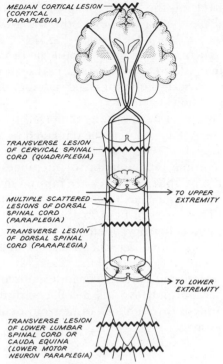

MEDIAN CORTICAL LESION
(CORTICAL
PARAPLEGIA)

TRANSVERSE LESION
OF CERVICAL SPINAL
CORD (QUADRIPLEGIA)

TO UPPER
EXTREMITY

MULTIPLE SCATTERED
LESIONS OF DORSAL
SPINAL CORD
(PARAPLEGIA)

TRANSVERSE LESION
OF DORSAL SPINAL
CORD (PARAPLEGIA)

TO LOWER
EXTREMITY

TRANSVERSE LESION
OF LOWER LUMBAR
SPINAL CORD OR
CAUDA EQUINA
(LOWER MOTOR
NEURON PARAPLEGIA)

Fig. 13-12. Central nervous system lesions causing paraplegia and quadriplegia.

ing blood to the brain (thrombosis) or is carried by the bloodstream (embolism).

The causes of paraplegia and quadriplegia can be divided into:

1. Selective degeneration of corticospinal tracts (amyotrophic lateral sclerosis, posterolateral sclerosis, Friedreich's ataxia).

2. Multiple scattered lesions (multiple sclerosis).

3. Transverse lesions of spinal cord.

    a. Congenital (spina bifida with myelomeningocele).

    b. Compression (abscess, tumor).

    c. Transection (fractured vertebrae, bullet).

4. Bilateral cortical cerebral lesions (hemorrhage, meningioma).

Causes of Lower Motoneuron and Muscle Paralysis

In lower motoneuron paralysis, a single lesion may produce involvement of one or several nerves of one limb, causing monoplegia.

A single lesion involving the lower spinal cord or the cauda equina may cause flaccid paraplegia. However, the diseases that affect the lower motoneuron and the muscle fiber (Fig. 13-9) may be more or less widespread and frequently have paraplegic or quadriplegic distribution. Since, in most infectious or systemic diseases, involvement is more or less symmetrical, the hemiplegic distribution is exceptional following such conditions.

The anterior horn cells can also be damaged by occlusion of the anterior spinal artery. The roots can be damaged by a tumor, herniation of intervertebral disk, bony spurring into intervertebral foramina (spondylosis) or chronic inflammation of meninges (arachnoiditis). The plexus and the peripheral nerves are injured mainly by trauma, although sometimes a tumor, an abscess or a surgical procedure may damage a nerve. The causes of neuropathy are multiple, and not all are known. Vitamin deficiency, metabolic disturbances (diabetes), poisons (heavy metals and other chemicals) as well as poor blood supply (ischemia) may cause neuropathy.

Muscle diseases causing paralysis include: muscular dystrophy, a hereditary disorder and polymyositis, a collagen disease. Myasthenia gravis leads to paralysis through lack of neuromuscular transmission of the nerve impulse.

Causes of Sensory Loss

Proprioceptive pathways are damaged in tabes dorsalis and in combined sclerosis. Pain and temperature sensation is lost in leprosy by nerve involvement and in syringomyelia by damage to sensory pathways in the spinal cord. Since sensory and motor pathways in the central nervous system and in the peripheral nerves are in close vicinity most lesions of this structure will affect both motor and sensory pathways and lead to a combination of motor and sensory loss.

Causes of Incoordination

Incoordination of the lower extremities is disabling. It leads to a peculiar, unsteady gait called *locomotor ataxia*. Proprioceptive nerve fibers can be involved in many disorders, e.g., in tabes that affects the posterior roots and in combined sclerosis (posterolateral sclerosis), which leads to degeneration of the nerve fibers in the posterior columns. In all these instances, we speak of spinal ataxia.

The cerebellum and its pathways can be affected by the same lesions as the brain (tumor, abscess, vascular disorder, etc.). This involvement leads to cerebellar ataxia.

Causes of Involuntary Motions

Chorea, or St. Vitus' dance (Sydenham's chorea), follows rheumatic fever. Chorea can be hereditary also (Huntington's chorea). *Athetosis,* a peculiar writhing motion of the extremities associated with grimacing, is caused frequently by brain damage due to lack of oxygen in fetal blood during childbirth. *Dystonias* are characterized by twisting movements of the trunk and the limbs. They can be hereditary (dystonia musculorum deformans) or secondary to encephalitis.

All these involuntary motions are due to involvement of basal ganglia of the brain. A very common basal ganglion lesion causes *Parkinson's disease,* which is characterized by constant tremor and rigidity of the trunk and the limbs. It may follow encephalitis or carbon monoxide poisoning or may be due to arteriosclerosis.

PROGNOSIS OF NEUROLOGIC IMPAIRMENT

Prognosis means prediction of the future of the patient. The future is always difficult to foresee and, therefore, physicians prefer to indicate it in the most general terms, such as, good, fair or poor. However, such a general statement gives very little guidance for the management of a disabled person. Since considerable effort and investment are involved on the part of the patient and persons concerned with rehabilitation, it is important to have as precise a knowledge as possible of the patient's future and potential. The following questions must be answered:

1. What is the prognosis of the pathologic process: recovery, stabilization, progression, recurrence?

2. What is the prognosis of the over-all function of the individual with a given neurologic disability? Will he deteriorate through development of secondary disabilities? Will he improve functionally with the help of appliances and substitutive functions?

3. What degree of improvement or deterioration is to be expected?

4. What is the time sequence of improvement and deterioration? The 3rd and the 4th questions apply to the neurologic as well as to over-all functional changes.

Factors Determining Prognosis
Factors Determining Neurologic Recovery or Deterioration

These factors are essentially inherent in the disease or injury causing the neurologic impairment. In some instances, the neurologic prognosis can be well predicted. There are several possible patterns of evolution.

Progressive Neurologic Disease. If the disease is known to be progressive and fatal, the final prognosis is obvious, yet the exact degree and timing of the progressive impairment are not always certain. Some disorders, such as the muscular dystrophies and muscular atrophies, are continuously progressive, though the rate of paralytic involvement varies from time to time. Other diseases, such as multiple sclerosis, cause bouts of disability that may be followed by remissions. However, successive bouts of multiple sclerosis leave the patient more and more disabled.

Acute Neurologic Impairment Followed by Recovery. Some neurologic diseases deliver the hardest blow to the nervous system at once, or within a few hours or days. Then, gradual recovery occurs. Such may be the case in poliomyelitis, Guillain-Barré syndrome, stroke or brain injury. If the neurologic recovery is complete, the patient had only transient neurologic impairment; if the neurologic recovery is incomplete, the patient is left with a residual neurologic impairment.

Factors Determining the Over-all Functional Improvement or Deterioration

With a stabilized or residual neurologic impairment, the over-all function of the patient may remain stationary, deteriorate or improve. The prognosis depends on the following factors: (1) the total number and disabilities present, (2) the development of secondary disabilities and (3) the resources of the individual.

The Total Number and Nature of Disabilities Present. If the neurologic impairment consists only of paralysis, the functional prognosis is better than if, in addition, the patient has ataxia and blindness. By careful weighing of all disabilities, the experienced person is able to foretell the functional potential.

The Development of Secondary Disabilities. The possibility of development of secondary disabilities due to disuse or misuse was pointed out in Chapter 3. It should be mentioned again that these disabilities can be prevented largely by proper management.

The Resources of the Individual. Given an equal number and nature of disabilities, individual patients still have different potentials for rehabilitation. This will depend on their physical stamina and general health and strength, as well as on their determination and motivation to achieve improvement. It is not possible to indicate a general rule for the prognosis of these factors. However, they frequently become evident early in the course of rehabilitation.

Prognosis for Overall Function in Hemiplegia, Paraplegia and Quadriplegia

Hemiplegia. The patient with a complete residual hemiplegia becomes ambulatory and self-caring unless prevented from doing so by additional disabilities. Most often, he will require a short leg brace for the hemiplegic leg and sometimes a long leg brace. Frequently, the hemiplegic patient uses a cane. He becomes able to use public transportation as well as to drive a car.

Paraplegia. The paraplegic patient becomes self-caring and independent in the wheelchair. Some paraplegic patients may also become ambulatory with long leg braces and crutches. Paraplegic patients need specially modified automobiles for transportation if travel is to be independent.

Quadriplegia. The quadriplegic patient, unless the involvement of the upper extremities is minimal, requires an attendant. Whatever activity he is capable of carrying out for himself depends on the degree of involvement of the upper extremities. Usually, the typical quadriplegic whose disability is caused by transection of the cervical spinal cord can feed himself, write, wash his face and upper body and wheel his chair. He usually needs some help with dressing and with transfers to and from the wheelchair.

Prognosis for Rehabilitation in Progressive Neurologic Disease

It is true that if one looks toward some final goal, rehabilitation in progressive disease is a losing battle. However, in rehabilitating the person with progressive disease, one must not focus on a final state of rehabilitation but strive for a status of functional ability that can be maintained for a given period of time. If a patient with multiple sclerosis has paraplegia as his present disability, he should be at the same functional level as a patient whose paraplegia is a residual disability due to spinal cord injury. If, after a new bout of multiple sclerosis, the patient develops ataxia, his functional potential will be diminished in accordance with his new additional disability. In the same way, the patient with amyotrophic lateral sclerosis and paraplegia should be considered just as any other paraplegic until marked weakness in his upper extremities occurs. At that point, he may be managed as a quadriplegic.

While it may be desirable in a stationary residual disability to push the patient to his maximal performance, it is advisable to choose a submaximal level in the patient with progressive disease, in order to leave some margin for neurologic deterioration without immediately changing the status and organization of the patient's set-up and without causing discouragement or despair.

REFERENCES

1. Brain, Lord and Walton, J. N. (ed.): Brain's Diseases of the Nervous System, 7th Ed. London: Oxford University Press, 1969.
2. Chusid, J. G. and McDonald, J. J.: Correlative Neuroanatomy and Functional Neurology, 15th Ed. Los Altos, Ca.: Lange Medical Publications, 1973.
3. Licht, S.: Stroke and Its Rehabilitation. New Haven: Elizabeth Licht, 1975.

14

Disabling Conditions Due to Neurologic Impairment

As it was pointed out in Chapter 13, neurologic disability depends on the structure that is damaged. The best known structure of the brain anatomically and physiologically is the corticospinal or pyramidal tract that originates in the motor cortex, traverses the cerebral hemispheres and the brain stem and continues into the spinal cord. Unilateral damage to this tract results in hemiplegia. The other structures concerned with motor function have been grouped under the term extrapyramidal system. This system includes, among others, the cerebellum and its pathways and the basal ganglia and their pathways. Disturbances of the cerebellar system lead to incoordination of motion, while disturbances of basal ganglia lead to involuntary movements. No specific structure has been isolated as related solely to the function of the mind. Nevertheless, diffuse, widespread or severe involvement of the brain may lead to organic mental impairment.

The subjects to be discussed in this chapter are:

A. Hemiplegia
B. Incoordination
C. Involuntary movements
D. Organic mental impairment

They are grouped into one chapter because patients with brain involvement may have one, several or all of these disabilities.

Section A. Rehabilitation of Hemiplegic Patients

Definitions. Hemiplegia is paralysis of one half of the body. Patients may have a right or a left hemiplegia, according to which side of the trunk and which limbs are involved. Cranial nerve involvement may be on the same side or on the opposite side of the trunk and the extremities (crossed hemiplegia). If no voluntary motion is possible on the hemiplegic side, the hemiplegia is complete; if some voluntary motion is present, the hemiplegia is partial (hemiparesis). Frequently, hemiplegia is associated with additional neurologic disabilities.

CAUSES (PATHOGENESIS)

Upper motoneuron hemiplegia (the most frequent "stroke") is due usually to a lesion in one cerebral hemisphere.

Major cause: cerebral vascular accident, i.e., thrombosis of a cerebral or extracranial artery, hemorrhage in the brain or cerebrospinal space, or embolism.

Other causes: brain tumor, brain abscess, head injury (contusion, hemorrhage), brain surgery, including carotid artery ligation.

An infrequent cause is a lesion of the spinal cord, e.g., unilateral pyramidal tract involvement in amyotrophic lateral sclerosis, multiple sclerosis, or hemisection of spinal cord by injury (Brown-Séquard syndrome).

Lower motoneuron hemiplegia (exceptional) may occur in poliomyelitis. All other lower motoneuron diseases tend to have symmetrical manifestations.

PROGNOSIS

For recovery from paralysis:

1. If complete recovery occurs, it is accomplished usually within 2 months. In this case, the hemiplegia is transient.

2. If complete recovery does not occur, the patient is left with a residual hemiplegia that may be complete or incomplete. In addition to paralysis, sensory defects may and frequently do add to the residual disability. If there is progression of neurologic abnormality and increasing paralysis, usually an expanding lesion or additional cerebral vascular disorder is responsible.

For functional improvement of the hemiplegic patient:

1. If hemiplegia is the only disability, the patient with complete residual hemiplegia can become ambulatory and self-caring within 4 weeks. He will have to wear a short leg or long leg brace and possibly walk with a cane, at least initially.

2. If additional disabilities are present, the prognosis covers a wide spectrum of functional levels, ranging from complete self-care to full dependence on nursing care. These levels of functional capacity and needs for medical and nursing services will be discussed.

REHABILITATION TECHNIQUES FOR THE HEMIPLEGIC PATIENT

For several reasons, hemiplegia is placed first among neurologic disabilities to be discussed. It is the most common and most widespread of all neurologic disorders affecting all age groups from infancy to the aged although it occurs most often in later life. Hemiplegia also offers the most complex problems of rehabilitation, because often brain involvement gives rise to many additional disabilities, because prognosis is difficult to assess and because often the elderly patient has few resources and little to motivate him positively toward recovery.

In order to present the approach to this problem as clearly as possible, the first part of the section will be devoted entirely to the techniques used to rehabilitate patients whose only disabilty is hemiplegia. The second part will be concerned with the effects of additional disabilities and the modifications of basic techniques which are then required.

REHABILITATION OF PATIENTS WHOSE ONLY DISABILITY IS HEMIPLEGIA

These patients, following completed strokes may have total residual hemiplegia or may retain or recover some function (partial residual hemiplegia). We shall first describe the rehabilitation techniques for:

Total Residual Hemiplegia

The rehabilitation goals are: (1) achievement of mobility and ambulation, (2) achievement of self-care, (3) psychosocial adjustment to disability and (4) prevention of secondary disability.

Achievement of Mobility and Ambulation
Principles. Delay in achieving mobility and self-care is often due to the erroneous opinion that these functions can be restored only after some motion returns to the paralyzed limbs. Therefore, it is most important to act according to the basic principle of rehabilitation, i.e., working with what the patient has left. In hemiplegia, this comprises the uninvolved half of the body. Even if there is no return of voluntary function in the paralyzed limbs, the hemiplegic patient is potentially capable of moving about in bed, of transferring from bed to chair, to wheelchair and toilet, and of ambulating independently.

Surprisingly, moving about in bed requires greater strength and effort than transfer and ambulation. Initially, to facilitate moving in bed, the patient needs side rails and overhead trapeze for support, but eventually, he will be able to move about and come to a sitting position without these supports. Transfers from bed to chair or from bed to commode can be carried out easily by bearing weight on the uninvolved leg and by using the uninvolved hand for support. However, ambulation requires use of both legs and the ability to stand and balance on each of them.

If the hemiplegic lower extremity does not recover voluntary function, nevertheless it frequently retains or recovers reflex function. When the patient is upright and puts weight on the hemiplegic lower extremity, the muscles in this extremity contract reflexly and stiffen it. The hip and the knee are stiffened in an extended position that is useful for walking. However, the ankle is usually forced into plantar flexion and inversion by the same extensor reflex. This position is undesirable because it deprives the patient of a flat and stable weight-bearing surface. Therefore, the plantar flexion and inversion must be corrected by bracing. Thus, the hemiplegic lower extremity is transformed into a stiff but stable support that can be moved in all directions from the hip by trunk motions. Here again, motion is achieved with the trunk muscles of the uninvolved side.

Since more strength is needed to move a heavy body than a light body, relative strengthening can be achieved by weight reduction. Overweight patients should reduce rapidly and maintain weight at a minimum consistent with good health. Weight should be controlled by a specified caloric intake and frequent weighing.

The course of events leading to restoration of mobility and ambulation can be divided into four phases according to the progress the patient makes in the use of his lower extremities: a non-weight-bearing phase or bed phase; a unilateral weight-bearing or stand-up phase; and bilateral weight-bearing phases (i.e., stair-climbing phase and cane-walking phase).

The first two phases of rehabilitation can be achieved by using only the uninvolved parts of the body, but the third and the fourth phases require the use of the hemiplegic lower extremity. However, strength, skill and balance of the uninvolved leg determine the efficiency of hemiplegic ambulation.

Bed Phase.   The bed phase constitutes the initial period of the care of the hemiplegic patient during the time he is bedfast for any reason. In the uncomplicated hemiplegic patient, it should last from less than 1 to 3 days. The duration of bed phase varies greatly in complicated hemiplegia. Restoration of mobility is started during the bed phase. It consists of selection and preparation of the bed, orientation of the patient and initiation of a hemiplegia bed exercise program.

Selection and Preparation of Bed.   In order to allow the patient some degree of mobility, the mattress must be firm and smooth—firm so that the patient does not sink into a hollow and get stuck, and smooth so that he can glide and slide himself upward and downward and from side to side. The bedclothes should be supported by a footboard to allow the patient to move his legs freely and prevent his feet from getting caught under the sheets. Side rails as well as one or two overhead trapezes are needed to give the patient supports he can grasp with his uninvolved hand. It is best to have a high-low bed that can be adjusted to a height convenient for nursing care as well as to the height required for stand-up exercises and transfer. If a high-low bed is not available, the patient may be treated initially in a high bed, but should be transferred to a bed of proper height when he has reached the stage of sitting on the edge of the bed.

Orientation of the Patient.   Immediately after the stroke, the patient may be entirely unable to displace himself in bed and may feel quite helpless. It is important to reassure him that some function will return on the hemiplegic side, but it should also be pointed out that in the meantime it is most important to strengthen the uninvolved side. Often, the patient will rebel at the thought that nothing is being done for the hemiplegic limbs and resent the exercises prescribed for the uninvolved side. It is best to explain to him in simple terms the site of the pathology and to indicate the possibility of some return of voluntary function within a relatively short time. However, he must be further reassured that even if there is no return whatsoever of voluntary function, he will still be able to care for himself and to walk within 4 to 6 weeks, provided he puts in the necessary effort during this time. He should be informed that any form of treatment to the involved side of his body cannot possibly have any influence on the return of function and that any measure carried out to that side is done only to prevent secondary disability. It might also be pointed out that strengthening and frequent use of his uninvolved limbs will indirectly help to hasten whatever spontaneous recovery of function may occur on the involved side.

The patient should then be familiarized with the plan of rehabilitation. He should be told that gradual strengthening of the uninvolved side will parallel progression from bed to standing to walking. The role of reflex function and the purpose of the leg brace should be explained. The schedule of exercises should be discussed with the patient, and he should be given ample opportunity to express his opinions and to be assured that his desires and opinions are receiving proper consideration. At this stage, it should also be explained to him how his mobility and ambulation program will be integrated with the other phases of rehabilitation and with his daily activities, such as eating, voiding, defecating, bathing, dressing, exercising, entertaining visitors, resting and participating in recreation.

Bed Exercise Program.   Bed exercises are used to strengthen the uninvolved side, to enable the patient to change position in bed, to prepare him for increasing self-care and finally, to achieve transfer ability.

These exercises are very strenuous for the acute hemiplegic. They are initiated immediately after the stroke. If they are delayed because bed rest is considered advisable for diagnostic or medical reasons, disuse weakens the patient. Furthermore, they are strenuous because of the difficulty of moving one's body in bed with the use of only one leg and one arm. Therefore, it is necessary to make exercise periods brief. In order to achieve some strengthening with brief exercise periods, the exercises must be repeated frequently. It is important also to progress gradually from the easiest bed exercises to the more strenuous ones as the patient's strength increases.

The exercises should be carried out at least 3 or 4 times a day, preferably more often. They should be done when the patient is well rested. The duration of each exercise period and the progression toward more strenuous acts will depend on the patient's tolerance. If the exercises are administered properly and the patient is cooperative, there should be daily increase in strength and endurance.

The bed exercises may be divided into three groups according to their difficulty, and are described in detail in the box (page 225). During all these bed exercises, the hemiplegic arm must be in a protected position. The patient should be dressed in shorts and a sweatshirt or other suitable clothing. The bedclothes should be out of the way.

The beginning exercises are the most easily accomplished and consist of the patient learning to turn to either side and to pull himself to a sitting position with his uninvolved hand. The turning exercises become more difficult in the intermediate stage when the patient turns to an angle beyond 90 degrees, learns to slide up and down in the bed and to push his paralyzed leg to the edge of the bed with his uninvolved leg. The advanced exercises help to prepare the patient for the next phase of the rehabilitation program; the stand up phase. He learns to slide sideways in bed, to come to a sitting position on the edge of the bed and, while sitting, to move up and down the edge of the bed. We must repeat that the exercises are strenuous and should be conducted in several brief periods when the patient is well rested.

BED EXERCISES
Beginning Exercises

1. Turn over to the paralyzed side by grasping the side rail (Fig. 14-1).

2. Turn over to the uninvolved side by grasping a low side rail or the mattress.

3. Pull up into half sitting or sitting position by grasping the overhead trapeze.

Intermediate Exercises

1. Turn to either side beyond an angle of 90 degrees.

2. Scoot up and down in bed by grasping the bar at the head of the bed and helping with the neck and the uninvolved leg (Fig. 14-2).

3. Push the paralyzed leg toward the edge of the bed with the uninvolved leg (Fig. 14-3).

Advanced Exercises

1. Scoot sideways in bed grasping a side rail. The moving is done with the use of leg, neck and shoulder.

2. Sit up on the edge of the bed, after lifting the paralyzed leg over the edge of the bed.

To come to a sitting position on the side of the bed the patient rolls to the side, lifts his paralyzed foot to the edge of the bed by placing his uninvolved foot under the paralyzed ankle. If the patient is to sit on the same side of the bed as his paralyzed side, he will push himself up with his uninvolved hand placed beside the paralyzed shoulder and at the same time push his legs over the edge of the bed, swinging to a sitting position. His feet must then be placed firmly on the floor for balance.

If the patient is to sit on the side of the bed opposite his paralyzed side, he turns to that side, pushes up with the uninvolved forearm, pushes up fully extending the arm, at the same time as he moves his legs over the edge of the bed, swings to a sitting position and places his feet firmly on the floor.

On either side the patient sits up by forcefully pushing up with the uninvolved arm and at the same time pushes the legs over the edge of the bed, using both legs as a counterweight to balance the weight of the upper body and raise it.

3. Move along the edge of the bed by having the uninvolved arm on an overhead trapeze or bar and the foot on the floor.

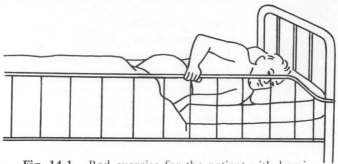

Fig. 14-1. Bed exercise for the patient with hemiplegia: turning to the paralyzed side.

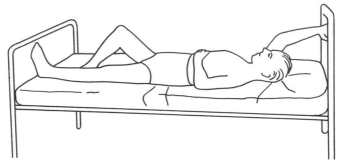

Fig. 14-2. Bed exercise for the patient with hemiplegia: sliding up and down in bed.

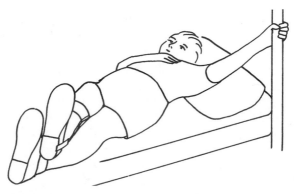

Fig. 14-3. Bed exercise for the patient with hemiplegia: moving the legs over the side of the bed. The paralyzed leg is carried by the uninvolved leg.

Concomitant Measures. During the bed phase, measures must be taken for prevention of secondary disabilities (positioning hemiplegic extremities and range of motion exercises) and certain simple self-care procedures are started (feeding, bathing the upper part of the body, use of urinal, writing, use of telephone, etc.).

Stand-up Phase. The stand-up phase starts ideally as soon as the patient has acquired the ability to move himself unassisted into a sitting position on the edge of the bed. It is characterized by the use of the uninvolved lower extremity for stand-ups and transfers and includes bracing of the involved lower extremity in preparation for the walking phase. For the hemiplegic patient this activity is considerably easier than the bed exercises. For this reason, it sometimes may be appropriate to assist him in getting into a seated position on the edge of the bed and start the stand-up exercises before the bed phase has been completed. Often, this accelerates the rehabilitation program.

Stand-up Exercises. The equipment for stand-up exercises is simple: a chair to sit on and a stable object that the patient can grasp for support. The latter may be the bed, the back of a heavy chair or a bracket attached to the wall (Fig. 14-4). In a hospital, group stand-up exercises, which usually stimulate patients toward greater effort, can be done around a parallel bar (Fig. 14-5). The chair must have armrests, and the seat height must be adjustable by means of blocks, cushions or adjustable legs. Since the main objectives of the stand-up exercises are to strengthen the trunk and the uninvolved lower extremity and to develop standing balance, the patient should stand up by using the uninvolved leg and *not* by pulling with the arm.

While standing, he should develop balance on one leg by leaning forward and to each side, doing a knee-bend and getting up on his toes and down again. He should not be assisted, for if he is, there is no way to grade the effectiveness of the exercise. Assistance should be avoided for psychological reasons as well. Each time a patient can carry out a task or exercise unaided, his morale is boosted. Each time he has to be helped, he is reminded of his disability.

It is important to begin this program with exercises requiring minimal effort, so that the patient can do the exercise by himself. For this reason, the initial chair height may be as high as one and one half times the patient's leg length. At this height, the patient merely leans against the edge of the seat and can get up with ease. As soon as 10 stand-ups can be done with ease, the seat height should be lowered 1 or 2 inches (3 to 5 cm.) until he can stand up readily from ordinary chair height. Hemiplegic patients need brief but frequent periods of exercise. There should be at least six stand-up sessions a day. A convenient way to schedule this program is to have the patient sit in a

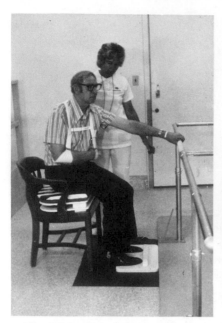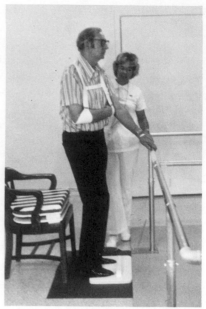

Fig. 14-4. Stand-up exercise: The patient sits in a chair, the height of the chair being adjusted by seat risers to the number of inches prescribed in the patient's program. The chair faces a railing, on which the patient places the uninvolved hand, palm down, fingers extended to preclude pulling at the rail. The patient's shoes are positioned, toes 5 inches away from the line of the rail, pointed straight forward and spaced 5 inches apart. The feet are blocked in this position if necessary.

The chair is placed so that the fronts of the patient's knees are directly above the toe caps of the shoes, with the patient sitting well forward in the chair.

Upon instruction from the attendant nurse, the patient rises to a standing position without pulling at the rail (which may be used only for balance and stability) and without lunging forward. Upon instruction, the patient sits again slowly.

This cycle is repeated 10 times, at 30-second intervals during each exercise period.

chair 3 times a day for meals and to do stand-up exercises before and after meals. Ten stand-ups at the rate of two per minute are sufficient for each session. Usually, the amount of exercise required for effective rehabilitation is more exercise than the patient was performing before the onset of disability. Frequently, he will demonstrate or complain of fatigue during the program. The person administering the exercise must judge the degree of fatigue and decide at what point to reduce the program. When the patient has mastered the stand-up technique and can arise with ease from a chair of standard height, he has the strength and the balance needed for gait training.

Frequently, one sees a patient who, unable to get up from a sitting position by himself, is hoisted to his feet by two nurses or therapists and made to ambulate with their support. This is detrimental to the patient; it prevents him from developing strength and balance and

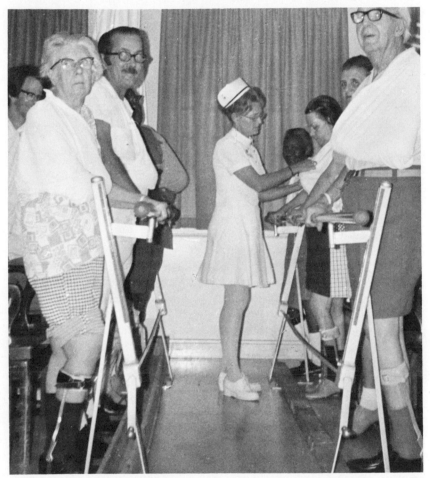

Fig. 14-5. Stand-up exercises. Group therapy for hemiplegic patients. The paralyzed arm is supported by a sling to prevent development of painful shoulder.

Disabling Conditions Due to Neurologic Impairment   229

leads to misuse complications. It is also of little value, as level walking is a poor exercise compared with stand-up exercise.*

Bracing of the Involved Leg.   After 1 or 2 weeks of stand-up exercises, the majority of patients with complete residual hemiplegia develop sufficient extensor spasticity in the involved leg to support their weight, even if the leg had been completely flaccid immediately after the stroke. These patients should be provided with a short leg brace with a 90-degree posterior stop to prevent plantar flexion and an outer T-strap to prevent inversion of the foot (Chap. 5). Those few patients who do not develop extensor spasticity within the first 2 or 3 weeks should be provided with a long leg brace prior to gait training.

One-Legged Transfer.   As soon as the patient is capable of carrying out stand-up exercises adequately from the edge of the bed, he is ready for transfer activities. The transfer is carried out by standing up, pivoting on the uninvolved leg and sitting down on a new seat. A simple transfer from bed to chair can be carried out very early. Initially, the transfer should be done with the uninvolved hand grasping a rigid support. Later on, the patient may transfer by holding an arm of the chair to which he transfers (Fig. 6-6).

Concomitant Activities During the Stand-up Phase.   The ability to transfer from bed to bedside chair and commode increases the scope of self-care activities. The patient may use the commode rather than a bedpan, and he may take his meals while seated in a chair instead of in bed. The time he sits up in a chair must be limited (not more than 1 hour), since the chair-fast patient is even more immobilized than the bed-fast patient. The ability to transfer also gives him access to a wheelchair. The hemiplegic patient can propel himself in a standard wheelchair by using the uninvolved hand on one wheel and the uninvolved foot on the floor or by using a one-arm drive wheelchair. The uncomplicated hemiplegic patient who masters stand-up exercises and transfers can become ambulatory in such a short time it does not seem worthwhile to spend time to become skilled with the wheelchair. It is better to spend available time exclusively for exercises and activities improving ambulation since there is danger of fostering dependence on the wheelchair. However, the patient with additional disability, who cannot become ambulatory or whose ambulation ability is considerably delayed, can profit greatly by learning how to handle a wheelchair. This not only increases his mobility and independence, but also contributes to the strengthening of the uninvolved side.

Step-up Phase.   During bed and stand-up activities, the patient does

*Hirschberg, G. G.: The use of stand-up and step-up exercises in rehabilitation, Clin. Orthop. *12*:30, 1958.

not have to depend on his involved leg. However, for walking it is necessary to lift the uninvolved leg off the ground and momentarily support a large part of the weight on the involved leg. In the patient who has no voluntary motion on the paralyzed side, the ankle must be supported by a short leg brace and the knee maintained either by spasticity or by bracing. Development of stability is the main problem. This is best achieved by stair-climbing or step-up exercises.

Advantages of Step-up Exercises. It is commonly assumed that stair-climbing is more difficult than level walking for the hemiplegic, as it is for patients with many other disabilities. However, this is not so. Since the hemiplegic patient steps up initially with the uninvolved leg that has been strengthened by stand-up exercises, the effort involved is no problem. Furthermore, the flexed uninvolved lower extremity placed in a higher and forward position gives him a more stable base for standing. The patient is also less afraid to climb stairs than to walk on the level because the rise of the steps gives the patient the sensation of being less far from the ground (Fig. 14-6). All theory aside, one needs but to place a hemiplegic in front of a staircase, explain to him what to do, and be surprised by the ease with which the patient climbs the stairs.

In addition to its greater ease, stair-climbing has considerably greater exercise value than walking on the level. It teaches the patient to lift his feet, to lead with the uninvolved leg, to raise his body with the uninvolved leg and to take small even steps. Coordination and control of gait are automatic. Stair-climbing exercise also continues to strengthen the uninvolved side.

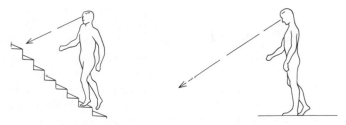

Fig. 14-6. Psychological effect of stair-climbing. The rise of the steps gives the patient the sensation of being less far from the ground and, indeed, his fall would be blocked by the stairs. When stair-climbing is done with the added safety of a hand on the banister, there is much less hazard than that involved in walking on the level.

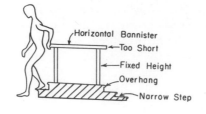

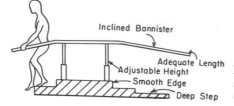

Fig. 14-7. Comparison of exercise staircases, constructed improperly (*top*) and properly (*bottom*).

Technique of Step-up Exercises. The exercise steps can be easily constructed but require certain special features. The step width should be greater than the shoe length. There should be no overhang that would catch the toe of the paralyzed foot. A handrail or banister should extend beyond the bottom step (Fig. 14-7).

There are three heights of stairs used in prescribed stair-climbing exercise. Just as stand-up exercises are graded by changing the height of the chair, stairs are graded by the height of the risers. Ordinarily, the 2-inch (5-cm.) stairs are used first. There are three steps with 2-inch (5-cm.) risers. A rail encloses the sides and the top of the stairs. The patient stands with his uninvolved side next to the rail. His uninvolved hand is placed on the rail ahead of his body, both feet flat on the floor at the foot of the stairs.

The exercise consists of two phases: (1) stepping up with the uninvolved leg, (2) placing the involved leg next to it.

The first phase is difficult, because the patient does not trust his involved leg to support him. His uninvolved leg seems glued to the floor. Initially, he may have to use his elbow and forearm on the banister to perform a step-up. If he wears a long leg brace, the step-up is usually easier than if he has to rely on spasticity for stability.

Placing the involved leg beside the good one may at first present a problem, particularly if the hemiplegic leg is flaccid. A 1- to 2-inch (3 to 5 cm.) lift under the shoe on the good side will greatly facilitate this phase.

Initially, he should go upstairs forward and downstairs backward. Later on, he will turn about and walk down forward (Fig. 14-8).

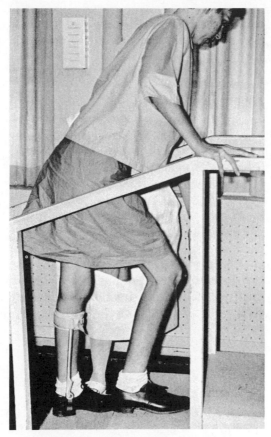

Fig. 14-8. Stair-climbing exercises.

CLIMBING STAIRS	DESCENDING STAIRS BACKWARD	DESCENDING STAIRS FORWARD
1. Place hand on rail 2. Lift uninvolved foot to first step. 3. Step up 1 step. 4. Bring hemiplegic foot up beside uninvolved foot. 5. Repeat procedure for subsequent steps, always leading with uninvolved foot.	1. Stand with both feet on the top step, hand on rail at the side. 2. Step down 1 step backward with hemiplegic foot. 3. Bring uninvolved foot down beside the hemiplegic foot. 4. Move hand downward on rail. 5. Repeat the same procedure for subsequent steps, always leading with the hemiplegic foot.	1. Place hand on rail ahead of body. 2. Lift hemiplegic foot and step down 1 step, descending slowly under control of uninvolved leg. 3. Bring the uninvolved foot beside the hemiplegic foot. 4. Repeat the same procedure for subsequent steps, always leading with the hemiplegic foot.

The procedure for climbing upstairs is:
1. Place hand on rail ahead of body, over center of first step.
2. Lift uninvolved foot to first step.
3. Step up one step.
4. Bring hemiplegic foot up beside uninvolved foot.
5. Repeat to top of stairs.

If the prescription states that the patient is to proceed backward down the stairs, the procedure is:
1. Stand with both feet on the top step, hand on rail at the side.
2. Step down one step backward with hemiplegic foot.
3. Bring uninvolved foot down beside hemiplegic foot.
4. Move hand downward on rail. Repeat.

If the prescription requires the patient to go down the stairs forward, the procedure is:
1. Turn at the top of the stairs and face downstairs, with both feet on top step.
2. Place hand on rail ahead of body.
3. Lift hemiplegic foot and step down one step.
4. Bring uninvolved foot beside hemiplegic foot. Repeat.

If voluntary motion returns, the patient can then use an alternating step-up.

As we indicated earlier in this chapter, stair climbing or step-up exercises are designed to provide the patient with the opportunity to develop the stability necessary for him to regain his ability to ambulate. When used with handrails and properly constructed exercise steps, stair climbing exercises are much less hazardous than walking on level ground and provide the additional advantage of offering a considerably greater exercise value. The patient learns to lift his feet, to lead with the uninvolved leg and to momentarily support a large portion of his weight on the involved leg. He will also automatically develop coordination and the ability to control his gait.

After 1 or 2 weeks of stair-climbing exercises, most patients will climb stairs without difficulty. Then they are ready for cane walking.

Cane-walking Phase.   After completion of the step-up phase, many patients with uncomplicated hemiplegia will be able at once to ambulate with a cane and find their own gait without specific instruction. When gait training is necessary, one should not try to impose a normal gait on the hemiplegic patient. The purpose of the cane is to replace the banister of the previous phase to give additional stability while the good leg is off the ground. The cane gaits are explained and illustrated in Figures 14-9 through 14-11. Gaits 1 and 3 are three point gaits, but the most efficient cane gait is the 2-point cane gait in

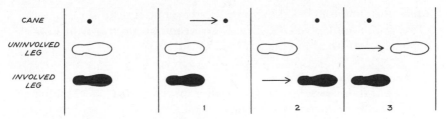

Fig. 14-9. Cane gait No. 1:
1. Advance uninvolved hand with cane, 1 shoe length ahead of toes and about 6 inches out to side from uninvolved toes. Lean on the cane.
2. Advance hemiplegic foot 1 shoe length (heel even with uninvolved toe). Shift weight to hemiplegic foot and cane held by uninvolved hand.
3. Advance uninvolved foot through to 1 shoe length ahead of hemiplegic foot. Repeat.

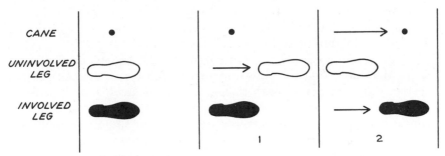

Fig. 14-10. Cane gait No. 2:
1. With weight on the hemiplegic foot and the cane, advance uninvolved foot 1 shoe length to bring heel even with the toes of the hemiplegic foot.
2. With all weight borne on the uninvolved foot, lift cane and hemiplegic foot off the ground simultaneously and advance them 1 shoe length beyond the uninvolved foot. Repeat.

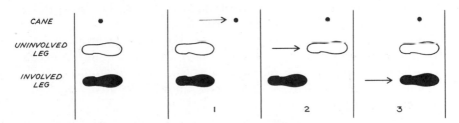

Fig. 14-11. Cane gait No. 3:
1. Advance uninvolved hand with cane forward approximately 6 inches ahead of toe and 8 inches out to side. Lean on the cane.
2. Advance uninvolved foot forward 1 shoe length, heel even with toe of hemiplegic foot.
3. Advance hemiplegic foot forward to match other foot. Repeat.

which the cane touches the ground at the same time and in the same plane as the uninvolved leg. The cane is then brought forward simultaneously with the hemiplegic leg (Fig. 14-10).

Achievement of Self-care

Restoration to self-care is a minor problem for the hemiplegic compared to restoration to mobility. Limiting discussion for the time being to the patient with complete residual hemiplegia who has no additional disabilities, self-care problems arise from the loss of function of one arm that affects all activities and from the paralysis of one leg that affects especially abilities to dress and to drive a car.

Upper extremity amputees have demonstrated that it is possible to carry out all self-care activities with only one arm. These activities include washing, dressing, feeding, driving a car, writing and many vocational pursuits. It is most important to direct the hemiplegic patient toward independence in self-care immediately without building up hopes for the recovery of the involved arm. This should be done even when the dominant side is paralyzed.

If the nondominant side is paralyzed, there is no serious problem. If the dominant side is involved, nearly all self-care activities can be carried out immediately with the nondominant arm though at first they will be slow and awkward. Of course, handwriting will require considerable practice and therefore should be initiated as promptly as possible. Usually, the patient needs much encouragement and should be given the benefit of whatever instruction is available.

Eating Activities.   Eating activities are easily carried out with one hand. Since pushing food such as peas onto a fork may become a nuisance, this difficulty can be remedied by a plateguard (Fig. 7-2). If stabilization of the plate or bowl is a problem, the use of a suction cup or a clamp is of value. Cutting meat, particularly steak, usually requires two hands; therefore, it is necessary to serve the patient meat cut into bite-size pieces or to provide food which can be cut with the edge of a fork, possibly a sharpened edge.

Toilet Activities.   The hemiplegic has no difficulty brushing his teeth, combing his hair or washing his face. Shaving can be done with one hand by using an electric razor. A woman's hairdo must either be suitable for one-handed grooming or she must have a friendly helping hand.

Shower and tub bath present problems both in terms of safety of transfer and in reaching to wash lower extremities. To wash and dry the involved leg, the hemiplegic must be seated. He should use a wooden captain's chair in the shower and a stool in the bathtub. For safe transfer to and from the bathtub, a bathtub rail (Fig. 7-5) is advisable.

In using the toilet bowl, only dressing problems are involved, since transfer is assumed to be routine.

Dressing Activities. Dressing can be facilitated by using clothes suitable for the hemiplegic. Buttons and zippers should always be in front; front fastening brassieres are available or can be made. All clothing should fit loosely and have wide sleeves and trouser legs; clothing that has to be pulled over the head should be avoided. If a man wears a long leg brace, the trouser leg on this side may have a zipper placed on the inside by which it can be opened.

When shirts, blouses or coats are put on, the hemiplegic arm should be placed first into the sleeve. Trousers, shorts and panties have to be put on in a lying or sitting position. First, the leg opening is pulled over the hemiplegic leg; then, the uninvolved leg is inserted into the other opening. If the patient is in a back-lying position, he raises his buttocks off the bed by pushing down with his good leg and at the same time pulls the garment up to his waist. If seated, he stands up to complete the dressing. A trouser belt can be buckled easily with one hand. For putting on socks or stockings, the patient lifts the hemiplegic leg with his hand, and crosses it over the good leg so that the foot can be reached. Getting the shoes on can be facilitated by a long-handled shoehorn, and the difficulty of tying the laces with one hand can be avoided by using elastic shoelaces.

Care of the Hemiplegic Upper Extremity. One of the self-care responsibilities for the hemiplegic is taking care of the involved arm. This includes the maintenance of useful range of motion (to permit dressing and bathing) and protection against injury.

To maintain range of motion, three exercises are carried out each morning in back-lying position and repeated 3 times. In addition, when the patient's condition permits, pulley exercises are carried out, as indicated below.

Exercise for Shoulder and Elbow Range of Motion (Fig. 14-12). The patient should be instructed to do the following:

1. Hold the wrist of the weak arm.

2. Pull the weak arm up as far as possible until the elbow is straight.

3. Carry the arm back alongside the head until it reaches the surface of the bed.

4. Lift the hand up and carry it forward to the starting position.

Exercise for Pronation and Supination (Fig. 14-13). Instruct the patient to:

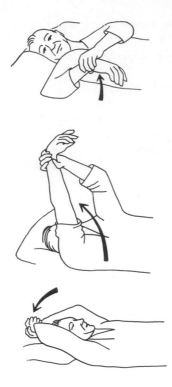

Fig. 14-12. Exercise to maintain range of motion of the shoulder and the elbow in hemiplegia.

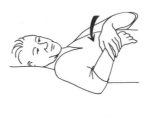

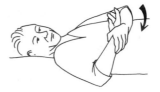

Fig. 14-13. Exercise to maintain range of motion of pronation and supination in hemiplegia.

1. Grasp the palm of the hemiplegic hand with the uninvolved hand.

2. Rotate the hand from the palm down to the palm up position.

3. Repeat.

Exercise for Wrist and Finger Range of Motion (Fig. 14-14).   Instruct the patient to:

1. With the good hand, bend the fingers of the weak hand into the palm.

2. Place hands palm to palm and straighten the weak fingers with the good fingers; then pull the hand back keeping the fingers straight.

Upper Extremity Exercise with Overhead Pulley.   The equipment is set up as shown in Fig. 14-15, and the patient is instructed to do the following:

1. Sit in the chair facing away from the pulley.

2. Pull the cuff down in front of you.

3. Pick up the paralyzed hand and slip the hand through the cuff so that the cuff is around the wrist.

4. Reach up and grasp the trapeze bar with the uninvolved hand.

5. Slowly pull down on the trapeze bar until the paralyzed arm is raised as high as you can raise it above your head.

6. Let the paralyzed arm down slowly as the other arm is raised. Continue alternately to pull the paralyzed arm up and slowly let it down. Repeat 10 times, twice daily.

To prevent injury to the shoulder, the arm should be kept in a sling until it becomes spastic. Many varieties of arm slings have been designed for the hemiplegic. The sling must prevent gravitational pull of the weak arm on the shoulder joint. It must support the hand and wrist in a slightly elevated position to prevent swelling and deformity. Finally, the patient himself must be able to apply the sling properly. The simplest sling is one made from a triangular piece of cloth (Fig. 14-16). The patient simply slips it over his shoulder and places the hemiplegic arm into it.

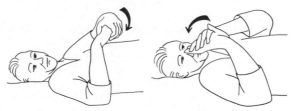

Fig. 14-14. Exercise to maintain range of motion of the wrist and the fingers in hemiplegia.

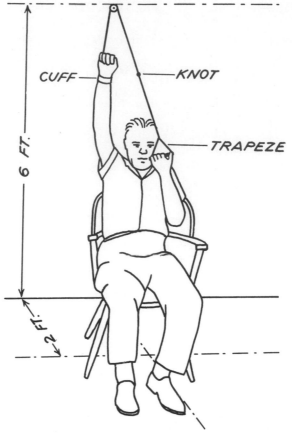

CUFF — KNOT

— TRAPEZE

6 FT.

2 FT.

Fig. 14-15. Pulley for range-of-motion exercise for hemiplegic upper extremity. This is an active exercise to be carried out by the patient to whom the following instructions are conveyed:

Equipment: Clothes line, approximately 7 feet; pulley, with ring or hook or other overhead attachment; trapeze bar which can be improvised from short dowel or pipe; wrist cuff made of flannel, leather or other material; chair.

Tie 1 end of the line to the trapeze bar. Measure up the line 17 inches and make a simple knot. Put the free end of the line through the pulley. Tie the end of the line to the cuff so that the total length from trapeze bar to lower end of cuff is 6 feet. Hang the pulley on the hook. Face the chair directly away from the hook, with the center of the chair (where patient will sit) 2 feet from the wall. This set-up is the same for either arm.

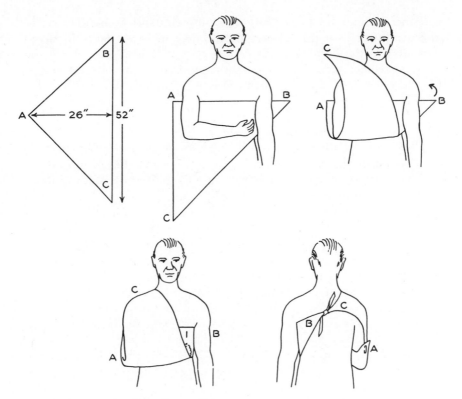

Fig. 14-16. Application of arm sling:
  1. Use triangular cloth with base of 52 inches.
  2. Place over chest so that side AB crosses both axillae and side AC is on the hemiplegic side of the body.
  3. Place the hemiplegic arm on the sling across the chest with the elbow bent at a right angle.
  4. Fold the corner C of the sling over the hemiplegic shoulder and tie it in back to corner B which is brought around the uninvolved axilla.
  5. Bring the right angular corner A forward around the hemiplegic arm and attach it to the front portion of the sling with a safety pin.

Miscellaneous Activities. *Writing.* As was pointed out, writing with the nondominant hand requires a great deal of practice. It is best to start with large printed letters, progressing to smaller print and then to script.
Handling Money. The patient places wallet or coin purse on a table, then removes money with one hand.
Driving a Car. If the patient has a right hemiplegia and no voluntary leg function, the brake and the gas pedal should be transferred to the

left and activated by the left foot. An automatic shift is mandatory for the hemiplegic; steering always should be done with the uninvolved arm even if the hemiplegic arm has some function. A knob on the steering wheel facilitates sharp and sudden turns. A hemiplegic should not be prevented from driving a car unless he has other disabilities.

Psychosocial Adjustment to Disability

The patient with complete residual hemiplegia, even if he recovers function sufficient for everyday activities, is nevertheless not always satisfied. While some patients adjust rapidly to their disability and are grateful that despite severe paralysis they are able to get around and take care of themselves, there are others who remain unhappy and are unwilling to accept anything less than complete neurologic recovery. These patients will not accept the short leg brace. They would rather walk with a more labored, more awkward and more insecure gait and take the risk of falling and becoming injured. They will go to considerable expense and effort in the attempt to restore function to the hemiplegic upper extremity. They will be supported in this endeavor by well-meaning relatives, physicians and physical therapists.

The physical management of the patient has a great deal to do with his final psychosocial adjustment. The patient who becomes ambulatory and self-caring rapidly, despite persistent paralysis, is more likely to accept the residual disability than a patient who has been poorly rehabilitated and requires assistance in walking and in daily activities. Well-intended consolation to help the patient over the initial shock by telling him that it takes "a long time" before neurologic recovery occurs may give temporary encouragement. On the other hand, it may foster his later search for a nonexisting remedy. While the psychological approach must vary with the individual, frankness will give the best results with the majority of patients. Frankness means telling the patient that, initially, neurologic recovery cannot be predicted. However, if no appreciable motion has returned after 2 months, one should not expect recovery of useful function.[1] Usually, it is the upper extremity that especially concerns the patient, since the lower extremity may be utilized even without neurologic recovery.

When physical management is adequate and all the benefits of prompt, well-ordered rehabilitation have been achieved, the outcome depends largely on psychological rather than physical factors. These psychological factors are determined by the mental abilities of the patient and his emotional status. Both intellect and affect, i.e., mental ability and emotion, are frequently affected in cerebral vascular disease. Therefore, the determining characteristics of the individual are his basic psychological qualities as influenced by the physical damage due to disease and the impact of that damage on his personality. Considering the nature of cerebral infarction or hemorrhage and the common residua of strokes, it is remarkable how many persons can succeed in making an adequate or even excellent adjustment if given the benefit of rehabilitative treatment.

The types of brain damage chiefly responsible for failure of rehabilitation are those that cause disturbances of orientation, memory and integrated thinking. These symptoms of organic deterioration cannot be dealt with easily, and they often defy the most skillful management. However, it is important to be sure that apparent evidence of organic mental syndrome is in fact due to pathology of the nervous system. All too often the syndrome is mimicked by functional changes that result from isolation, unsatisfactory management or frank neglect.

At times, it is difficult to distinguish between organic mental changes affecting intellect and those affecting communication (Chap. 8). In dealing with the patient, it is most important to assume that he understands, and to talk or gesture consistently and intelligently. Nothing is lost if the patient cannot comprehend. If he can comprehend and he is dealt with in a demeaning way, by making references to him in the third person (e.g., "He doesn't do anything for me."), or by voicing complaints about untidiness or incontinence, only unfavorable consequences can result. Depression following the catastrophe of paralysis and aphasia hardly requires supplementation by careless speech or action by medical personnel.

Often, the patient with hemiplegia as the sole disabilty makes good social adjustment. This can be assured if he has a family that either spontaneously or with guidance offers him needed psychological support. The isolated person, without family or friends, faces a most difficult problem. In such event, especially for the elderly patient, discharge to a nursing or boarding facility may be the only or best solution. The elements of discharge planning have been discussed in Chapter 11.

Vocational rehabilitation, in respect to gainful employment, is a consideration among those patients who are still of working age. Many patients with hemiplegia return to their accustomed work, even despite permanent paralysis. Others can succeed in vocational retraining. The services of official agencies should be sought whenever an apparently mentally competent hemiplegic, otherwise eligible for employment, cannot return to his job or find satisfactory work.

Common Secondary Disabilities of the Hemiplegic.   These can be divided into those occurring in the uninvolved portion of his body and those occurring in the paralyzed lower extremity, the paralyzed upper extremity and the face.

The Uninvolved Portion.   Unfortunately, the uninvolved parts of the stroke patient are most frequently overlooked. Doctors, nurses and therapists pounce on the hemiplegic extremities and massage them, stretch them, try to exercise them. Meanwhile, the uninvolved side of the body progresses in its very disabling secondary disability, namely, disuse atrophy of the muscle. Frequently, after several weeks of bed rest, with treatment of the hemiplegic side in vain expectation of return of function, the stroke patient has become so weakened on the uninvolved side that he is not only hemiplegic but quadriplegic. The later the fight against disuse is started, the more difficult it is to win. As was pointed out previously, the hemiplegic patient has great difficulty in moving himself in bed and thus lies still and does not use his uninvolved side unless urged and enabled to do so. The increasing weakness of the uninvolved side not only has the bad physiologic effect of weakening but also has tremendous psychological effect by impressing on the patient the hopelessness of the situation. He is conscious of getting weaker rather than stronger.

Frequently, the secondary disability of disuse atrophy precedes the defect due to stroke in elderly persons. Their inactivity is induced culturally or is due to other disabilities. Therefore, it is most urgent to institute a program of strengthening the uninvolved side by an adequate bed exercise program. It should be pointed out again that *the functional prognosis of the hemiplegic patient depends on the function in the uninvolved side and not on the function in the hemiplegic side.*

The Hemiplegic Lower Extremity.   The common secondary disabilities of this limb are: pressure sores, contractures and back knee (genu recurvatum).

Usually, *pressure sores* develop either on the heel or, if the hemiplegic extremity is externally rotated, on the outer malleolus. Very poorly managed hemiplegic patients may also have pressure sores in the sacral area from lying on their backs.

The most common *contractures* in the lower extremity result from external rotation of the hip and flexion of the knee and the hip. These occur if the patient is allowed to lie with the paralyzed leg and thigh unsupported and with the knee flexed. If some noxious stimulus of the lower extremity (such as a bedsore) causes flexor spasticity, the tendency toward contracture is increased. Once well established, these contractures are practically impossible to reverse. The patient with hip and knee flexion contractures cannot become ambulatory at all and at best will be condemned to a wheelchair for life. The patient with fixed external rotation contracture of the hip will walk with a considerable limp and an outward rotated leg, leading to instability of gait.

At times weakness of the internal rotators permits external rotation at the hip during walking. This deformity can be remedied by a rotation spring (Fig. 14-17) attached to a pelvic band above and to the short leg brace below. This spring forces the leg and thigh into internal rotation when the knee is extended. A knee joint in the spring permits the patient to flex his knee.

If the patient was not provided early with a short leg brace with a 90-degree posterior stop, he may develop a plantar flexion contracture (heel cord shortening) at the ankle. This handicaps walking and may lead, in addition, to back knee deformity. If this contracture is pronounced, surgically lengthening the heel cord is the simplest remedial measure.

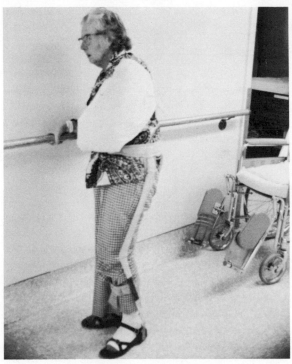

Fig. 14-17. Rotation spring.

Disabling Conditions Due to Neurologic Impairment 245

Back knee deformity has already been labeled a misuse phenomenon (Fig. 14-18). Usually, it does not occur in patients who have no return of voluntary function. It results from good quadriceps strength associated with hamstring weakness. During the initial stage, patients with this type of motor recovery do not rely on the quadriceps for weight-bearing but use it to force the knee back into a locked position. Because of the combination of weak posterior muscles (hamstrings) and also some sensory impairment, they stretch the posterior ligaments and force the knee into hyperextension. Since they have no control over the range between full extension and hyperextension, the knee tends to snap backward suddenly with each step, further increasing the instability. Finally, these patients who initially walked well start to walk very poorly and begin to fall. The back knee disability is very difficult to correct in the advanced stage. It can usually be

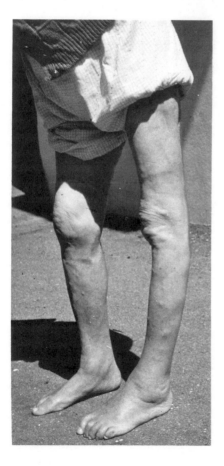

Fig. 14-18. Back knee deformity.

detected during the stair-climbing phase. The patient should be advised to keep the knee slightly flexed. This habit can be reinforced by fixing the posterior stop of the short leg brace at 10 or 15 degrees of dorsiflexion. If possible the patient should climb stairs by leading with the hemiplegic leg.

In the advanced stage the back knee deformity may require the use of a long leg brace and, if associated with heel cord shortening, lengthening of the achilles tendon.

The Hemiplegic Upper Extremity. There are also two secondary phenomena that disable the upper extremity. These are contractures and painful shoulder.

Contractures of fingers, wrist and elbow occur commonly when no voluntary function returns but the arm becomes very spastic. These contractures are not an obstacle to voluntary function since there is none, but they are cosmetically undesirable, and they also interfere with dressing and other self-care activities and therefore should be avoided.

The *painful shoulder* can probably be attributed essentially to misuse. Painful shoulder occurs not only in patients who do not recover voluntary function but may occur also in stroke patients with all grades of recovery of voluntary function in the upper extremity. It is probably due to a combination of factors, the most important of which is some type of trauma to the paralyzed shoulder or the neck. This may ocur while the patient is turned in bed or while he is transported to and about the hospital or lifted onto the commode. Frequently, the paralyzed arm dangles unsupported or, if initially supported, is dropped suddenly, causing a ligamentous injury to the shoulder joint. As sensation returns, the shoulder becomes painful, and the end-result may be a frozen shoulder.

Some elderly patients have suffered from shoulder pain before, and injury produces a recurrence of pain. All elderly persons have a certain degree of cervical osteoarthritis, and development of a painful shoulder may be due in part to a cervicobrachial syndrome. To prevent development of a painful shoulder, the shoulder must be protected.

The Face. The facial palsy of the hemiplegic, though not of great functional importance, may lead to disfiguring contractures of facial muscles. This may also interfere with eating.

Prevention of Secondary Disabilities. The prevention of secondary disability by passive range of motion exercises, positioning and other exercises has been discussed in Chapter 3. Here, only the specific problems or the specific measures for the hemiplegic patient will be pointed out. The measures for the prevention of disuse atrophy in the uninvolved side were also discussed in the chapter on mobility and ambulation. It will be necessary to mention some details on positioning of the hemiplegic patient, protection of the hemiplegic shoulder, on prevention of back knee deformity and facial disfigurement.

Special Positioning Problems of the Hemiplegic.   The danger of bedsores as well as hip or knee contractures is minimal in the uncomplicated hemiplegic because of his early stand-up activity. However, it is wise to use the positioning procedures routinely in all hemiplegics. Maintenance of the hemiplegic leg in normal position, that is, avoidance of external rotation, is achieved by sandbag or a sandbag gutter.

Protection of the Hemiplegic Arm and Shoulder.   Protection of the hemiplegic arm in bed is a difficult problem. The best answer to date is the most careful support of the arm during all movements and displacements of the patient and use of a triangular sling in bed.

Support of the hemiplegic arm while sitting or exercising in an upright position is necessary to prevent subluxation of the shoulder joint and a traumatizing pull on the whole neck-shoulder region by a flail arm. Several types of slings have been devised, none entirely satisfactory. The sling may be discarded only after the development of considerable spasticity or of some voluntary shoulder shrugging ability.

Prevention of Back Knee Deformity.   During the bed phase, a small pad or roll under the knee is always indicated for a paralyzed leg when the patient is in a back-lying position. This will prevent an early stretch on the posterior structures of the knee. In the hemiplegic the back knee problem is not only a matter of weakness but of sensory loss. It will show up only when weight is borne on the hemiplegic leg, that is, at the step-up and cane-walking phases. If the hemiplegic leg is completely flail, a long leg brace is needed anyway, and a special posterior popliteal band can prevent back kneeing within the brace. If the patient has spasticity or voluntary power of the quadriceps, a special back knee brace may be used that has a free knee joint for flexion and a posterior stop to prevent hyperextension. A reversed thigh band exerts pressure anteriorly, while a high calf band is the posterior pressure part. This back knee brace can be attached to a short leg brace as an extension.

Prevention of Facial Disfigurement.   The patient with marked facial palsy should be provided with cellophane tape, adhesive tape or other facial splints to prevent contracture of facial muscles. Massage, stretching and electrical stimulation may also help to prevent facial deformity.

Bladder and Bowel Program. *Bladder rehabilitation routine* to promote spontaneous voiding:

1. Remove indwelling catheter, if used.
2. Catheterize twice daily for residual urine until residual is less than 100 ml.
3. Schedule voiding every 2 hours initially and increase to every 4 hours.

Bowel rehabilitation routine to establish regular bowel evacuation:

1. Administer adequate fluids.
2. Give high residue diet. Give prune juice before breakfast where ordered.
3. Schedule a regular time for defecation.
4. Place a glycerin suppository at least 2½ inches (6 cm.) into rectum, against rectal mucosa, ½ hour before defecation time.
5. Place patient in sitting position on toilet or commode.

Partial Residual Hemiplegia (Hemiparesis)

For the hemiplegic patient with complete residual paralysis, it is obvious that the rehabilitation effort should be directed mainly toward the uninvolved side. Does this apply also to patients who initially have only partial paralysis or to those who recover some function? If the patient has very little paralysis, he may not need any rehabilitation. However, if he is in need of rehabilitation, it should be applied essentially to the uninvolved side. It is a misconception to assume that an extremity weakened by central upper motoneuron paralysis can be strengthened by exercise. Usually, this weakness is caused not by diminished muscle strength but rather by paucity of voluntary motor impulses from the brain and by spasticity.

Recovery of useful function in the affected arm does not occur frequently, and return of voluntary motion does not necessarily mean that the patient will be able to use the arm for functional activities despite optimal rehabilitation. In patients with long-standing hemiplegia who initially have had inadequate management, physical therapy may lead to functional improvement by restoration of range of motion and strength. In these cases, neurologic recovery had occurred but had been masked by secondary disabilities, such as contractures or atrophy.

Paradoxically, rehabilitating the hemiplegic patient with partial function on the affected side is more complex and more difficult than rehabilitating the patient with complete paralysis. Although the partially paralyzed patient has the same or even greater potential for ambulation and self-care, he is less likely to accept leg bracing and

Disabling Conditions Due to Neurologic Impairment 249

one-handed self-care training. The physician and the therapist will be inclined to let him walk with inadequate preparation. Back knee disabilities are found frequently in these patients. Often, endless hours of therapy are wasted on the patient with partial paralysis of the upper extremity. It requires expert knowledge to determine the true functional prognosis of these hemiparetic limbs, and requires considerable power of persuasion to convince the patient and his family of this prognosis.

REHABILITATION OF THE HEMIPLEGIC PATIENT WITH ADDITIONAL DISABILITIES

In view of the infinite number of possible additional disabilities occurring in hemiplegia, one cannot be as precise in dealing with this subject as in the discussion of patients who have hemiplegia without other impairment. First, the common additional disabilities will be indicated. Second, their influence on prognosis and management of the hemiplegic condition in itself will be analyzed. Finally, consideration will be given to the management of the additional disabilities per se.

Classification of Additional Disabilities

The additional disabilities of the hemiplegic patient can be divided into three groups: concomitant, subsequent and pre-existing disabilities.

Concomitant Disabilities

Concomitant disabilities are caused by the same brain pathology that causes the hemiplegia. Therefore, they are primary disabilities. The most common concomitant disabilities occurring with hemiplegia are: aphasia (essentially in cases of involvement of the left hemisphere), agnosia and apraxia, homonymous hemianopsia, cerebellar ataxia, disturbances of balance, hemianesthesia, disturbances of consciousness and other organic mental changes.

Subsequent Disabilities

The disabilities that occur after the stroke are secondary to the paralysis and to the management of the patient. These disabilities can and should be avoided. Disabilities that result from disuse are: muscle atrophy and weakness, osteoporosis, contractures of the lower extremity (contracture of the hip in external rotation, of the knee in flexion, and shortening of the heel cord), contractures of the upper extremity (frozen shoulder; elbow, wrist and finger flexion contractures), pressure sores, urinary incontinence (from patient neglect and use of indwelling catheters) and mental and psychological deterioration (from lack of attention and social contact).

Disabilities resulting from misuse are painful shoulder (caused by injury or manipulation of the shoulder), back knee deformity (caused by premature ambulation) and various fractures caused by falls, improper exercise or improper handling of the patient.

Pre-existing Disabilities

The possible pre-existing disabilities are innumerable. They may be related to the stroke, such as peripheral vascular disease, hypertension and diabetes, or they may be entirely independent. The pre-existing disability may be the result of an illness that dominates the clinical picture, such as severe heart disease. In other instances, the pre-existing disabilities are not obvious, and one must look for them. These cryptic disorders may be musculoskeletal—for example, disabilities such as osteoarthritis, difference in length of limb, scoliosis or deformities from old fractures. Though apparently insignificant, such minor musculoskeletal impairments may interfere with ambulation and self-care ability if they are not corrected, or at least taken into account in the treatment of a patient.

Prognosis of Hemiplegia with Additional Disabilities

Additional disabilities may worsen the prognosis for rehabilitation solely because the physician shies away from an early rehabilitation program or finds himself unable to institute it. Adequate knowledge of the rehabilitation program of the hemiplegic patient coupled with imagination and determination can overcome this impasse. The prognosis will then depend only on the degree of physical impairment caused by these additional disabilities.

Some of these disabilities do not interfere with the rehabilitation program, and the patient becomes self-caring within 4 weeks, as in the case of disability limited to hemiplegia. Other disabilities may prolong the rehabilitation program, but the patient can achieve the same goal of ambulation and self-care. Certain additional disabilities interfere with ambulation, but the patient may still become self-caring with use of a wheelchair. In a few instances, the additional impairments are such that the patient will require permanent nursing care. Even in these cases, rehabilitation may help to give the patient a certain amount of self-care ability and a somewhat richer life.

The three categories of patients whose additional disabilities influence the prognosis for rehabilitation following hemiplegia are:

(1) the ambulatory self-caring patient requiring more than 4 weeks' rehabilitation, (2) the self-caring nonambulatory patient and (3) the nonambulatory nonself-caring patient.

The Ambulatory, Self-caring Patient Requiring More Than 4 Weeks' Rehabilitation

Disabilities can prolong the course of treatment either by delaying the onset of rehabilitation or by slowing the program.

Disabilities that delay the onset of the rehabilitation program are either acute illness, in which activitiy is impossible or contraindicated, or disturbances of consciousness to the extent that the patient is unable to cooperate. While the patient recovers from illness or regains sufficient consciousness to cooperate, a maintenance program must be instituted to prevent deterioration and occurrence of secondary disability.

Disabilities that tend to slow the rehabilitation program are:
1. Obesity
2. Excessive weakness of the uninvolved side
3. Low exercise tolerance as a result of cardiovascular or respiratory impairment
4. Communication disturbances
5. Minor problems of balance

In all five instances, ambulation and self-care will eventually be possible, though the rehabilitation time will be longer. The patient should not be written off as impossible to rehabilitate.

The Nonambulatory, Self-caring Patient

The disabilities interfering with ambulation but not with self-care are major disturbances of balance and coordination. For example, severe cerebellar ataxia may prevent the patient from becoming ambulatory independently but will not prevent him from walking if he can hold on to a fixed object, nor will it prevent him from wheeling his chair or transferring from the wheelchair to other places. In general, all patients who can acquire good stand-up ability but cannot walk without support are included in this group.

The Nonambulatory, Non-self-caring Patient

The disabilities that require permanent nursing care are of three types:
1. Severe organic mental disturbances
2. Severe illness that interferes with effort
3. Multiple disabilities that lead to involvement of the nonhemi-

plegic side to the extent that the patient cannot achieve stand-up ability

Influence of Additional Disabilities on the Management of Hemiplegia

Perhaps the most important principle in the management of hemiplegic patients with troublesome additional disabilities is that of carrying out the program described for hemiplegia despite the presence of additional disabilities. This requires some courage, some imagination and, above all, the knowledge of how to go about it. The more rapidly this hemiplegia program can be carried out, the better is the prognosis for functional recovery since deterioration is minimized. Although it is not always possible to make an early prognosis for ability to ambulate, the rehabilitation program must be geared from the very beginning toward the development of stand-up ability. In most instances, the program can be started immediately, with special attention to additional disabilities that tend to impede it. In a few instances, it is necessary to delay the rehabilitation, and patients have to be placed temporarily on maintenance programs.

Immediate Institution of Hemiplegia Program Despite Additional Disabilities

The disorders that tend to interfere with immediate rehabilitation are communication disturbances, weakness or obesity and difficulty in balancing. As was pointed out in the section on prognosis, these troubles may prolong rehabilitation but should never discourage it.

Communication Disturbances. As in rehabilitation generally, the principle of dealing with communication problems is to utilize what the patient has left (Chap. 8). If the patient is deaf, one should communicate with him by writing and gestures. If the patient has aphasia and alexia, one should communicate with gestures. If, in addition, he has visual impairment, one can still communicate by touch and tactile directions. Substitution of gestures for speech is tedious and time consuming and increases the number of nursing hours required for the individual patient, but usually it is effective, since the rehabilitation program for hemiplegia as outlined is very simple.

Whenever there can be compensation for communication deficits, it should be done immediately so that the patient's whole potential can be used. The use of needed eyeglasses and functioning hearing aids throughout the day should be routine. The patient with hemianopsia should be approached from the side of the intact visual field. While these recommendations appear obvious, they are rarely carried out because appliances are not ordered or nurses and therapists are not instructed as to how to manage the patient's communication problems.

Strength or Weight Problems. In cases of excessive overweight or marked weakness of the uninvolved leg, one-legged stand-up exercises may be feasible only if the seat is extremely high, so that the patient is nearly standing and practically leans against the chair. Severe reducing diets as low as 200 calories per day, or even temporary starvation, may lead to rapid weight reduction (Chap. 2). Frequent but short exercise periods will help to strengthen gradually the uninvolved extremity. It is important that progress be made in weight reduction and strengthening and that the stand-up exercise program is carried out properly despite the difficulties. The patient should be weighed every other day if he is on a reducing diet and should lose weight constantly. The desired rate of weight loss is a matter of medical judgment. The gain in strength can be noted by the fact that the patient becomes able to stand up from gradually lower chair heights and stands up with greater ease.

Balance Problems. If the patient has difficulty in maintaining balance on one leg, he should be given the opportunity to hold securely to a firm support. If he tends to fall to the hemiplegic side, his chair should be placed lateral to the support, so that his arm is stretched nearly sideways when he supports himself. Exercises in balancing while seated and in changing position while seated also hasten recovery of balance.

While ability to balance will improve with practice, it may never become sufficient for independent walking. Therefore, once the patient has achieved stand-up and stair-climbing ability, one must decide whether his balancing ability is sufficient to permit cane walking. If it is not, the program will be geared toward self-care with use of a wheelchair. If it is, the patient should be started out with a 3-point cane gait. Patients with function in the hemiplegic arm may use a small walker or walkerette (Fig. 6-14).

Maintenance Program

A maintenance program is needed only in cases of disturbances of consciousness or severe illness. It is designed to prevent the aftereffects of disuse and misuse while the patient is unable to undergo the stand-up program. If the patient is bedridden, proper positioning and frequent change of position will prevent contractures. He should be turned on the abdomen and to either side for change of position.

He should also spend time in a chair to have hips and knees flexed and should spend some time weight bearing on a tilt table with hips and knees straight.

The greatest difficulty is the maintenance of strength in the uninvolved parts of the body. Frequently, the patient who is unable to carry out the standard program is unable to carry out bed exercises and therefore loses strength at a rapid rate. Whenever possible, self-turning, self-feeding and self-dressing will help to maintain strength.

Approach to Associated Disabilities Per Se

What should be done about some of the associated disabilities themselves? Should the aphasic receive speech therapy? Should the patient with a painful shoulder receive physical therapy, and the deaf patient learn speech reading (lip reading)? Should the patients be offered counseling, social work and recreation? When faced with the many disabilities and problems of the patient with complicated hemiplegia, the physician must make a judicious choice of the difficulties to be dealt with first. Any measures that remedy disability without excessive demand on the patient's time and energy should be instituted promptly. These include such things as hearing aid, eyeglasses, proper medication and a reducing diet.

Next come measures needed to prevent secondary disabilities, for example, passive range-of-motion exercise to prevent a frozen shoulder. In addition, high priority should be given to factors that interfere with the stand-up program. For instance, if the ability to stand up tends to be delayed by psychological difficulties, intensive counseling is indicated. Otherwise, these services and therapies would best be delayed until the patient has achieved stand-up ability, since he does not have the time or the energy to receive them while engaged in the standard program. Similarly, certain diagnostic and therapeutic procedures for associated conditions may best be postponed if the patient's health will not be jeopardized by delay.

Obviously, there is no rule as to how to proportion the various rehabilitation activities. Often, a patient becomes involved in too many activities to achieve optimum benefit from the program. This is true particularly in rehabilitation centers where all of the staff would like to participate in the treatment of every patient. For this reason, hemiplegic patients frequently do better at home, where an attendant or a member of his family may be trained to guide him in a program directed toward independent ambulation and self-care.

SUMMARY

A program of rehabilitation in hemiplegia should be concerned mainly with the uninvolved side, with the goals of ambulation and self-care.

To prepare for ambulation, exercises for the uninvolved side must be vigorous, progressive, unassisted, of short duration and repeated frequently. This is best achieved by a program of stand-up exercises. When he begins to walk, the patient should retain his specific hemiplegic gait pattern and not attempt to simulate a normal gait.

The patient should be trained in self-care activities with use of the uninvolved arm. The hemiplegic upper extremity should be protected against secondary disabilities.

The presence of associated disabilities should not distract the staff from carrying out the program to achieve stand-up ability, ambulation and self-care. A rigid schedule of priorities must be established in the face of multiple problems.

Section B. Incoordination

Incoordination is a disturbance of motor function in which smoothness and precision of motion are disturbed. Normal smoothness and precision of motion depend on extremely sensitive coordination of many muscle groups. Motor coordination requires and is regulated by constant sensory feedback of many data concerning tension in muscles, position of joints and the position of the body and the limbs in relationship to each other and in relationship to gravity. The data are derived from the vestibular apparatus of the inner ear and from the retina as well as from proprioceptive sensory connections with joints and muscles. This sensory feedback is integrated principally in the cerebellum and coupled by cerebellar pathways with the motor tracts. Coordinated motion may be disturbed by many factors. Muscle paralysis, mechanical joint disturbances, pain, involuntary movements and many other causes may interfere with coordinated movements. However, the disabilities discussed in this section are those related to impairment of either cerebellar function or of proprioception. The term ataxia is used here for disturbances of these two functions. One may distinguish cerebellar ataxia, spinal ataxia and peripheral nerve ataxia (ataxic form of peripheral neuropathy).

CAUSES

Cerebellar Ataxia

1. Specific involvement of cerebellar pathways
    a. Isolated: cerebellar agenesis, cerebellar atrophy
    b. Combined with other structures: spinal-cerebellar degenerations (e.g., Friedreich's ataxia), multiple sclerosis
2. Involvement of cerebellar pathways in random lesions
    a. Traumatic brain injuries, cerebral palsy
    b. Space-occupying lesions
    c. Vascular lesions, particularly of the brain stem

Spinal Ataxia

This results from disease of the posterior columns of the spinal cord. It occurs in tabes dorsalis and combined (posterolateral) sclerosis.

Peripheral Nerve Ataxia

This may occur in many forms of peripheral neuropathy if proprioceptive fibers are involved.

PROGNOSIS

The ataxia may be progressive as in Friedreich's ataxia and other spinal cerebellar degenerations. It may remain stationary as in certain congenital ataxias. There may be improvement as in ataxias due to vascular lesions of the brain and to head injuries. In these cases, ataxia usually improves over a long period of time, which means from 1 to 2 years or possibly longer.

REHABILITATION OF THE PATIENT WITH INCOORDINATION

Incoordination may involve the upper extremities, the lower extremities and the trunk.

In *upper extremity involvement,* the patient is greatly handicapped in all activities of daily living and is unable to do fine work. If the ataxia is severe, the patient may need assistance with some of these activities. Usually, he manages to carry out self-care activities but with considerable delay and with great frustration because of frequently unsuccessful attempts to carry out a motion. While feeding himself, food is often splattered around.

Simple measures to improve hand activity and self-care activities are proper stabilization of the trunk and possibly the elbow, the use of adapted equipment such as plates with suction cups, food guards, special drinking cups with spouts to prevent spillage, and a multitude of other devices (Chap. 7). More drastic measures such as attaching a weight to the upper extremity or restricting motion by braces that allow movement in only one plane frequently prove to be more of a handicap than a help. Since incoordination is aggravated by nervous tension, use of tranquilizers to induce relaxation may be helpful.

Lower extremity ataxia interferes with locomotion. In spinal ataxia the disability is less severe than in cerebellar ataxia. Spinal ataxic gait is quite characteristic. The patient raises his legs higher than necessary and throws them out with greater force than is necessary. The apparent lack of motor control actually is due to impaired or absent position sense. In this type of ataxia the gait can be considerably improved if the patient keeps his eyes fixed on his lower extremities. This is practiced in the so-called Frenkel exercises originally designed for tabetics. Stair-climbing exercises are helpful also.

In cerebellar ataxia of the lower extremities the gait pattern may be more disturbed, and sometimes wheelchair locomotion is the only possibility, particularly if ataxia of the trunk is associated with ataxia of the lower extremities. If the cerebellar ataxia is moderate, the patient may walk with a walker. If his upper extremities are not particularly involved in incoordination, he may possibly walk with Canadian crutches. The use of vision as a prop or substitute for joint and muscle sense does not produce spectacular improvement in cerebellar ataxia, but continued practice frequently leads to gradual improvement.

Frenkel Exercises

These exercises are carried out while the patient is lying, sitting, standing or walking. Exercises for only the latter three positions will be described here.

Exercises in Sitting Position

1. The patient is seated in a comfortable chair. Both feet are placed firmly on the floor upon traced footprints. The patient raises each knee alternately and places the foot back exactly on the traced footprint.

2. The patient stands up and sits down slowly without dropping into the chair, preferably without using his hands for support.

Exercises in Standing Position

For these exercises, parallel bars are needed. On the floor space between the bars, footprints are traced at regular step intervals. The patient places one foot on the footprint in front of the base position, then on the footprint in back of the base position and then returns the foot to the base position. The exercise is performed alternately with both legs.

Walking Exercises

1. Two parallel lines are traced on the floor, and the patient is asked to place first one foot then the other exactly on the appropriate line while walking.

2. Footprints are traced on the floor at regular step intervals, and the patient is requested to place each foot exactly on the appropriate footprint while walking forward.

In all coordination exercises the patient is requested initially to look at his feet as well as at the places where he is supposed to put them. Later on, he gradually should attempt to find his mark without visual assistance.

Section C. Involuntary Movements

As the name implies, involuntary movements are movements of the head, the trunk, or the limbs occurring spontaneously and purposelessly.

TYPES OF INVOLUNTARY MOVEMENT

The most common involuntary movements are tremors that are rhythmic motions of a segment of the body. They may exist at rest as in Parkinson's syndrome (rest tremors) or they may occur only on voluntary motion as, for example, in multiple sclerosis (intention tremor).

Other involuntary motions are named for the syndromes in which they occur. Choreiform movements occur in chorea, or St. Vitus' dance. Athetoid movements occur in athetosis, a syndrome characterized by writhing motions of hands and wrists and grimacing of the face. Dystonic movements occur in dystonias, which consist of slow but strong muscular contraction causing twisting of a part of the body.

REHABILITATION OF PATIENTS WITH INVOLUNTARY MOVEMENTS

Rehabilitation of the Patient with Parkinsonism

Parkinsonism is a syndrome caused by damage to the basal ganglia. It occurs most commonly as a late sequel to epidemic encephalitis or as a consequence of diminished blood supply to the brain due to arteriosclerosis. A type of parkinsonian syndrome is seen also following carbon monoxide poisoning. The typical case of postencephalitic parkinsonism is gradually progressive. The patient suffers from a number of disabilities.

The tremor which is the most obvious one and has given the disease the name of *shaking palsy* may initially exist only at rest and subside when the patient carries out a motion. However, as the disease becomes more severe, the tremor of parkinsonism interferes with ambulation and hand activity, and the patient may become severely disabled and require nursing care.

A second disability encountered in patients with parkinsonism is muscular rigidity. This is a stiffness of muscles and is characterized by resistance to active and passive movement. It differs in certain features from the spasticity described in patients with spastic paralysis. Rigidity is more constant and more uniform in distribution than spasticity. It is as marked in flexors as in extensors and does not tend to produce involuntary motions as do the pseudospontaneous spasms in spasticity. Nevertheless, rigidity is a severe disability; it causes considerable slowness of motion of the patients with parkinsonism, and movement requires great effort. Therefore, patients tend to become immobilized and to develop contractures.

A maintenance regimen for a patient with parkinsonian rigidity consisting of passive range of motion of all joints twice daily may considerably prolong the patient's ability for independent locomotion and self-care.

The third disability of the patient with parkinsonism is disturbance of standing and walking balance. He may have a tendency to fall backward (retropulsion), to the side (lateropulsion) or forward (propulsion). This may make independent ambulation for patients very hazardous since they are easily subject to falls and fractures. The use of a walker or a wheelchair is not too helpful since the upper extremities are as badly or more involved than the lower extremities. However, the patient with balance problems should not be prevented from walking entirely but should walk with an attendant who can prevent falls. Once the patient with parkinsonism has ceased to ambulate, he develops contractures and pressure sores very rapidly and becomes a nursing care patient without further possibility of rehabilitation.

Other disabilities that occur in advanced parkinsonism are urinary incontinence requiring an indwelling catheter, difficulties of speech and swallowing and troublesome hypersalivation.

The most effective medication for symptomatic relief is L-Dopa. Other useful medications are Atropine-like drugs such as trihexyphenidyl hydrochloride (Artane) and benztropine mesylate (Cogentin). Surgical destruction of a portion of the basal ganglia is useful in relieving tremor.

Rehabilitation of the Patient with Intention Tremor

Intention tremor is commonly seen in multiple sclerosis, hepatolenticular degeneration, Friedreich's ataxia and other cerebellar diseases. Intention tremor occurs only during voluntary motion and prevents the patient from carrying out a coordinated movement. It interferes greatly with hand activities and activities of daily living. Management is the same as that of incoordination described in Section B.

Rehabilitation of the Patient with Athetosis

Athetosis is seen most commonly in that form of cerebral palsy in which damage to the basal ganglia has occurred. Athetosis may be found also in brain injuries of the adult. Although athetoid patients are frequently able to ambulate with an awkward and dancing gait, they are often handicapped in hand activities. Mental retardation in children with athetoid cerebral palsy is exceptional and in contrast to the spastic forms of cerebral palsy. Therefore, the rehabilitation potential is more promising.

Unfortunately, exercises and bracing are rarely useful for functional improvement of these patients. Often, their status is improved to a considerable extent by adjustment to their involuntary movements. This allows them to carry out some acts that take advantage of the motions and some that can be done in the interval between involuntary motions. There is also some promise that surgical destruction of basal ganglia may help many of the patients with athetosis by diminishing the involuntary motions much as tremor is diminished in parkinsonism.

Conditions in which involuntary movements are the only disorder are uncommon causes of severe disability. However, involuntary motions may contribute to the disability of patients with parkinsonism and multiple sclerosis who are also suffering from other neurologic disabilities.

Section D. Organic Mental Impairment

Definition. Organic mental impairment is defined as any impairment of mental function caused by organic disorder of the brain.

Although this book is not concerned with rehabilitation of the mentally ill, it is necessary to discuss briefly some of the conditions in the category of mental impairment that are caused by damage to the brain. It is particularly important to be familiar with some of the forms of organic mental impairment that may occur in association with the motor disabilities due to brain damage described in previous sections. For example, in the patient with head injury, in patients who have suffered strokes and in some patients with parkinsonism, organic mental impairment is a frequent concomitant disability. On the other hand, organic mental impairment is common in elderly patients even without impairment of motor function. Then, it is generally referred to under the rather vague term of senility.

Unfortunately, very little is known about the precise localization of mental functions within the brain. It is also very difficult to classify the disabilities and manifestations of organic mental impairment since they occur frequently in association with each other and also simultaneously with psychological disturbances that further complicate the clinical picture. An attempt will be made to present those aspects of organic mental impairment that are of importance in the rehabilitation of the severely disabled and of the elderly patient.

CAUSES

The standard medical nomenclature distinguishes two major groups of organic mental impairment: the acute brain syndrome, which is caused by metabolic disturbances of brain function and the chronic brain syndrome, which is caused by loss of brain cells due to a pathologic process. Either the acute or the chronic brain syndrome may be associated with psychosis.

Some of the common metabolic disturbances causing organic mental impairment are:

1. Local circulatory embarrassment by a space-occupying vascular or inflammatory lesion. Such local metabolic disturbances are common immediately following a head injury, brain surgery or stroke.

2. Impaired cerebral metabolism due to lack of oxygen from a systemic cause such as congestive heart failure, respiratory failure or severe anemia

3. Impaired cerebral metabolism of toxic origin as seen in uremia, acidosis and lead encephalopathy

The chronic brain syndrome or loss of brain cells may be caused by:

1. Degenerative diseases such as Alzheimer's disease

2. Generalized arteriosclerosis of the brain with subsequent cortical atrophy

3. Numerous focal brain lesions such as those that occur after repeated vascular accidents or in certain severe head injuries

The separation of the two major groups of organic mental impairment is not always clear-cut in the elderly or severely disabled patient. For instance, after head injury there may be hemorrhage and edema causing early metabolic disturbances, but also cell destruction that may cause permanent damage and produce a chronic type of brain syndrome. Similarly, in the elderly stroke patient there may be an acute type of brain syndrome present initially that results eventually in chronic mental impairment, particularly if several strokes have occurred. In addition, the elderly stroke patient often has concomitant heart failure, emphysema, uremia or anemia, and the acute or chronic nature of the mental disturbance cannot always be distinguished immediately.

Furthermore, the mental impairment is rarely entirely due to organic disease. In addition to the psychosis that could be associated with organic syndromes, the elderly patient with chronic or acute brain syndrome may have many reasons for psychological disturbances as a consequence of his physical and mental disability and his precarious socioeconomic situation.

PROGNOSIS

Organic mental impairment may be progressive, stationary for long periods, or it may improve. Progressive organic mental impairment is found in degenerative disease such as Alzheimer's disease and Huntington's chorea, in progressive arteriosclerosis or in recurrent cerebral vascular accidents.

The disabilty may remain stationary in the patient with a brain injury after the acute brain syndrome has subsided. Generally, improvement occurs in metabolic brain disturbances once the metabolic disturbance has been corrected. Improvement may occur also in chronic brain syndromes by adjustment of the patient to his environment and by resolution of psychological components of his mental disturbance.

CLINICAL TYPES OF ORGANIC MENTAL IMPAIRMENT

Organic mental impairment can be classified into the following groups: (1) disturbances of consciousness, (2) disturbances of communication, (3) disturbances of memory and thinking, and (4) emotional impairment.

Disturbances of Consciousness

These are frequently subdivided according to the degree or level of consciousness, e.g., coma, stupor, and so forth. Usually, periods of unconsciousness are transient but at times patients remain unconscious for many years, following head injuries, for example.

Disturbances of Communication

While some disturbances of communication are caused by abnormalities of motor function or of the special senses, a certain group of communication disabilities are due to deficits in mental function. Such is the case in the agnosias, the apraxias and in disturbances of integration (Chap. 8).

Disturbances of Memory and Thinking

These manifestations of mental retardation characterize patients with senility or organic mental syndromes. The typical disabilities in the later group are disorientation as to time and space, impairment of memory and judgment and diminution of attention span. These patients form a large group of the elderly disabled population. Frequently, the organic mental syndrome is associated, at least in stroke patients, with disorders of communication or disorders of emotion. Such disabilities may be due entirely to a metabolic cause that is reversible, or entirely to cortical atrophy that is irreversible, or partly to one and partly to the other, in which case they are subject to some improvement but not to full recovery.

Emotional Impairment

This may take many forms. For purposes of management three types are distinguished: the apathetic or depressed patient, the irritable patient and the anxious patient. It is impossible to say whether these emotional patterns are entirely due to psychological factors or whether they are due to psychological factors associated with organic disorders. The apathetic patient shows no spontaneous interest and must be prodded to perform his activities of daily living and his exercises. The anxious patient who is very commonly also a patient with communication disabilities and with poor attention span is the opposite of the apathetic patient. He is very eager to perform exercises and activities but frequently tends to do things too fast and with poor planning. He falls behind in his achievement and activities of daily living and locomotion. The irritable patient poses a rehabilitation problem mainly because of his lack of cooperation. He is irritated and annoyed by the rehabilitation program and the hospital routine. Such patients frequently become querulous and quite angry. This pattern of behavior is also common in patients with communication disabilities.

MANAGEMENT OF PATIENTS WITH ORGANIC MENTAL IMPAIRMENT

Management of the Comatose Patient

Obviously, this patient is unable to cooperate in a rehabilitation program, and his management is entirely passive. To maintain his nutrition, nasogastric feeding or gastrostomy may be necessary. Sometimes his airway is in jeopardy, and a tracheostomy must be performed. In all instances, the unconscious patient is subject to the disuse phenomena of contracture and pressure sores and must be subjected to the routine of positioning and passive range of motion described in Chapter 3. An indwelling catheter may also be needed to keep the patient dry.

Management of the Disoriented Patient

The disoriented patient (senile patient, patient with organic mental syndrome) may cooperate fairly well with a simple rehabilitation program. His management includes, first, the restoration of proper brain metabolism. This means the correction of possible heart failure, anemia, metabolic disturbances, and so forth. Many patients in this category become entirely clear mentally after better oxygenation of the blood or elimination of toxic substances. In many other instances, there is a considerable improvement in mental function after these factors have been corrected.

The psychological management of these patients, once the metabolic factors have been corrected, consists of two phases: (1) the patient must be given an adequate amount of stimulation and (2) he must not be subject to excessive demands. It is an interesting finding that the elderly disabled patient with mild senility who is kept in bed and to whom no attention is paid gradually becomes incontinent, more withdrawn, more disoriented and more confused. As soon as this same patient is involved in a daily routine that brings him in contact with other people and requires activity, his attention span, memory and orientation improve considerably, and frequently adequate function is restored.

On the other hand, if the activity is overdone and if this patient has to meet many people and engage in varied activities in different places, his disorientation may increase again. For optimum mental function it is therefore necessary to exercise judgment about permissible changes of environment and variety of social intercourse to avoid overstimulation. Social contacts may later be increased very gradually. The rule of management of these patients with organic mental syndrome is parallel to the rule of strengthening of the patient with muscle weakness. If the exercise is too violent, it is damaging by misuse and if the exercise is insufficient, it is damaging by disuse.

Management of Emotional Disturbances of the Senile Patient

While a proper psychological approach is helpful, often it is insufficient in itself to achieve rehabilitation of the patient. However, the use of pharmacologic agents as adjuncts to rehabilitation may cause definite improvement in his attitudes and activities. The apathetic or depressed patient may be benefited by an array of antidepressive drugs. Alerting stimulants such as methylphenidate (Ritalin) and dextroamphetamine sulfate (Dexedrine) are frequently very effective. However, if the depression is associated with anxiety, some of the newer mood-elevating drugs such as Tofranil may be of value. Both anxious and irritable patients may be benefited by tranquilizers. Frequently, use of small doses of phenothiazines is sufficient to improve performance. In cases of severe irritability high doses of chlorpromazine (Thorazine) or promazine (Sparine) may sometimes be used.

CONCLUSION

Since rehabilitation involves active participation of the patient, the combination of mental impairment and physical disability constitutes a most difficult problem of management. However, as one proceeds with proper evaluation and identifies the disabilities, one may find very often that the prognosis is better than it seemed at first, and persistent effort often leads to gratifying results.

It goes without saying that consultants in clinical psychology and neuropsychiatry may provide both diagnostic and therapeutic assistance in the management of these difficult problems. Specialized testing may reveal the presence of parietal lobe disorders causing not only apraxias but also defects of interpretation and integration.

REFERENCES

1. American Medical Association: Current Medical Information and Terminology. Chicago: AMA, 1971.
2. Bard, G. and Hirschberg, G. G.: "Recovery of Voluntary Motion in Upper Extremity Following Hemiplegia." Arch. Phys. Med. & Rehab., 45:567, 1965.
3. Hirschberg, G. G.: "Use of Stand-up and Step-up Exercises in Rehabilitation." Clin. Orthop, 12:30, 1958.
4. Hirschberg, G. G., Bard, G. and Robertson, K. B.: "Technics of Rehabilitation of Hemiplegic Patients." Am. J. Med., 35:536, 1963.
5. Licht, S.: Stroke and Its Rehabilitation. New Haven: Elizabeth Licht, 1975.
6. Pesczynski, M.: "Exercises for Hemiplegia," in Licht, S.: Therapeutic Exercise, 2nd Ed. New Haven: Elizabeth Licht, 1965.

Disabling Conditions Due to Neurologic Impairment (Continued)

Section A. Paraplegia

Definition. Paraplegia is a paralysis of both lower extremities.

CAUSES OF PARAPLEGIA

Paraplegia is a common disability in chronic neurologic disorders. It can result from a number of causes that may be grouped as follows:

A.   Upper motoneuron lesions
   1. Transverse lesions of the spinal cord
     a. By injury
       (1) Transection by displaced vertebral fragments in fractures of spine: e.g., automobile accidents, falls
       (2) Transection or disruption by foreign bodies: e.g., bullets, shell fragments, knives
     b. By compression
       (1) Slow compression: e.g., tumor, varicosities, constrictive arachnoiditis, cervical spondylosis
       (2) Rapid compression: e.g., collapsed vertebrae, extruded intervertebral disk, epidural abscess
     c. By infection: e.g., transverse myelitis, tuberculosis, syphilis, viral infections
     d. By vascular occlusion
       (1) Thrombosis or hemorrhage: e.g., arteriosclerosis of the arteries of the spinal cord
       (2) Embolism
     e. By congenital deformity: e.g., spina bifida with meningomyelocele
   2. Parasagittal lesions of the brain (adjacent to sagittal fissure)

     a. Parasagittal tumors: e.g., meningioma, compressing right and left motor cortex

     b. Hemorrhage from the sagittal sinus. This is most common as a birth injury, producing spastic cerebral palsy

  3. Diseases involving motor tracts

     a. Multiple sclerosis

     b. Combined sclerosis

     c. Amyotrophic lateral sclerosis

B. Lower motoneuron and muscle lesions

  1. Diseases involving the anterior horn cells

     a. Acute anterior poliomyelitis

     b. Progressive spinal muscular atrophy

  2. Lesions of nerves and nerve roots

     a. Polyneuritis

     b. Guillain-Barré syndrome

     c. Cauda equina and conus lesions

  3. Muscular dystrophy

PROGNOSIS

1. Recovery or progression of paralysis

  a. The paraplegia may remain stationary: e.g., complete traumatic transection of the dorsal spinal cord.

  b. There may be gradual recovery: e.g., Guillain-Barré syndrome.

  c. There may be gradual progression: e.g., multiple sclerosis, progressive muscular atrophy.

2. Functional prognosis for the patient with residual paraplegia depends on: the extent of involvement of motor function and additional involvement of other than motor functions.

  a. Prognosis when motor function alone is involved (example: poliomyelitis). These patients are handicapped in ambulation and in self-care involving the lower extremities. If paralysis is limited to the lower limbs, the patient can walk with long leg braces and crutches with a 4-point or a swinging crutch gait. If there is also considerable trunk involvement, crutch walking becomes more difficult. Then, the patient will need a pelvic band and may be limited to swinging crutch gaits. He may prefer to use a wheelchair most of the time.

  b. Prognosis for a patient with complete transection of the spinal cord (example: traumatic transection). In addition to lower extremity paralysis, these patients have loss of bladder control and of sensation. They are subject to pressure sores and urinary tract infections. Functionally, they can often perform as well as poliomyelitis paraplegics, although they have to use a swinging gait and are handicapped by sensory loss and spasticity. The patient with a cauda equina or conus lesion causing flaccid paralysis can swing or use a 4-point gait. For the patient with a mid-dorsal spinal cord lesion, crutch-walking becomes strenuous; for one with a high dorsal lesion it becomes an athletic feat. The higher the spinal cord lesion the less the patient walks and the more he uses a wheelchair. Usually, self-care is possible for the patient with a spinal cord injury, although dressing and bathing activities are slowed down considerably.

   c. Prognosis for the paraplegic with additional disabilities. The presence of additional neurologic disabilities considerably worsens the functional prognosis. The association of ataxia with paraplegia as seen in multiple sclerosis or Friedreich's ataxia makes ambulation impossible at an early stage. Additional mental retardation in spastic cerebral palsy may even handicap independent self-care.

A precise evaluation of all disabilities and establishment of an accurate and clear-cut prognosis are necessary to assure a practical rehabilitation program and optimal results.

REHABILITATION TECHNIQUES FOR THE PARAPLEGIC PATIENT

Introduction

The most common causes of paraplegia are lesions of the spinal cord. The age distribution of paraplegics now ranges from infancy to middle age. There are very few elderly paraplegics because, until recently, the life span was shortened by infections and urinary tract complications. As methods of care improve, the paraplegic may survive to old age.

In contradistinction to the wide spectrum of prognoses in hemiplegia, often the fate of the paraplegic can be pinpointed on the basis of evaluation data. In general, self-care from a wheelchair with or without ambulation on braces and crutches is the rehabilitation goal. Because of this uniformity of objective, the rehabilitation program has become remarkably standardized. In fact, rehabilitation to locomotion and self-care is the lesser problem of the paraplegic patient. His major problem is the fight against secondary disabilities and complications, such as pressure sores, urinary tract infections and stones and excessive spasticity. Since these patients are in a younger age group than hemiplegics, greater emphasis is necessarily placed on vocational rehabilitation.

A clear picture of rehabilitation techniques for paraplegics is shown by the example of a patient with traumatic transection of the dorsal spinal cord due to injury. The clinical course of such a patient comprises two stages: an initial period of flaccid paralysis (spinal shock) followed by a second stage of gradually developing spasticity which reaches its maximum in several weeks or months.

First Stage.   During the initial period where there is flaccid paralysis, all nervous function is abolished below the level of the lesion. In the lower extremities there is neither voluntary nor reflex motion. There is also complete loss of sensory function below the level of the lesion. There is no sensation in bladder or bowel, and sexual function is absent. Bladder and bowel musculature is flaccid, and these viscera are easily distended. Some intestinal peristalsis may persist. At this stage the patient needs an indwelling catheter and is dependent on enemas for elimination. The complete immobility and lack of sensation in the lower half of the body lead readily to formation of pressure sores.

Second Stage.   After several days or weeks, reflex activity becomes exaggerated, and spastic paralysis ensues. There is stiffness and pseudospontaneous spasm in the lower extremities. Either flexion or extension spasm may predominate. These are associated with feelings of discomfort or pain in the lower extremities. The bladder becomes spastic and small, and there is also spasticity of anal and vesical sphincters. Flexor spasticity, if predominant, tends to lead to flexion contractures.

Rehabilitation Program.   The rehabilitation program for paraplegia can be subdivided into 5 phases: (1) mobility and locomotion, (2) self-care, (3) bladder and bowel program, (4) psychosocial program and (5) the vocational rehabilitation program.

Restoration to Mobility and Locomotion

In the example under discussion—traumatic dorsal spinal cord injury—an initial period of enforced immobilization in bed may be necessary. This is the case particularly if a fracture dislocation of the spine has occurred. The bed phase should be as brief as care of the fracture will permit. It is followed by the wheelchair phase. The patient may be started on the parallel bar phase while still learning wheelchair activities. As in the case of hemiplegia, speed in carrying through the restoration of mobility is of the greatest importance in the prevention of many secondary disabilities, including depression and loss of will to work toward rehabilitation.

Paraplegic Bed Phase

The bed phase starts on the day of the spinal cord injury and may last from a few days to several months according to the immobilization required by the injury. In most instances of spinal cord injury due to fracture of the spine, the patient may be sitting up with a brace or a corset within 3 to 4 weeks. The program includes: preparation of the bed, orientation of the patient, positioning, bed exercises and trunk support.

Special Beds Versus Regular Beds. In view of the need for frequent change of position as well as immobilization of the spine, the Stryker frame (Fig. 6-3) is frequently used initially. The Circ-Olectric bed (Fig. 6-4) is preferable because it affords a greater variety of positions. A patient with spinal cord injury may be cared for initially in a regular bed provided that he is turned with great care. The vertebrae are well stabilized by many ligaments, and as long as the patient remains horizontal, further bony disruption is not likely. The bed should have side rails, and an overhead trapeze should be available. There should be a space between the end of the mattress and the footboard to allow room for the toes in face-lying position and the heels in back-lying position. (Fig. 15-1).

Orientation of the Patient. In the early phases of a spinal cord injury there is always the possibility of partial or complete neurologic recovery. The patient should be aware of the fact that this recovery, if it occurs, will be spontaneous and that treatment of the paralyzed extremities cannot influence it. He should be so well informed of the dangers of disuse that he will understand the importance of participating, at least mentally, in his positioning and disuse prevention program. He should be encouraged to assume responsibility for requesting the nurses to turn him at proper intervals. It should be emphasized that disuse phenomena are most likely to occur during the flaccid paralysis stage.

Positioning. The main purpose of the early positioning program is the prevention of pressure sores. Because of complete lack of sensation and muscular flaccidity, the danger of pressure sores is greatest at this stage. The details of positioning were described in Chapter 3. It should be stressed that the face-lying position is the safest for prevention of pressure sores and respiratory complications. It can be main-

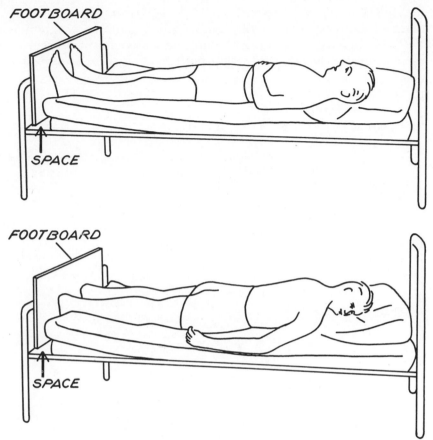

Fig. 15-1. Bed for the paraplegic patient, illustrating use of footboard.

tained up to 3 or 4 hours if the knees are protected properly. Back-lying periods should not exceed 1 hour and side-lying periods 2 hours for the average patient.

The time spent in each position must be governed by the need for prevention of pressure sores. It should be prescribed by the physician in the form of a precise schedule including all therapeutic and nursing procedures. Routine orders such as: "may dangle," "ambulate," "up in chair as tolerated" or "turn every 2 hours" are ineffective or even harmful. Think of the paraplegic who "tolerates" 6 hours' sitting in a chair and ends up with bilateral ischial pressure sores.

The change of position schedule varies with each individual patient according to need and tolerance. Following is a sample schedule for change of position of a severely impaired patient. Let us assume that because of flaccid paralysis, sensory loss, heavy body weight and lack of substantial fat padding, the maximum time for pressure over the sacrum, trochanters and ischia must be limited to ½ hour at a time.

Day Schedule:

7:00-7:30	Bed Bath
7:30-8:00	Chair (breakfast)
8:00-9:00	Bed—
	½ hour right side-lying
	½ hour left side-lying
9:00-9:30	Commode (bowel training)
9:30-10:30	Bed—
	½ hour back-lying
	½ hour Fowler's position
10:30-11:00	Tilt Table
11:00-12:00	Bed (face-lying)
12:00-12:30	Chair (lunch)

Afternoon Schedule:

12:30-3:00	Bed—
	½ hour right side-lying
	½ hour back-lying
	½ hour left side-lying
	1 hour face-lying
3:00-3:30	Tilt Table
3:30-4:30	Bed—
	½ hour right side-lying
	½ hour left side-lying
4:30-5:00	Chair (dinner)
5:00-7:00	Bed—
	½ hour right side-lying
	½ hour Fowler's position
	½ hour left side-lying
	½ hour back-lying

Night Schedule:

7:00-10:00	Face-lying
10:00-11:30	½ hour right side-lying
	½ hour back-lying
	½ hour left side-lying
11:30-2:30	Face-lying
2:30-4:00	½ hour right side-lying
	½ hour back lying
	½ hour left side-lying
4:00-7:00	Face-lying

During the bed phase, the use of a tilt table (Fig. 15-2) or of a tilted position in a special bed (Fig. 6-4) affords a good change of position which puts some pressure on the feet. However, one should guard against orthostatic hypotension (Chap. 3) by using a scultetus binder or a body corset as well as lower extremity bandages. As the patient becomes adjusted to the upright position, bandages can be removed.

The tilting and weight-bearing program helps to prevent pressure sores, adapts circulatory dynamics to the upright posture and also promotes better urinary drainage and development of extensor spasticity that is desirable in crutch-walking. It is claimed that demineralization of the bones of the lower extremities is somewhat diminished by weight-bearing. A major benefit of the tilting and standing program is the psychological lift derived from the upright position.

Technique for Use of the Tilt Table. A tilt table resembles a stretcher which can be tilted gradually from a horizontal to a vertical position. A footboard at the lower end prevents the patient from sliding down

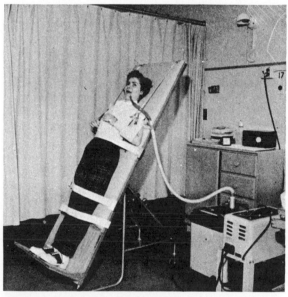

Fig. 15-2. The tilt table is used not only in rehabilitation of paraplegic patients but also, as illustrated, for quadriplegic patients. In the figure, the patient is using a positive-pressure attachment from a portable respirator for assisted breathing. (Tilt table, Med-Tek, Berkeley; Respirator, Thompson Respiration Products.)

Disabling Conditions Due to Neurologic Impairment   275

and allows weight-bearing. The patient may be strapped to the table top across the pelvis, knees, and chest as needed. He should not be immobilized more than necessary, and should perform some exercise activity during the standing period. The angle of tilt is determined by the desired amount of weight-bearing and tolerance of erect position. It is usually between 45 and 80 degrees.

In most patients for whom the tilt table is indicated, i.e., patients with paralysis or who have been at bed rest for long periods, the tilted position must be established gradually over a period of days or weeks. Once the patient is used to the tilt table, he may remain in the maximum tilt position, up to 1 hour, two or three times daily. Tilt table treatment is begun as follows:

1. Bandage the patient's lower extremities tightly with elastic bandages and apply a tight abdominal binder (scultetus).

2. Place the patient on a flat tilt table and fasten the straps across the pelvis, knees, and chest or abdomen.

3. Apply a blood pressure (BP) cuff to the arm and record the BP.

4. Tilt the table 30 degrees and take BP every 2 or 3 minutes.

a. If the patient feels faint or dizzy and the BP drops, return to flat position and start over, raising the table only 20 degrees. (If the patient complains of dizziness but BP does not drop, encourage him to stay up and proceed as below.)

b. If the patient feels all right but the BP drops, watch closely. After a few minutes the BP may rise and stabilize slightly below the patient's normal pressure. Do not increase tilt but maintain a 30 degree tilt for 15 to 30 minutes. If the BP continues to drop, the patient will soon feel dizzy and should be returned to the flat position.

c. If the patient feels all right and the BP maintains itself for several minutes, increase tilt by another 15 degrees.

5. Continue procedure until the patient tolerates the desired tilt. Then gradually eliminate bandages and abdominal binders.

6. The routine of blood pressure and pulse measurement may be discontinued when the patient tolerates the upright position.

Bed Exercises.   During the period when the patient's spine needs to be protected, the bed exercise program is very limited. Its purpose is to maintain and increase strength in the upper extremities. Dumbbell exercises in back-lying and face-lying positions are indicated. Of particular importance is the strengthening of elbow extensors and shoulder depressors needed for future transfers and crutch-walking.

If the spine is less vulnerable or protected by a body corset, the patient may start on exercises which increase bed mobility. These consist of moving about in bed and of turning by holding onto the bed frame, the side rails and the overhead trapeze. At this stage, the patient may also practice to position and flex his lower extremities passively with his hands. Change of position on his own initiative helps to prevent pressure sores and contractures and diminishes the feeling of helplessness.

During the final stage of the bed phase, he must learn to get into sitting position on the edge of the bed and perform seated push-ups. This forms the transition to the wheelchair phase.

APPLICATION AND CARE OF THE FULL-LENGTH CANVAS BODY CORSET

A. Application of Corset

1. With patient in left side-lying position, place the gathered left side of the corset well under the patient so that the steel stays are aligned with the lumbar lordosis.

2. Spread out the right half of the corset and roll the patient over to the right.

3. Spread out the previously gathered left half of the corset, and turn the patient onto his back. The spine should be in the center between the steel stays.

4. Tighten the straps in the following manner:

   a. First the lowest straps, which should be just above the pubis, should be tightened very snugly.

   b. Tighten the remainder of the straps progressively less snugly from below upward. The uppermost strap should allow the easy insertion of a hand between the epigastrium and the corset.

B. Care of Corset: Method of Laundering

1. Remove steel stays from pockets, marking the top portions of their outer surfaces in order to replace them in their proper positions.

2. Place corset in hot water with mild soap suds for 15 minutes. Do *not* use detergents or bleaches. Do *not* use washing machine or dryer.

3. Scrub both sides of corset with stiff bristle brush.

4. Rinse 3 or 4 times in tepid or cool water.

5. Spread out well and straight to dry, either hanging or on a flat surface. Do *not* put in a dryer. Do *not* iron.

6. When dry, replace steel stays.

Trunk Support. Whether or not there is a fracture of the spine which requires bracing, the patient with a mid-dorsal transverse lesion of the spinal cord requires a trunk support initially in order to sit up or stand. A full-length canvas body corset (Fig. 15-3) with heavy steel stays in the back is commonly used. The corset has advantages over a brace because it can be worn in bed without discomfort and without risk of causing pressure sores. It allows for somewhat greater trunk mobility and at the same time protects against orthostatic hypotension when the patient is stood up. The corset may be prescribed early during the bed phase. Thus, it will expedite active exercises and at the same time afford greater protection to the fracture site of the spine. In a mid-dorsal or higher spinal cord lesion, a trunk support should always be provided before the wheelchair phase is begun. It may be discarded later when the trunk musculature becomes spastic.

Concomitant Activities of the Bed Phase. The following activities should also be conducted during the bed phase.

1. Bowel training.

2. Bladder program—indwelling catheter to be irrigated twice daily (Chap. 15, Sect. D).

3. Bed self-care: feeding, washing.

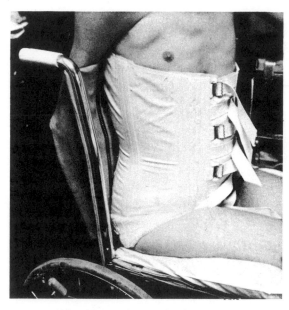

Fig. 15-3. Canvas body corset.

Paraplegic Wheelchair Phase

This phase includes the prescription and procurement of the proper wheelchair and training in wheelchair transfer and other wheelchair activities.

The Wheelchair.   By the time the patient is ready for the wheelchair, it should be ready for him. The paraplegic patient needs a Universal-type folding wheelchair with removable arms, upholstered armrests, footrests with heel loops and legrests. The chair should have a 3- or 4-inch (8- to 10-cm.) foam rubber cushion or an air cushion. The height and the width of the chair should correspond to the patient's dimensions (Chap. 6).

The Non-weight-bearing Transfer.   Initially, the paraplegic should be instructed in all three methods of non-weight-bearing transfer. He should learn to transfer on the same level from bed to chair, bed to wheelchair, wheelchair to toilet, and so forth. He should also be able to transfer to a higher and a lower level by the push-up method. Later, he should also practice non-weight-bearing transfers from wheelchair to car and car to wheelchair. The toilet should be provided with proper supports eventually to permit a weight-bearing as well as a non-weight-bearing transfer (Chap. 6).

Other Wheelchair Activities.   One activity, the importance of which cannot be stressed too greatly, is the periodic push-up to prevent ischial pressure sores. These push-ups should become an automatic, habitual routine to be done every 20 to 30 minutes. The patient should push himself up from the armrests or from the wheels so that the buttocks completely clear the seat. He should stay up, out of contact with the seat for 60 seconds (Fig. 15-4). Initially, a small timing device with a buzzer may be used to remind him to push up at regular intervals.

The second activity of importance is, of course, wheeling forward, backward and turning. Later, the patient should practice wheeling up and down ramps. Wheeling with skill is a matter of practice. Finally, he should learn to get from the locked wheelchair to a floor mat or to the floor and back into the chair. In connection with transfer to the car, he should also learn to fold and place the wheelchair into the car whether he does so when seated in the driver's seat or while he stands braced at the side of the car.

Concomitant Activities of the Wheelchair Phase.   The following activities should also be conducted during the wheelchair phase.

1. Tilt table program may be continued.
2. Bowel program: use of suppositories and commode.
3. Bladder program: use of rubber urinal for male paraplegics;

Disabling Conditions Due to Neurologic Impairment   279

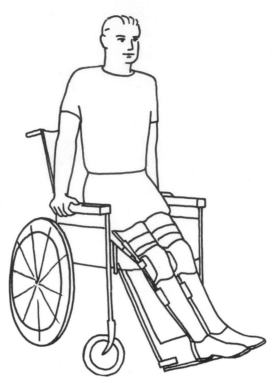

Fig. 15-4.   Wheelchair push-up.

for females, indwelling catheter with leg bag or diaper and plastic panties.

    4. Self-care activities: feeding, dressing and toilet activities from wheelchair.

    5. Ascending and descending stairs by seated push-ups.

    6. Home visits for week ends.

    7. Explanation of prognosis for sexual function.

Paraplegic Standing Phase

    The importance of the upright position was mentioned in connection with the tilt table procedure. Every paraplegic has the potentiality of getting into the upright position independently and even of ambulating with crutches if the lower extremities are braced properly. The procedures of bracing and crutch-walking are as follows:

Bracing.   Providing the patient with lower extremity braces serves several purposes. The braces help to maintain the lower extremities in position and help to control involuntary motion due to spasticity.

They permit weight-bearing transfer; they enable the patient to stand up periodically to help to prevent hip-flexion contractures and ischial pressure sores. Braced and standing in parallel bars, the patient can stretch his spastic trunk and lower extremity muscles and thus diminish spasticity. Finally, braces are needed for ambulation.

For proper support the paraplegic with a mid-dorsal lesion requires long leg braces with a pelvic band (Chap. 6). Eventually, the band may be discarded. Despite the considerable weight of these braces (10 to 15 lbs. [5 to 8 Kg.]), patients should be encouraged to wear them and carry out parallel bar exercises with braces even if they do not wish to become crutch-walkers.

Parallel Bar Exercises.   The parallel bar program replaces the tilt table for weight-bearing and upright position as soon as adaptation to standing is assured. Three types of exercises can be carried out in the parallel bars by the paraplegic patient: stretching exercises, balancing exercises and exercises to strengthen the upper extremities.

Stretching Exercises.   The purpose of the exercises is to counteract contractures and diminish spasticity. Essentially, they are a trunk hyperextension stretch and a trunk flexion stretch (Fig. 15-5A).

Balancing Exercises.   These exercises facilitate weight-bearing transfers and activities in standing position. They are a preparation to crutch-balancing and crutch-walking. While the knees and the ankles are well stabilized by the braces, the pelvis is stabilized only laterally by the pelvic band. Flexion is still possible. For balancing, it is necessary to stand with completely extended hip joints. This requires a slight dorsiflexion at the ankle and a compensatory hyperextension of the trunk so that there is continuous concavity from the heels to the occiput, and the abdomen points forward (Fig. 15-5B). Initially, these exercises are to be done with corset on; later, the corset should be discarded.

Strengthening of Upper Extremities.   This is done by push-ups with a triple maneuver: elbow extension, shoulder depression and trunk rotation around the shoulder joint to gain maximum elevation (15-5C).

Weight-bearing Transfer (described in Chap. 6).   After the knee joints of the braces have been locked, the patient gets into standing position by the push-up or pull-up method. He then pivots into the new seat. If sitting in a low chair, he may need assistance.

Concomitant Activities.   The following activities should also be conducted during the stand-up phase.

1. Self-care activities with braces: putting on long leg braces with pelvic band; dressing with long leg braces.

2. Wheelchair activities with long leg braces.

Disabling Conditions Due to Neurologic Impairment   281

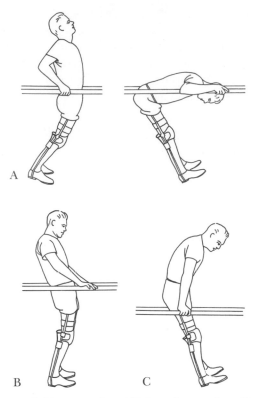

Fig. 15-5. Parallel bar exercises. (A) Stretch exercises. (*Left*) Hypertension stretch. (*Right*) Flexion stretch. (B) Balancing in parallel bars. (C) Maximum elevation push-up.

Paraplegic Crutch-Walking Phase
Crutches Versus Wheelchair. In the initial enthusiasm about rehabilitating the paraplegic, crutch-walking was considered as being essential even though for the average paraplegic with a mid-dorsal lesion it is about 8 times as strenuous as regular walking. If the lesion is high or the patient is overweight or elderly, crutch-walking becomes too strenuous to have practical value. Very frequently, paraplegics start out as enthusiastic crutch-walkers and end up using only the wheelchair and not even wearing their braces. There is no harm if a paraplegic chooses and prefers wheelchair locomotion. However, one must not conclude that a patient who will not walk does not need braces and can dispense with parallel bar exercises. As was pointed out before, these exercises are important for disuse prevention. If they are carried out properly, the patient can always become a

crutch-walker if he decides to do so. Therefore, he may be discharged from the hospital after completing the parallel bar phase.

Training in crutch-walking goes through three phases: crutch-balancing, crutch-walking and crutch elevation.

Crutch-balancing. Initially, the patient may use underarm crutches or he may begin immediately with Canadian-type forearm crutches which are the most suitable ones for the paraplegic (Fig. 15-6).

For crutch-balancing, the patient should assume the balanced stance and:

1. Elevate both crutches and replace them into the same spot.

2. Elevate both crutches and place about 12 inches (30 cm.) forward.

3. Elevate both crutches and place them 12 to 18 inches (30 to 45 cm.) behind the heels.

It may take 1 or 2 weeks to perfect this maneuver. However, when the patient can do this well, crutch-walking will be easy, and his crutch stability will be good. He should feel safe standing on crutches and be

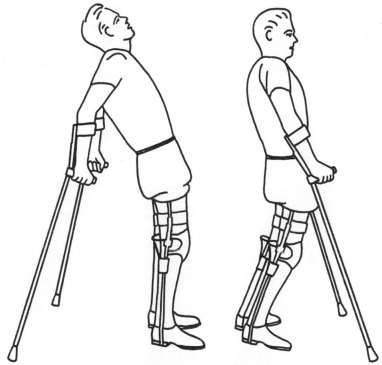

Fig. 15-6. Crutch-balancing.

Disabling Conditions Due to Neurologic Impairment 283

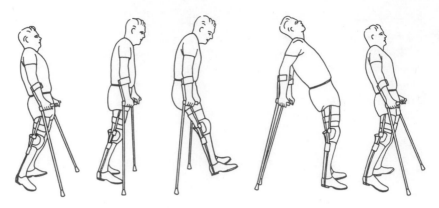

Fig. 15-7. Swing-through gait.

able to lose and recover his balance forward, backward and sideways before crutch-walking is started. He should also be able to raise one crutch briefly and replace it while balancing on the other.

Crutch-walking.   Since in a complete mid-dorsal lesion both legs are paralyzed and cannot be moved independently, the patient uses the swing-to and swing-through gaits (Chap. 6). If he is capable of good crutch-balancing, it is best to start immediately with the swing-through gait (Fig. 15-7). It consists of a forward swing with a push-up bringing the legs in front of the crutches. By arching the back the patient stands balanced with the crutches behind him. After a brief stop the crutches can be brought forward as was done in crutch-balancing. During the swing-through, considerable momentum is required. This not only carries shoulders and feet in front of the crutches but continues to carry the pelvis forward after shoulders and feet have stabilized and helps achieve the arched position.

Crutch Elevation.   This includes getting up from a chair with braces and crutches, getting up from the floor into standing position with braces and crutches and stair-climbing with braces and crutches.

Restoration of the Paraplegic to Self-care

Toilet and Dressing Activities

Difficulty with toilet and dressing stems from impairment of mobility of the paraplegic, from the need to carry out these activities in the wheelchair and from the encumbrance of appliances. Developing a fixed routine will facilitate and accelerate dressing and toilet procedures.

The paraplegic starts the day by transferring to the wheelchair completely undressed. He wheels himself into the bathroom and transfers to a wooden bench or stool in the shower. From this seat he must be able to reach the faucets and the soap so that he can take a shower in a seated position. His towel must be within reach outside the shower so that he can dry himself. After the shower he transfers back into the wheelchair and wheels himself to the washstand for shaving, grooming and oral hygiene.

Dressing is begun by putting on socks and long leg braces. With the knee joint at right angle, the thigh bands of the brace are pushed under the thigh with one hand while the other hand elevates the thigh, grasping it near the knee. The foot is then placed into the shoe, the front buckles of calf band and thigh band are closed, and the knee pad is buckled over the knee. Next, the rubber urinal is applied, and the urinal bag is attached to one calf.

Putting on undershirt and shirt is no problem, but shorts and trousers (panties for women) require a special technique. If done in the wheelchair, the patient places the opening of his shorts at the feet and pulls one leg of the shorts over each foot. The same is done with the trousers, and the trouser legs are gathered up between the shoe and the knee. Then, the paraplegic locks his braces and comes to a standing position. While holding himself with one hand (on bedpost, wall bracket or parallel bar), he pulls the trousers up with the other hand and fastens the belt. Then he sits down and finishes dressing.

If the procedure is too strenuous or if the paraplegic does not wear his braces, he can put on his shorts and trousers while lying on the bed. First, he transfers from the wheelchair to the bed. In sitting position he pulls on his shorts, then pulls the trouser legs over his feet and as high as possible. Then, he assumes a side-lying position and pulls the free half of the trouser top over his upper hip. He turns to the other side and pulls up the other half of the trouser top and buckles his belt. Putting on trousers is so complex an act that the paraplegic will use help whenever it is available. In this case, he stays in the chair, pushes himself up from the armrests, and the assistant pulls the trouser top over his hips.

Eating and Miscellaneous Activities

Since both upper extremities are intact, eating is no problem. However, the patient must wheel himself close to the table. Since the sides of a wheelchair may not fit under the table, he may have to remove them. Special desk arms are designed to fit under a desk or a table.

Of the other common activities only driving a car requires special equipment. There are several types of hand controls available.

Special Problems of the Paraplegic Patient

In addition to restoration to mobility and self-care, the paraplegic with a mid-dorsal spinal cord lesion has a number of special problems. In fact, while for the hemiplegic the most important problems are solved once he is ambulatory and self-caring, the principal problems of the paraplegic begin at this point. They are the continued regulation of bladder and bowel function (Chap. 15, Sect. D), and the prevention of contractures, urinary tract infections and stones (Chap. 2). Since these problems are dealt with in detail in other places, as indicated, the following additional problems—spasticity, pressure sores, sexual problems and psychosocial adjustment—will be discussed in this section.

Spasticity

Definition.   As was pointed out in Chapter 13, upper motoneuron lesions lead to spastic paralysis. Essentially, this means that voluntary motion is abolished while reflex function is maintained or heightened. This gives rise to a number of clinical manifestations: resistance to passive stretch that manifests itself as stiffness, involuntary reflex motions or spasms in reponse to an apparent stimulus or to a stimulus that is not obvious. The latter are called pseudospontaneous spasms. Sometimes, response to stretch triggers a rhythmic shaking called clonus. All these manifestations are grouped under the term spasticity.

In hemiplegics, spasticity has proved an asset, stabilizing the leg by the extensor reflex and supporting the upper extremity by flexor spasticity. In spastic paraplegics, spasticity may have beneficial as well as detrimental effects but frequently the latter outweigh the former.

Beneficial Effects of Spasticity.   *Disuse prevention.*   By its frequent involuntary motions, spasticity prevents muscle atrophy, osteoporosis and also pressure sores, since it causes frequent change of position and succeeds in pumping blood through compressed areas.

Maintenance of Blood Pressure.   Trunk spasticity elicited by the upright posture as a postural reflex counteracts orthostatic hypotension.

Supportive Effect.   Trunk spasticity also has a stabilizing effect and obviates the need for a body corset. At times, extensor spasticity of the lower extremities may permit a weight-bearing transfer of the unbraced patient.

Maintenance of Body Image.   The bulging and moving muscles of the patient with spastic paralysis give him a greater feeling of bodily completeness than the marked atrophy and flailness of flaccid paralysis.

Detrimental Effects of Spasticity.   From the practical standpoint, the detrimental effects outweigh the beneficial ones if the spasticity is excessive.

1. Involuntary motion may interfere with rest, normal mobility and skilled work. It also interferes with crutch-walking and causes falls. Violent contact with furniture or other objects due to spasm may cause contusions and lacerations of the lower extremities.

2. Spastic reflex resistance to passive motion interferes with mobility by causing stiffness. This may interfere with self-care, vocational activities and proper positioning and may lead to pressure sores and contractures.

3. The disuse phenomena developed with spasticity form a vicious cycle. Pressure sores, bladder infection and bed rest aggravate flexor spasticity. Persistent severe flexor spasticity of the hips and knees makes it impossible to mobilize the patient, and often he develops more pressure sores, more urinary tract infection and true flexion contractures. In such cases, drastic measures to abolish spasticity must be taken as soon as possible.

Measures to Combat Spasticity. *Preventive Measures.* Usually, excessive spasticity is caused by strong sensory stimuli from skin or viscera. When a patient complains of excessive spasticity, one should first look for such causes as pressure sores, urinary calculi or infections, and tight shoes, clothes or braces and eliminate any of these as promptly as possible. Often, excessive spasticity subsides when the offending cause is removed.

Physical Measures. Physical measures to combat spasticity are: physical activity or active exercise, passive stretching and restrictive bracing. The former two are by far the most commendable since restrictive bracing carries the danger of aggravating spasticity by sensory stimulation and by causing pressure sores. Nevertheless, while the hemiplegic is usually successfully restricted by his short leg brace, the paraplegic may be relieved from the effects of spasticity by wearing his long leg braces all day. Restrictive bracing is effective if the spasticity is not excessive.

Antispastic Drugs. At the present time there has been no satisfactory drug available to counteract spasticity in the paraplegic without adverse effect on his sensorium. During the night or for the bedridden patient with mild spasticity, drugs may be of some assistance. In severe spasticity, surgical measures may be required.

Surgical Measures. Essentially, the surgical approach to spasticity means transforming the spastic paralysis into flaccid paralysis by creating a lower motoneuron lesion. The most comprehensive approach is that of destruction of all motor fibers in the spastic portion of the body or, at least, in the lower extremities. This can be done by destroying all lumbar and sacral roots either by injection of alcohol or phenol into the subarachnoid space or by cutting all motor roots surgically (anterior rhizotomy). More selective surgical approaches to spasticity consist of cutting certain nerves or even by cutting or lengthening the tendons of certain muscles.

Pressure Sores

The pathogenesis, clinical appearance and prevention of pressure sores were discussed in Chapter 3. Frequently, a paraplegic with sensory loss develops a pressure sore despite precautions. Usually, pressure sores from lying occur in the initial phase following spinal cord injury. They are located over the sacrum, the femoral trochanters or the heels. Sitting may cause ischial pressure sores in the paraplegic who forgets to do his push-ups. Finally, pressure sores in various places may be caused by clothes or braces.

Usually, conservative treatment leads to gradual healing. Pressure or injury to the involved area must be completely avoided. Protective foam rubber pads may be indicated for certain areas; otherwise, there should be no change in the patient's program.

As soon as sloughing starts, sugar dressings should be applied as described on page 290. There may be a prolonged period of sloughing. Usually, débridement is not necessary. Daily hydrogen peroxide irrigations and sugar dressings are continued after all necrotic tissue has sloughed off. Gradual healing will occur. After the ulcer cavity has filled with granulation tissue, the surface may need touching with silver nitrate once weekly to keep the granulation below skin level.

Surgical treatment is needed in specific complications, such as abscess formation or osteomyelitis. In recurring ischial pressure sores, part of the ischial tuberosities may be removed. Plastic surgery for closure of large ulcers by skin flaps is rarely necessary. Dangers of this procedure are the complications arising from prolonged bed rest required for healing of the grafts.

Sexual Problems

The male paraplegic may have occasional, temporary erections and sometimes priapism. Frequently, however, erections are brief. Usually, orgasm occurs, but diminished sensation limits satisfaction. Male paraplegics usually are sterile, because ejaculation generally occurs into the bladder. Female paraplegics are capable of childbearing.

Psychosocial and Vocational Problems

The psychosocial and vocational rehabilitation programs must be integrated with physical rehabilitation. Timing depends on the attitude and the personality of the patient, his family, social relationships, intelligence, aptitudes and capabilities, among other things. Social case work, vocational counseling, group therapy, recreational therapy and psychotherapy may be required in varying degrees according to the problems presented by the individual patient.

In general, the program may be schematized as follows:

During the Bed Phase:
1. Orientation of the patient: information, support, assistance in acceptance of reality.
2. Orientation of family: social case work with patient and family.
3. Exploration of home conditions and vocational resources.

During the Wheelchair Phase:
1. Week-end leave for the patient for home visits.
2. Modification of the home to facilitate function.
3. Explanation as to changes in sexual function.
4. Beginning of vocational counseling.

Upright Phase:
1. Re-establishment of family and group relationships; visits home regularly on week ends.
2. Vocational retraining begun, if necessary.
3. Vocational training continued until satisfactory placement.

Other Types of Paraplegia

All of the preceding discussion of paraplegia was concerned with a patient with a complete transection of the mid-dorsal spinal cord.

Incomplete Lesions of the Spinal Cord

In cases of incomplete traumatic lesions or partial spinal cord involvement by disease, some voluntary motion of the lower extremities may be possible. In this case, the patient may not need any braces or he may need only short leg braces. He may be able to walk with 4-point and 2-point crutch gaits or even without crutches. His principal handicap may be spasticity rather than paralysis.

Lower Motoneuron Paraplegia

In flaccid paraplegia due to anterior horn cell, root or motor nerve involvement (poliomyelitis, Guillain-Barré syndrome) the patient has the advantage of retaining sensation and sphincter control. In these conditions, there is muscle atrophy and vasomotor disturbance leading to trophic changes. The management is the same as that of spastic paraplegia and frequently less difficult. These patients rarely have organic problems of urinary control or sexual activity.

Disabling Conditions Due to Neurologic Impairment 289

SUMMARY

1. Excluding additional disabilities, the rehabilitated paraplegic can live independently.

2. His method of locomotion (wheelchair or crutches) depends on the segmental level of paralysis, degree of spasticity and his own preference.

3. The crucial point of paraplegia management is not achievement of independence, which is easy, but prevention of pressure sores and urinary tract complications.

TREATMENT OF PRESSURE SORES WITH SUGAR DRESSING

1. Cleanse ulcerated area by irrigation with a syringe using full-strength, hydrogen peroxide solution.
2. Position the part so that the ulcer is horizontal.
3. Fill the ulcer to the skin margin with granulated sugar.
4. Cover the area generously with gauze or a perforated dressing.
5. Seal the edges with tape, preferably with wide transparent plastic tape.
6. Apply additional gauze or pad to absorb drainage.
7. Change dressing daily.

Section B. Quadriplegia

Definition. Quadriplegia or tetraplegia is paralysis of all four extremities. It includes the trunk and sometimes the neck. Paralysis of each extremity may be complete or partial, but all four extremities must show some paralytic involvement if the condition is characterized as quadriplegia. If all four extremities have become paretic or paralyzed by two separate attacks of hemiplegia, we speak of bilateral hemiplegia rather than quadriplegia.

CAUSES OF QUADRIPLEGIA

Upper motoneuron quadriplegia may be the result of:

1. Transverse lesions of the cervical spinal cord (e.g., traumatic transection).

2. Advanced degenerative disease involving the corticospinal tracts (e.g., multiple sclerosis).

3. Bilateral brain damage involving both corticospinal tracts (e.g., brain stem hemorrhage).

Lower motoneuron quadriplegia may be caued by:

1. Anterior horn cell disease (e.g., acute anterior poliomyelitis or progressive muscular atrophy).

2. Spinal root or nerve involvement (e.g., Guillain-Barré syndrome or polyneuropathy).

Muscular quadriplegia may be caused by:

1. Widespread disease of muscles (e.g., muscular dystrophy).

2. Defects of neuromuscular transmission (e.g., myasthenia gravis).

PROGNOSIS

Recovery or Progression of Paralysis

1. The quadriplegia may remain essentially stationary (e.g. complete traumatic transection of the cervical spinal cord).

2. There may be gradual recovery from quadriplegia (e.g. contusion of the cervical spinal cord or Guillain-Barré syndrome).

3. There may be gradual progression of the quadriplegia (e.g. multiple sclerosis or progressive muscular atrophy).

Functional Prognosis of the Quadriplegic Patient

This varies with the degree or completeness of paralysis. It is worst if, in addition to trunk, neck and extremity paralysis, there is also paralysis of the diaphragm and all the muscles innervated by cranial nerves. The motor functions of the patient may be almost nil. This means that he will need mechanical assistance for breathing and require feeding through a nasogastric tube. He will have practically no means of communication. Fortunately, such horrible disability is extremely rare. However, patients have survived whose only motor function during the early phase of convalescence was the ability to open and close the eyes, which made possible some means of communication. If all cranial nerves are intact, at least the patient will be able to speak, swallow and move his neck. This gives him the possibility of managing mouth-activated devices that may lead to an unexpected number of useful functions. The functional prognosis of a patient with a transverse section of the spinal cord at the 6th cervical segment will be described in detail. As more function of the upper extremity is preserved, the functional prognosis approaches that of the paraplegic patient with a high spinal cord lesion.

REHABILITATION TECHNIQUES FOR THE
QUADRIPLEGIC PATIENT

Introduction

Of course, details of the rehabilitation program depend on the potential functional abilty of the quadriplegic patient. It was pointed out that this varies greatly. Even if involvement of the cranial and the respiratory nerves is excluded, the variations of functional potential are still much greater than those of the paraplegic because of the different grades of involvement of the upper extremities. Appliances for upper extremities have been devised that can harness the power of a single muscle or make use of a single motion to enable the patient to carry out a useful function. In order to provide the appropriate device for the patient and to enable him to use it, close cooperation of orthotists, nurses, therapists and physicians is required. Sometimes, surgical procedures may be helpful in increasing the function in the upper extremities with or without the use of appliances.

In order to describe the standard rehabilitation procedure for quadriplegic patients, the management of a specific quadriplegic is described. A transverse lesion of the cervical spinal cord at the C-5 or C-6 segment is not uncommon, and the rehabilitation of this type of spinal cord injury gives a fairly typical picture of the problems of the quadriplegic. Following this presentation, the rehabilitation problems of a more involved patient will be mentioned briefly.

Rehabilitation of a Patient with Traumatic Transverse Section of the Spinal Cord at the C-6 or C-7 Level

General Plan

A transverse section of the cervical spinal cord occurs in fractures or fracture dislocations of the cervical vertebrae. Two common causes of such fractures are automobile accidents and injuries that occur by diving into shallow water. Patients with such lesions initially have flaccid paralysis and gradually develop spasticity similar to that of spinal cord injuries at the thoracic level. Often, surgical exploration of the area is done shortly after injury, in an endeavor to relieve compression or remove bone fragments from the spinal cord. At times, prognosis may not warrant exploration. In either case, the neck will be immobilized by a brace, by plaster of Paris or by traction for a certain length of time. All too frequently the spinal cord is transected completely at the time of injury, and subsequent measures have no effect on neurologic recovery. At times, however, the initial injury may have caused only a contusion to the spinal cord, and the patient may recover nearly complete neurologic function. In this case, no rehabilitation is needed. Therefore, discussion will be limited to permanent complete transection of the spinal cord at the C-6 or C-7 segment.

It should be noted that injury to the cervical spine above the C-4 segment paralyzes the diaphragm and leads to death from asphyxia since artificial respiration usually is not immediately available. Any lesion below C-7 spares the upper extremity and causes paraplegia instead of quadriplegia. Therefore, the segmental margin in which quadriplegia occurs from spinal cord injury is rather narrow, involving only 3 segments, namely, C-5, C-6 and C-7. The patient with a transverse section at the level of C-6 has preservation of full shoulder motion and elbow flexion. He loses the ability to straighten the elbow and has complete paralysis of the wrist and the fingers. If the lesion is one segment lower, he will have preserved the ability to hyperextend his wrist.

In fracture or dislocation of a cervical vertebra, not only is the spinal cord damaged but also the nerve roots at this level. Therefore, the lesions may result in slightly different disabilities in the two arms depending on the degree of root damage. Except for the presence of the above-mentioned motions in the upper extremities, a patient with a transection of the spinal cord at the cervical level has complete paralysis of trunk, lower extremities, bladder and bowel.

The functional prognosis of such a patient is as follows:

1. Usually, he can learn to feed himself with a special feeding splint.

2. He will be able to perform some dressing and bathing activities.

3. He will be able to wheel his wheelchair if it has a special rim with projections.

4. He will be able to have his upper extremity function enhanced by appliances which will be described later.

Therefore, the patient with such a disability can never be entirely independent and thus needs an attendant at least part of the time. His rehabilitation will involve a bed phase and a wheelchair phase. The upright position will not be of functional value, but the quadriplegic should be placed in the upright position on a tilt table or a standing board for change of position and recreational and metabolic purposes.

Restoration to Mobility

Bed Phase. After the injury, the patient with quadriplegia commonly receives his initial care on a surgical ward or neurosurgical unit. Surgical exploration and débridement may be carried out with efforts at fixation of the fracture. Immobilization of the neck by traction or brace may have been prescribed and ordered to be maintained for a number of weeks. If such immobilization is necessary, a brace or a cast is preferable to traction, in our opinion, since they do not restrict the mobility of the whole patient as much as traction does. Let us assume that the bone injury is minor and requires no special attention and that the patient is transferred immediately to a rehabilitation service. Although the injured person may have potential for neurologic recovery, it is best to proceed with the rehabilitation program as if no recovery were to be expected.

Preventive Measures.   During the bed phase, the patient is exposed to two great dangers of secondary disabilities, namely, the formation of pressure sores and the occurrence of urinary tract infection. With present knowledge and technique, pressure sores can be prevented entirely, but not without meticulous, expert and time-consuming nursing, medical and rehabilitation care. During the bed phase, the danger areas for pressure sores are the lower back and the hips. Methods of positioning and turning are described in Chapter 15, Sect. A. The quadriplegic is best handled on the CircOlectric bed. This bed has advantages over the Stryker frame, since it allows positioning not only in the face-lying and back-lying positions but also in side-lying and semireclining positions.

The care related to the paralyzed bladder is described in detail later in this chapter. Initially, the patient is likely to have a flaccid bladder that will retain a very large amount of urine and become distended. Then, urine will be squeezed out of the bladder by pressure, causing incontinence of overflow. It is not desirable to allow the bladder to be distended to that extent. Therefore, the patient should either be catheterized at regular intervals or be provided with an indwelling catheter. After several weeks, the bladder will become spastic. Then, it will empty automatically but will still present the dangers of reflux into the ureters, residual urine in the bladder and urinary tract infection, all to be discussed in more detail.

Special Problems.   A special problem of the patient with a cervical spinal cord injury is the so-called mass reflex. This is a reflex connected with the emptying of the automatic bladder. There is simultaneous spasm of muscles of the extremities and frequently an attack of sweating and hypertension. The latter may lead to severe headache. Even in the presence of an indwelling catheter a mass reflex may be produced by the slightest catheter obstruction and create considerable discomfort for the patient.

Another special problem of the patient with a cervical spinal cord injury is that of heat regulation. Normally, the body is cooled by radiation when the outside temperature is below 70° F. and by sweating, that is, by the evaporation of sweat, when the outside temperature rises above 70° F. This reflex sweating in response to outside temperature is abolished in the patient with a complete transverse cervical spinal cord lesion. Therefore, on a warm summer day, these patients may develop high temperatures, not because of infection or illness but simply because of their inability to cool off by sweating. Frequently, these patients will try to cool themselves by drinking excessive amounts of water. If the physician and the nurse are aware of the deficit in heat regulation, they will cover the patient with a moist sheet and have a fan blow against it to reduce the body temperature and compensate for the loss of sweating function. It is both pointless and hazardous to treat this type of temperature elevation at random by antibiotics, and there is serious danger of water intoxication if the patient is allowed to drink as much as he pleases.

Wheelchair Phase.   Since wheelchair locomotion is the final goal of the complete quadriplegic, wheeling should be initiated as soon as possible. The quadriplegic has four problems in relation to wheelchair activities, resulting in handicaps that the paraplegic does not have. They are: (1) problems of blood pressure regulation, (2) problems of transfer, (3) problems of wheeling, (4) problems of push-up to prevent ischial pressure sores.

Problems of Blood Pressure Regulation.   It will be recalled that the patient with a cervical spinal cord lesion has more problems with visceral nerve phenomena during the bed phase than the patient with a dorsal thoracic spinal cord lesion. This is due to the fact that the level of his lesion is above the highest level of the sympathetic prevertebral sympathetic chain. By virtue of this, the sympathetic outflow is separated entirely from the regulatory centers in the brain stem and in the brain. Therefore, problems of heat regulation are encountered, and for similar reasons a problem of blood pressure regulation occurs. This manifests itself particularly when the patient is changed from a lying to a sitting position.

Gravity will tend to draw the blood toward the lower portions of the body, causing lack of blood supply in the brain. Normally, this is counteracted by muscular contraction of the blood vesels in the abdomen and the lower extremities. However, this reflex contraction is abolished or diminished in spinal cord quadriplegics, and the results are a sudden drop in blood pressure and fainting. Several measures are used to prevent the accumulation of blood in the lower extremities during the sitting or upright position. These are: (1) bandaging of the lower extremities with elastic bandages, (2) application of a scultetus binder to the abdomen as tightly as possible, (3) the use of full-length body corset drawn very tightly over the lower abdomen. In addition to these mechanical measures to prevent the accumulation of blood in the lower portion of the body, there is the physiologic method of very gradual adaptation to the upright position.

An aggravating circumstance is the initial complete flaccidity of the patient's abdominal muscles which may also be responsible, in part, for fall of blood pressure in the upright position. The hazard of hypotension tends to diminish once the patient becomes spastic. Since it is desirable to get the patient into the wheelchair as quickly as possible in order to accelerate rehabilitation, it is best to provide him immediately with a full-length canvas body corset (Fig. 15-3). This is not only useful in blood pressure regulation in the upright position but also for trunk stabilization, since there is complete flaccid paralysis.

Gradual adaptation to the upright position can be achieved by use of the tilt table or by positioning in the CircOlectric or other tilting bed or by using a reclining or semireclining wheelchair. The initial steps of elevation of posture must be taken with a blood pressure cuff on the arm for frequent determinations. It is imperative to be alert to a fall of blood pressure and to lower the patient to a horizontal position at the slightest indication of fainting; otherwise, he may suffer permanent brain damage from impairment of blood supply. Therefore, the gradual shift from the recumbent to the upright position is a rather delicate and dangerous procedure for the quadriplegic patient. As soon as he tolerates the semireclining or sitting position in bed without fainting or discomfort or tolerates standing on a tilt table at about 60 degrees without fall of blood pressure, he is ready to start wheelchair activity.

Problems of Transfer.   Unassisted transfer is extremely difficult for the quadriplegic patient for the following reasons:

1. Since both legs are paralyzed, he is not able to carry out weight-bearing transfer unless the lower extremities are braced. Even with braced lower extremities, the quadriplegic does not have adequate upper extremity function to lock and unlock the braces and to pull himself up to standing position while being stiff-legged. However, it is relatively easy for an attendant to assist a stiff-legged, braced quadriplegic in weight-bearing transfer by pulling him up to a standing position, pivoting him and letting him down to the new seat. For this reason, long leg braces are sometimes used with quadriplegic patients for the sole purpose of facilitating assisted transfer.

2. Because of paralysis of elbow extension, the quadriplegic lacks

push-up power for non-weight-bearing transfer, and because of paralysis of finger flexors he lacks pull-up power. Some patients obtain push-up power by shoulder depression. Other are able to grab an overhead sling, using the flexed elbow as a hook. Even for these athletes a fixed and accurate arrangement of the areas of support may be present. Therefore, in their own specially set up quarters they may be able to carry out unassisted transfers but cannot transfer independently to just any chair, toilet, car or other seat.

Problems of Wheeling.   Since the quadriplegic cannot grasp the rim of the wheel and has no leg power to propel his wheelchair, a rim with projections must be provided to allow him to hook his wrist behind the projections and push the wheel around by simultaneous elbow and shoulder flexion (Fig. 15-8). Backward wheeling can be achieved by locking the elbow and pushing down on a projection at the hind part of the rim (Fig. 15-9). It has become more common to provide the quadriplegic with a battery-powered electric wheelchair (Fig. 15-10). This offers an advantage for traveling longer distances but is not needed inside a home.

Problems of Push-ups.   In order to avoid the development of ischial pressure sores, quadriplegic and paraplegic patients must relieve the pressure on the ischium at intervals. This is best done by a push-up until all weight has been taken off the buttocks, maintaining this position for 60 seconds. Such push-ups should be repeated every ½ hour.

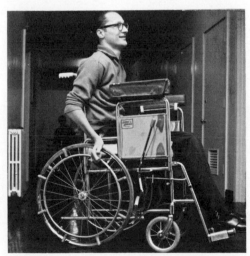

Fig. 15-8. Forward wheeling by quadriplegic patient using hand rim with projections.

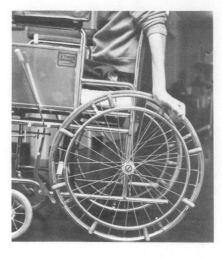

Fig. 15-9. Backward wheeling by patient with quadriplegia.

In view of the weakness of elbow extension, the quadriplegic is not able to carry out the push-up in the same fashion as the paraplegic. Possibly, he may lock his elbows and lift himself by shoulder depression, but this is very strenuous and may injure the elbow joints. A more satisfactory method is the push-up with elbow support. In order to permit such a push-up, the armrests on the wheelchair must be

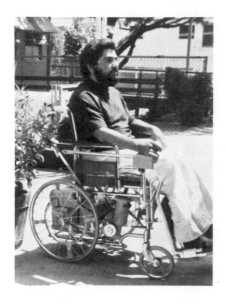

Fig. 15-10. Standard electric-powered wheelchair.

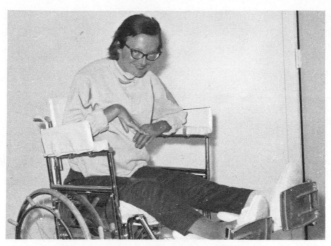

Fig. 15-11. Elevated armrests with rims.

higher than usual and must be provided with an outer rim to prevent the elbows from slipping off (Fig. 15-11). The patient takes the weight on the elbows and puts his head far forward, pivoting his body weight around the shoulders (Fig. 15-12). Thus, he is able to relieve pressure on the buttocks without great strain. As an additional safeguard,

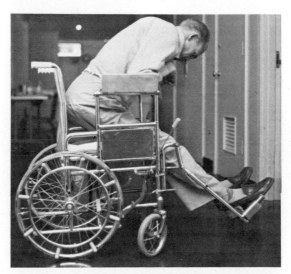

Fig. 15-12. Elbow push-up by quadriplegic patient to relieve pressure on buttocks.

Disabling Conditions Due to Neurologic Impairment 299

paraplegic and quadriplegic patients should use air cushions or sponge rubber pads on wheelchair seats. We have achieved the best decubitus prevention with cushions containing foam rubber, water and air.

Self-Care of the Quadriplegic Patient

Since self-care activities, such as feeding, dressing, washing and so forth, are essentially carried out with the upper extremities, the quadriplegic patient without any hand function appears to be particularly handicapped. However, with the help of three types of appliances, the patient may carry out a considerable number of activities. The three appliances to facilitate upper extremity function are:

1. A wrist-and-hand splint with a special clamp to hold a desired gadget (Fig. 15-13)

2. A terminal grasping device attached to a wrist splint (Handihook) and activated by a cable which is controlled by shoulder motion (Fig. 15-14)

3. A special splint (useful only for those patients who have maintained the ability to hyperextend the wrist) that embraces the thumb on one side and the index and middle fingers on the opposing side and is activated in such a way that dropping of the wrist by gravity opens the grip between the thumb and the fingers, while hyperex-

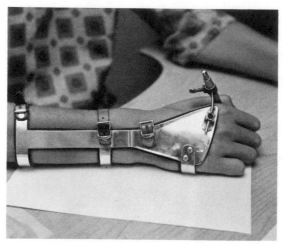

Fig. 15-13. Splint, showing attached pencil. Other objects or implements can be similarly attached.

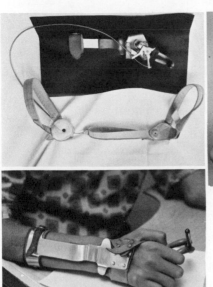

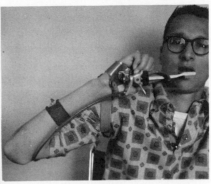

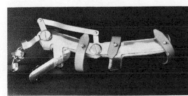

Fig. 15-14. *(Left, top)* Handihook, showing shoulder straps and cable-activated clamp (hook). *(Left, bottom)* Handihook used for holding a pencil. *(Right)* Handihook used for holding a toothbrush.

tending the wrist by the action of available muscle closes the thumb against the fingers, thus permitting the patient to grip (tenodesis splint) (Fig. 15-15).

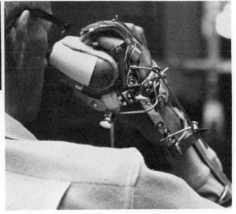

Fig. 15-15. *(Left)* Tenodesis splint. When the wrist is hyperextended, the thumb and the forefingers are approximated. Flexion, caused by gravity, releases the grasp. *(Right)* Tenodesis splint in use.

Rehabilitation of a Patient with Complete Quadriplegia

While, in the spinal cord, quadriplegic function above C-6 or C-7 is preserved and used for rehabilitation, a patient with complete quadriplegia may have no usable motor function at all. Complete quadriplegia occurs in brain injuries where the quadriplegia is spastic and in lower motoneuron diseases i.e., Guillain-Barré, progressive muscular atrophy, poliomyelitis) where the paralysis is flaccid. The rehabilitation of these patients is essentially based on the use of assistive devices.

A hypothetical case is described to convince the reader that even extensive paralysis may permit some degree of self-care and functional ability if rehabilitation is carried out with the appropriate equipment in a supportive environment and with patience and imagination. Let us assume that the paralyzed patient has preservation of function of the neck and the face, including the mouth, and slight flexor power in the right index finger. All the rest of his body musculature is completely paralyzed. What can he do?

Obviously, this patient is not able to feed, dress or bathe himself. He needs nursing care for these simple functions. If a bottle with drinking tube is stationed within his reach, neck mobility will permit him to take fluids whenever he wishes without having to call a nurse or an attendant. He may be set up with a reading rack and a book and turn the pages with a mouth wand that he can take from a nearby mouth wand stand and replace without having to disturb anyone. He can also use an automatic page-turner activated by a switch that he can

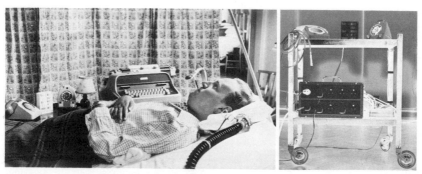

Fig. 15-16. *(Left)* Although he was paralyzed by poliomyelitis, this patient can carry on his business as a stockbroker. He is shown here using the Mark I, a British invention which enables him to telephone, type, operate a TV set, radio, light and bell by sucking and puffing on the tube in his mouth. (Photograph by John Jackson; copyright by the Polio Research Fund at Stoke Mandeville Hospital, England.) *(Right)* The "Breath of Life Machine."

operate with the only remaining function of the index finger. In fact, by using this index finger the patient can operate a micro-switch that sets in motion apparatus to subserve many purposes by means of an electronic device called a multicontroller. By putting different signals into the machine, that is, by pushing the button 1, 2 or 3 times or by giving a short signal and a long signal, he may turn on many appliances in his room and around him. He may turn the lights in the room on and off; he may draw or open the curtains; he may turn the radio or television set on or off; he may signal the operator on the telephone. The power of a single finger is almost limitless, thanks to modern electronics. A general purpose control device activated by the force of a breath (Fig. 15-16) was first developed in England.* There are now many variations of this principle.

SUMMARY

The quadriplegic patient rarely can achieve independence and usually requires attendant care.

His self-care ability varies from complete helplessness to complete self-care according to the extent of upper extremity involvement.

Most patients with transverse lesions of the cervical spinal cord can feed themselves by means of appliances and can wheel their chairs.

Progress in electronic controls, in upper extremity bracing and in surgical procedures for restoration of function serves constantly to improve the lot of the severely paralyzed and enables many of them to lead useful lives despite their considerable handicaps.

Like the paraplegic, the quadriplegic is subject to pressure sores and urinary tract complications.

Section C. Bulbar and Respiratory Paralysis

The term "bulbar paralysis" is a clinical designation for a variety of disorders that occur from transient or permanent pathology of the pontomedullary portion of the brain stem. Fortunately, it is possible to characterize the disorders resulting from pathologic lesions of this part of the brain stem without having to refer to the complex mechanisms of pathophysiology that are involved. Stated in the simplest way possible, the two phenomena with which clinicians and nurses are frequently concerned are disorders of respiration and of

*Kitchin, C. H.: The breath of life machine, pp. 73-75, Harpers, November, 1962.

swallowing, both of which depend on extremely intricate neuromuscular systems.

The kinds of disturbances encountered in clinical medicine which are grouped generally as bulbar paralyses are: disturbances in the rhythm, the depth, the rate and the effectiveness of respiration; paralysis of the vocal cords and related structures; partial or complete paralyses of the pharynx and the esophagus; paralysis of the palate; impairment of tongue motion; and many vasomotor visceral disturbances resulting from disorders of sympathetic and vagal innervation or visceral centers in the medulla. Disturbances of respiratory function are by all odds the most important threats to life.

The pathologic lesion causing central respiratory paralysis need not be located in the special centers in the medulla that control respiratory drive. Rhythm and depth of respiration may be disturbed by lesions elsewhere in the central nervous system or by abnormal pressure within the subarachnoid space. Lesions of the cervical motor nerve cells in the anterior horns or their axons interrupt neural pathways to the diaphragm, the most important muscle of respiration. Lesions producing lower motoneuron paralysis of the chest, the neck and especially of the abdominal muscles may also cause serious impairment of breathing function. The wide variety of pathogenesis of respiratory impairment deserves detailed consideration, but for the purposes of this chapter the impairments due to lesions of the medullary respiratory centers and those due to lesions of the motor cells of the spinal cord will be considered concurrently, since they have much in common from the standpoints of disability and management.

CAUSES OF BULBAR AND RESPIRATORY PARALYSIS

Anterior Horn Cell Disease

The bulbar nuclei of the cranial nerves are the equivalent of the anterior horn cells in the spinal cord. They may be involved in progressive muscular atrophy, amyotrophic lateral sclerosis and poliomyelitis.

Guillain-Barré Syndrome and Neuropathies

While not involving the nuclei within the central nervous system or the motor nerve cells of the spinal cord, the poorly understood Guillain-Barré syndrome is characterized pathologically by lesions of the motor roots and motor axons and leads to paralysis very similar to that of poliomyelitis. Frequently, the paralysis starts in lower extremities and progresses gradually upward within hours or days to involve respiratory muscles. This progression is characteristic of Landry's ascending paralysis, now thought to be the same disease as Guillain-Barré syndrome.

Toxic neuropathies also may cause respiratory paralysis, for example, thallium poisoning, botulism or curare poisoning. The neuromyopathy due to tetanus toxin may cause death from hypertonicity of respiratory muscles, which can halt breathing as effectively as paralysis.

Bulbar Lesions

The region under consideration is very vulnerable in the event of hemorrhage, injury or tumor since this portion of the brain stem is inaccessible to surgery and too confined to allow adequate expansion for tissue survival when the pathologic process is accompanied by swelling or growth of the lesion.

Pseudobulbar Palsy

It is important to differentiate between paralyses and other defects due to involvement of pontomedullary areas and pseudobulbar palsy which is a result of cortical or subcortical lesions, usually in association with hemiplegia. Usually, pseudobulbar palsy results from multiple small areas of arteriosclerotic damage in the cerebrum. Either the cortex or pathways leading from the cortex to the bulbar centers may be involved.

The clinical manifestations usually are disturbances in motion of the tongue, the muscles of mastication, the swallowing muscles and the apparatus for phonation. Often, chewing, swallowing and speaking are impaired. Palatal motions may be sluggish; the muscles of the mouth may be relaxed, and the mouth may remain partially open; food is poorly moved about in the chewing process and often escapes from the mouth; excessive salivation may occur. The facial expression is masklike, with open drooling mouth, and is most pathetic in appearance. The vocal cords are not involved in pseudobulbar palsy, and rarely is there any threat to life. Prognosis depends on the nature and the course of the underlying disease.

MANAGEMENT OF THE PATIENT WITH BULBAR AND RESPIRATORY PARALYSIS

Often, patients with pontobulbar disorders are transferred to rehabilitation facilities as soon as their prognosis for survival is established. In order to treat them successfully, knowledge of the pathophysiology of pontobulbar lesions is essential. Furthermore, clinical management of these disorders involves techniques applicable to seemingly quite unrelated syndromes. For example, the problems of an adequate airway, of artificial respiration, of tracheobronchial drainage and of nasogastric feeding—all of these, which are of extreme importance in treatment of the pontobulbar paralytic, may also be essential in the management of individuals who have suffered severe cerebral vascular accidents, brain and cord injuries, lesions of the upper airway, myasthenia gravis or respiratory failure of any type.

For the purposes of this manual, less emphasis will be placed on disease entities than on clinical observations leading to diagnosis and determination of disability. The methods of management that will assure survival and make rehabilitation possible will then be discussed. Necessarily, management of acute manifestations will have to be considered since acute crises in respiration and other vital functions may occur in the course of rehabilitation and require immediate care. Some patients treated in acute care facilities before transfer for rehabilitation must continue to receive respiratory assistance, special feeding and careful medical supervision in addition to rehabilitative therapy. Clinical observations made periodically during the diagnostic phase of treatment have to be continued throughout the rehabilitation phase in order to determine if and when respiratory assistance can be withdrawn and to what extent exercise or other modalities may be used to improve unassisted function.

Diagnostic Observations

A patient suspected of having a pontobulbar or an upper spinal lesion should be observed closely and frequently to determine:

Rate, Depth and, Particularly, Rhythm of Breathing. Intervals of apnea or variability in depth of breathing, especially total irregularity, strongly suggest involvement of respiratory centers.

Adequacy of Breathing. This is reliably determinable only by objective tests. Even the experienced clinician can be misled by seeing apparently vigorous respiratory motions which, when subjected to measurement of air flow, are found to be inadequate. If the hospital or institution where such a patient is observed does not have a respirometer or one of the respiratory meters now available, there will almost certainly be a basal metabolism machine that can be used to measure tidal volume and vital capacity. The soda lime container can be removed from the apparatus for the measurement of a few breaths and for determination of vital capacity. Graphic recording of breathing not only affords an opportunity to determine whether there is adequate air exchange but also detects irregularity of rhythm that usually occurs with lesions of the respiratory center. To test for disturbances of rhythm, the soda lime canister should not be removed.

If breathing is regular and even if tidal volume seems normal, the vital capacity observation is extremely important since it provides a rough index of respiratory sufficiency. On the basis of many observations in patients with poliomyelitis, it has been determined that patients whose vital capacity falls below 50 per cent of predicted normal, and certainly those with values below 35 per cent, must receive respiratory assistance to prevent exhaustion and eventual failure.

Reference should be made to the nomograms for predicted vital capacity and tidal air (Figs. 15-17 and 15-18). It should be emphasized that the tidal air values are useful only for rough regulation of pressures and breathing rates of mechanical respiratory equipment to maintain adequate air flow. Except when tidal volume is extremely low, one cannot rely on its measurement in determining adequacy of breathing. For this purpose, the vital capacity is very meaningful when it can be determined. Vital capacity tests are impossible in the

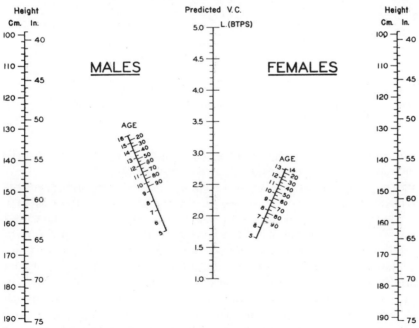

Fig. 15-17. Vital capacity nomogram. (After Collier, C. R., Ferris, B. G., Jr., and Affeldt, J. E.)

Disabling Conditions Due to Neurologic Impairment 307

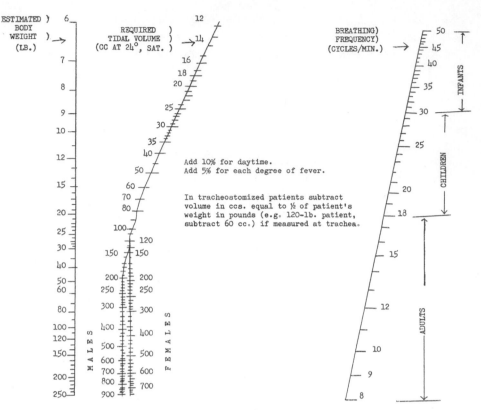

Fig. 15-18. Nomogram for determination of tidal air in tank respirator: required tidal volume vs. body weight and breathing frequency. (After Radford, E. P., Jr.: Appl. Physiol. 7:451.)

unconscious. Here, as in many severe pulmonary disorders, arterial blood analyses are required.

Patency of Airway. The vocal cords receive their nerve supply from the vagus nerves. If disease or injury destroy or impair a vagus nucleus on one side of the medulla or disrupt the recurrent laryngeal nerve, unilateral paralysis of the larynx ensues. Paralysis of the vocal cords or of a cord may be suspected if a flaccid soft palate (glossopharyngeal paralysis) is observed, if the voice has a nasal resonance and if there is gross wheezing in expiration. Listening to air flow by placing a stethoscope over the mouth is sometimes informative. If there is a question of bilateral flaccidity of the vocal cords, direct observation is essential. This is best performed by or in company with an anesthesiologist or laryngologist who is prepared to insert a cuffed endotracheal tube that can be used as artificial airway until a decision is made about the advisability of tracheostomy.

Paralysis of both vocal cords is a very infrequent cause of airway obstruction. It has been observed, however, in Guillain-Barré syndrome as well as in viral infections of the central nervous system. The commonest cause is the accumulation of secretions in the trachea. Undoubtedly, secretion is increased during the stress of respiratory impairment. Motor weakness associated with neurologic disease makes cough ineffective. Sitting patients up in bed when they have respiratory difficulty, a maneuver commonly used because it is helpful in cardiac dyspnea, causes secretions to accumulate in the tracheobronchial tree, and the common back-lying position also imposes mechanical obstruction since the major bronchi are then directed downhill.

Sometimes, secretions can be expelled if the patient is turned face down and "cupped." Manual respiratory assistance or back pounding sometimes helps. Accumulation of secretion may in itself be a sufficient indication for tracheostomy.

Palatopharyngeal and Esophageal Function

Paralysis of the palate is manifested by outflow of fluid through the nose when swallowing is attempted. Complete pharyngeal and esophageal paralysis makes swallowing impossible. When these manifestations of paralysis are suspected, swallowing tests should be made under radiographic control. An aspirating apparatus should be at hand to remove material from the upper airway if swallowing is grossly impaired. Usually, semisolid or solid food is handled more easily than liquid by a weak pharynx, but the danger of airway obstruction is greater.

Swallowing difficulty may be transient or prolonged. In either case, a nasogastric tube should be passed whether or not food is to be administered by this route. Even if intravenous fluid is used to sustain the patient during acute illness, the tube should remain in place to aspirate gastric secretion and prevent esophageal reflux with overflow of fluids and aspiration into the larynx. Especially when respiratory paralysis is suspected and an artificial airway is being considered, the stomach should be intubated and evacuated. Whenever a patient is intubated or a tracheal tube is installed, a soft cuff should be used and inflated to prevent or diminish aspiration of food into the lungs regardless of whether it is needed for respiratory purposes.

Other Visceral Phenomena

Clues concerning the extent of involvement of pontobulbar centers can be derived from observing the heart rate (vagal disease tends to increase the rate), disturbances of sense of taste, impairment of tongue motion and sensation and, rarely, unilateral disturbances of sweating. These observations, of course, apply to the conscious patient. In severe stupor or coma, pupillary changes, oculomotor phenomena and other reflexes are important. Usually when there is severe coma and evidence of a bulbar lesion, the prognosis is very grave.[4]

Acute Phase Treatment

The prognosis for rehabilitation as well as for survival depends on the skill and the wisdom shown in management of the acute and emergency phase of bulbar or bulbospinal disease. Accuracy of medical observation is essential, judgment is required about timing of emergency measures, and skill is required not only in the use of pharmaceutical, mechanical and other devices to save life, but also in providing reassurance and security that mitigate against the extreme psychobiologic damage that often persists throughout the life of seriously threatened individuals.

Obvious lack of confidence and self-assurance on the part of the physician and his staff, delay in the use of artificial respiration, failure to recognize the gravity of airway obstruction and other common errors of management may precipitate critical hormonal crises and acute anxieties that become more formidable problems than the organic disease as such. These warning statements are interposed in order to alert physicians and nurses to the magnitude of the emergency of critical respiratory problems.

There are numerous reports of the psychobiologic cataclysms that can follow mismanagement. These have been described as "hyposthenuric syndrome" or severe reactions to stress. Survival following near-asphyxia or threat of death may be accompanied by a syndrome of Cushingoid facies, acute acne or seborrheic dermatitis, hypertension, impaired ability of the kidneys to concentrate urine (hyposthenuria), exquisite hyperalgesia and extreme fear and anxiety. While this full-blown syndrome is seen only rarely and usually in young adults, various elements of it are frequently noted among patients of all ages, and hypertension or seborrhea, for example, may persist throughout life as stigmata of a frightful experience.

The Airway

Airway problems may occur in unconscious patients as well as in those with disease of the pontobulbar area of the brain. Tracheobronchial drainage should be promoted by using the face-down position and by careful aspiration of secretions from the oral and nasal pharynx. If these measures fail, the following indications for tracheostomy must be considered:

1. *Obvious impairment of the airway:* cyanosis, stridor or air hunger. These signs are already evidence of clinical neglect and are inexcusable in a patient who has been under observation. They are reasonable criteria only among patients to whom medical care has been inaccessible.

2. *Accumulation of secretions* that cannot be expectorated or swallowed. Usually, this is associated with palatopharyngeal weakness; it may be necessary to choose between frequent mechanical aspiration of secretions and tracheostomy to prevent asphyxia.

3. *Evidence of regurgitation and aspiration* of foodstuff or fluid into the lungs due to paralysis of the pharynx and the esophagus. Tracheostomy and cuffing of the tube are essential to prevent continued aspiration and infection of the lungs.

4. *Falling vital capacity,* especially in association with fulminating disease and clouding of consciousness. Change of mood or loss of orientation may be a very significant warning. Often, this is mistakenly thought to be due to cerebral involvement in nervous system infection.

5. *Vocal cord paralysis or spasm* manifested by marked change of quality of speech, expiratory stridor, and observable flaccidity of the cords.

6. *Constellation of symptoms,* suggesting severe pontobulbar disease, such as progressive impairment and irregularity of breathing, pulmonary edema, or other critical respiratory problems, especially if associated with swallowing dysfunction.

The technique and management of tracheostomy will be found in Chapter 17 (pp. 432-439).

Section D. Bladder and Bowel Paralysis

The bladder and the bowel are internal organs. As such, they are innervated by visceral (sympathetic and parasympathetic) nerves that mediate automatic function. However, in addition to autonomic innervation, the bladder and the bowel have sensory and voluntary motor nerve supply. Evacuation is influenced by conscious sensory awareness and voluntary sphincter control.

BOWEL FUNCTION IN NEUROLOGIC IMPAIRMENT

Normal Function

The contents of the bowel are propelled by peristalsis, the wavelike intestinal muscle contractions. When fecal matter reaches the rectum, it is stored there until defecation occurs. Rectal musculature is stimulated by distention with feces and is also subject to neural influences from the upper intestinal tract. Its contents may then be expelled reflexly, as occurs in infants. This occurs in many adults with impaired innervation. When nerve connections and neurologic function are intact, fecal expulsion can be postponed by voluntary inhibition of the reflex.

The rectum can then be emptied voluntarily at the appropriate time and place by relaxation of sphincter and contraction of abdominal and pelvic muscles. The sphincter, a circular muscle at the anal end of the rectum, maintains a continuously closed orifice until it is relaxed voluntarily.

Effect of Paralysis on Bowel Function

In the majority of neurogenic impairments of the bowel by spastic paralysis, flaccid paralysis or sensory loss, usually it is possible to regain bowel control through appropriate training. Since the bowel musculature has its own nerve centers within the intestinal wall, usually it is not affected greatly by damage to upper and lower motoneurons. In certain conditions, the bowel itself may become paralyzed at least temporarily (so-called paralytic ileus), but this is rarely the case in the impairments discussed here. Therefore, peristalsis is present or can be stimulated despite somatic paralysis.

The disabilities that occur in neurologic conditions are loss or impairment of: (1) sensation of fullness and awareness of evacuation of the rectum, (2) sphincter control, i.e., ability to inhibit or facilitate evacuation, (3) strength to produce intra-abdominal pressure and to expel the contents of the rectum. The latter results from paralysis of abdominal and pelvic muscles. Despite these three disabilities, evacuation of feces is possible by peristalsis provided the stool is soft. The objectives in restoring bowel function are to produce a soft stool, to maintain sufficient peristalsis to expel it and to have this occur at the desired time. The measures to accomplish these goals are called, rather inappropriately, "bowel training."

Bowel Management in Paralysis (Paraplegia)

A. *To obtain soft consistency of feces*
1. Diet: fluids freely, including fruit juices
2. Medications: stool softeners, wetting agents, no laxatives

B. *To maintain peristalsis*
1. Diet: adequate (See Chap. 2.)
2. Medications: bulk producers, e.g., methylcellulose; peristalsis stimulators: Dulcolax suppositories; avoid laxatives.

C. *To time evacuation*
1. Habit formation: use toilet at same time every day or every other day, preferably after breakfast, to take advantage of reflex stimulation. Conditioned reflex is established.
2. Initiation of bowel movement by patient. In upper motoneuron paralysis, devices such as a push-up and forward leaning or stroking the abdominal skin may aid emptying.
3. Initiation of bowel movement by suppository. A glycerin or Dulcolax suppository is placed in the rectum after breakfast. Evacuation occurs within 20 minutes to 1 hour. It is important to insert the suppository well beyond the internal anal sphincter, in contact with mucosa. If one suppository is ineffectual, two may be used, the first one to be inserted before breakfast, the second immediately after breakfast. Experience is needed to determine the interval between use of suppository and time to sit on the commode or toilet. For morale purposes, it is important to avoid soiling by too long a delay.

Complications of Bowel Paralysis

A. *Constipation and fecal impaction*
1. Symptoms: constipation may produce only vague discomfort. Often, impaction is followed by passage of ribbonlike stools or semiliquid discharge.
2. Management: the rectum should be examined with a gloved finger if impaction is suspected. The fecal mass must be broken up manually and removed by enemata. The occurrence of impaction is an indication of an inadequate bowel program.

B. *Fecal incontinence*
1. Causes: rarely, complete impairment of rectal and sphincter tone. Usually, incontinence is due to use, or overuse, of laxatives, excessive stimulant foods or poorly carried out bowel training.
2. Management: review program. Psychological aspects may need careful study. Persistence in bowel program, under confident supervision, usually is successful.

Disabling Conditions Due to Neurologic Impairment   313

BLADDER FUNCTION IN NEUROLOGIC IMPAIRMENT

Normal Function

Like the rectum, the bladder is under dual nervous control. The empty bladder fills slowly with urine conveyed from the kidney to the bladder by the ureters. Once the adult bladder has filled to approximately 500 ml., an emptying reflex is triggered. This reflex causes a contraction of the muscle inside the bladder wall which, if uninhibited, will force the urine out through the urethra until the bladder is completely empty. In the infant, this type of bladder emptying occurs automatically. In the adult, it is possible to inhibit the emptying reflex, at least for a certain length of time. As the bladder becomes more and more filled, the pressure becomes painful until the individual is unable to inhibit the emptying reflex, and the bladder then empties completely. As in the bowel, the bladder outlet, also called the bladder neck, is occluded by a circular muscle, the sphincter of the urethra. The external portion of the sphincter is under voluntary control. Unlike the bowel, when there is neurologic involvement of the bladder, control is *not* readily regained. In fact, bladder function is very sensitive to even slight degrees of neurologic impairment, and disturbances of urinary control may sometimes be the first signs of certain neurologic conditions.

Neurogenic Impairment of Bladder Function

Basically, there are two kinds of neurogenic impairment of the bladder: those in which the emptying reflex is abolished or diminished and those in which the emptying reflex is present or exaggerated, but voluntary control is lost.

Areflexic Bladder

If reflex function is abolished, the bladder continues to fill until it becomes greatly distended. The bladder muscle does not contract forcefully at any time. For this reason, the areflexic bladder is also called atonic or flaccid. This areflexia may be caused by injury to the motor branch of the reflex arc, as would occur in lower motoneuron disease, or by injuries to the sensory branch of the reflex arc, as occurs, for example, in tabes dorsalis and combined sclerosis. Areflexia also occurs immediately after spinal cord injury and may last for several weeks; however, reflex function returns eventually. Therefore, patients with spinal cord injuries at first have an areflexic or flaccid bladder and later develop a reflex or spastic bladder.

The clinical result of bladder areflexia is marked distention of the bladder that continues until urine is squeezed out through the sphincter by increased abdominal pressure. When the pressure reaches a breakthrough point, small amounts of urine dribble frequently from the urethra as the bladder continues to fill. This has been called overflow incontinence. Often, sensory loss accompanies the areflexic bladder so the patient does not become uncomfortable. In time, excessive distention damages the bladder musculature, the stagnant urine readily becomes infected, and the kidneys are ultimately endangered by back pressure of urine.

A patient with an areflexic bladder may sometimes be able to empty it satisfactorily by making pressure over the suprapubic area with both fists, the so-called Credé method. However, this does not always result in complete emptying, and the patient would be better advised to catheterize himself or be catheterized twice or more times daily. At times, one must resort to an indwelling catheter in order to permit complete emptying of the bladder.

The Automatic Bladder

In patients with transverse lesions of the spinal cord, the pathways for inhibition of the bladder reflex are interrupted and frequently, also, conscious sensation of bladder fullness is lost. However, since the reflex arc is intact, this bladder will contract once a certain degree of filling, approximately 500 ml., is reached and will then empty spontaneously and completely.

From the clinical standpoint, the patient with a spinal cord injury may have a bladder with ideal automatic function. In this case his essential handicap is due to the uncertainty of the emptying time of his bladder. Some paraplegics have a forewarning of urination time as the bladder fills completely, and they succeed often in developing methods of eliciting an emptying reflex. Pinching the thigh, pulling the thigh or the pubic hair or other stimuli are at times effective in initiating bladder contraction. However, once started, there is no way to inhibit reflex emptying and, therefore, the paraplegic has a relatively short time in which to reach a toilet after receiving a warning signal. He must be at a toilet or have a receptacle ready when he uses external stimuli. For all practical purposes, the paraplegic needs continuous protection against incontinence. The male paraplegic is well served by a rubber or plastic sheath into which the penis is inserted, and the urine flows through a tube into a rubber or plastic bag attached to the legs (Figs. 15-19 and 15-20). The bag must be emptied periodically to avoid overflow. For the female paraplegic there is no

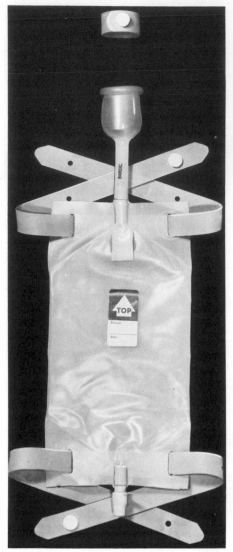
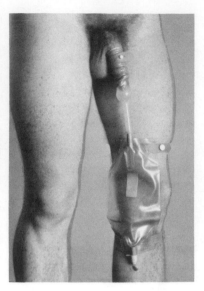

Fig. 15-19. Plastic sheath and bag for incontinent male. When used on patients with sensory defects, especially paraplegics and quadriplegics with spinal cord injuries, elastic adhesive should be substituted for the rubber strap supplied by the manufacturer. The rubber strap around the shaft of the penis may produce pressure sore. It is imperative to use elastic or ordinary adhesive tape to secure the sheath to the penis. (C. R. Bard, Inc.)

way to install a leak-proof attachment, and she must either wear a special type of diaper panties (Fig. 15-21) or use an indwelling catheter that empties into a bag urinal attached to the leg or wheelchair.

Many patients with spastic bladder do not have ideal automatic emptying. Often, they develop complications of the reflex mechanism. In upper motoneuron involvement, the reflex activity

Rehabilitation of Patients with Specific Disabilities

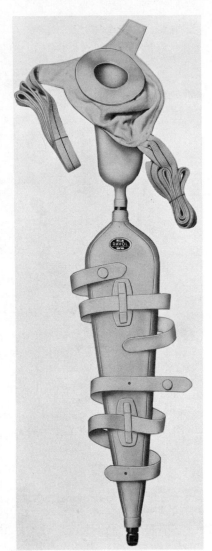

Fig. 15-20. Rubber incontinent appliance for males. This device is held in place by the ties which are placed around the lower trunk. The rubber appliance is somewhat more cumbersome than the plastic but has the advantage of not requiring a snug fit around the penis. Devices for incontinence must be selected on the basis of individual requirements and according to each patient's preference. (Davol Rubber Co.)

usually is hyperactive and somewhat incoordinated. After the emptying reflex is initiated and the bladder is emptied halfway, the sphincter may close suddenly, and residual urine remain in the bladder. In this way spasticity of the sphincter causes retention of urine that is an excellent culture medium for bacteria. When the spastic bladder muscle contracts while the sphincter does not open, the increased pres-

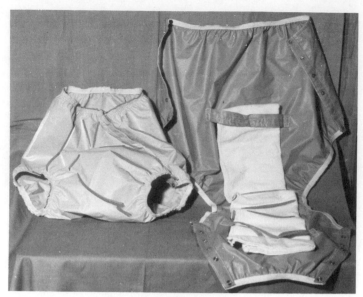

Fig. 15-21. Diaper panties.

sure causes structural changes of the bladder wall that lead to destruction of the valvelike orifices of the ureters. If this dissociation of muscle function persists, there will be a reflux of urine into the ureter and eventually to the kidney pelvis. Each time the bladder contracts this force will widen the ureter, put pressure on the kidney, cause infection to extend from the bladder to the kidney and finally destroy it.

Another reflex disturbance that occurs especially in quadriplegics, as was previously mentioned, is the mass reflex that leads to widespread spastic contraction, or rigor, as well as sweating, hypertension and severe headache each time the bladder empties.

While the patient with the ideal automatic bladder usually is better off than one with an areflexic bladder, this is not true for those who have very spastic bladders with residual urine, ureteral reflux or distressing mass reflex. Therefore, it is sometimes advisable to transform an automatic bladder into an areflexic bladder by section of the sacral nerve roots leading to the bladder or by destroying them chemically by injection of alcohol or phenol. Certainly, this is the best treatment for the uncontrollable mass reflex in the quadriplegic patient. For more conservative management of reflux and residual urine, the use of an indwelling catheter may be indicated.

Complications of the Neurogenic Bladder

In addition to the complications mentioned previously that are inherent in the areflexic or hyperreflexic bladder, both types of neurogenic bladder are subject to infection and to stone formation.

Bladder Stones

The pathogenesis of stones in the urinary tract has been discussed in Chapters 2 and 3. The same basic chemical and metabolic phenomena underlie formation of kidney, ureteral and bladder stones. However, the latter often are attributable principally to poor catheter management. The indwelling catheter has a small bag attached to it that is inflated inside the bladder to prevent the catheter from slipping out. Often, a thin shell of calcium salts deposits around the bag at the tip of the catheter. If the bladder is not irrigated properly and the catheter is not changed frequently, this shell may become large enough to slip off the catheter and remain in the bladder when the catheter is changed. More calcium is then deposited around it, and eventually a fist-sized bladder stone may develop. This stone reduces the capacity of the bladder, irritates the bladder mucosa and favors chronic, irremediable bladder infection.

Urinary Tract Infection

Infection of the urinary tract is the greatest and the most threatening problem of the patient with a neurogenic bladder. The causes leading to intractable bladder infection are multiple. The introduction of a foreign body that occurs during catheterization and especially the permanent maintenance of the foreign body in the bladder in the form of an indwelling catheter, invariably introduces bacteria. Normally, the sterility of the bladder is maintained by constant dilution with fresh urine and periodic complete emptying. The presence of residual urine creates a stagnant culture medium that leads to chronic infection. Residual urine as well as reflux are likely to extend the infection to the kidney pelves, causing at first acute and later chronic pyelonephritis. While the infection may initially respond to antibiotics or other antimicrobial medications, the invading bacteria soon become resistant to antibiotics, and persistent chronic infection of the urinary tract results. Certain bacteria, by their metabolism of urea, tend to make the urine alkaline which, in turn, favors stone formation in both the bladder and the kidneys. Stone formation in turn favors the maintenance of chronic infection of the kidney pelvis, which may lead to final destruction of the organ. Renal failure is a major cause of death of patients with neurologic impairment of the bladder.

Evaluation of the Neurogenic Bladder

The patient with neurogenic bladder impairment may complain of a variety of symptoms: he may have urinary retention or incontinence, urgency or frequency; he may complain of suprapubic pain and have bouts of chills and fever. The patient who wears an indwelling catheter or a rubber urinal frequently has no complaints at all, but his life may, nevertheless, be in jeopardy because stone formation and infection are destroying his kidneys.

Laboratory studies are essential to determine renal and bladder status. The levels of blood urea nitrogen or creatinine should be checked periodically, and cystography and intravenous urography should be carried out from time to time. Nurses can contribute a great deal in evaluating the state of the bladder. Recording the frequency and amount of voided urine in patients who have some voluntary control may provide the first indication of trouble. The measurement of residual urine, determined according to the method described below, should be done repeatedly for several days during the evaluation period to ascertain whether or not the presumably emptied bladder retains urine. Finally, the determination of bladder capacity, as also described below, is very helpful in the evaluation of bladder dysfunction. A bladder capable of holding over 500 or 600 ml. of slowly introduced fluid is probably an areflexic, atonic bladder, while a bladder holding 200 ml. or less is usually a small contracted bladder. Frequently, fibrous contraction is the end-result of maintaining continuous gravity drainage of the spastic bladder by means of an indwelling catheter. Usually, the automatic bladder will fill to about 300 to 500 ml. and then contract strongly, expelling urine around the catheter.

A more elaborate means of determining the state of reflex function of the bladder is cystometry, a method that records the intravesical pressure in response to the amount of fluid contained in the bladder. However, for most practical purposes, the information obtained by testing bladder capacity is adequate, and one can dispense with cystometry.

Method of Measuring Residual Urine

Equipment.   Catheter tray with appropriate urethral catheter; collecting vessel and graduate cylinder, 1000 ml.

Technique.   The patient voids, emptying the bladder as completely as possible without external pressure on the bladder. Immediately thereafter, the catheter is passed and the bladder is emptied of any urine that may still be present. This urine is collected, measured, and the quantity is recorded as "residual urine."

Method of Measuring Bladder Capacity

Equipment. Catheter tray with appropriate catheter, preferably Foley type; Kelly flask, 1000 ml. capacity, with connecting tubing, sterilized; clamp for tubing; collecting vessel and 500 ml. graduate cylinder; sterile normal saline solution or other isotonic solution suitable for bladder installation, 1000 ml.

Technique. The following procedures should be used to determine the bladder capacity.

1. Pass catheter with usual aseptic precautions.

2. Attach Kelly flask containing 1000 ml. irrigating solution to the catheter.

3. With the lower end of the Kelly flask held 12 inches (30 cm.) above the body level of the recumbent patient, open the tubing clamp to allow the fluid to run slowly into the bladder until flow ceases.

4. Read off the volume of fluid on the Kelly flask and record the amount that has flowed into the bladder.

5. Clamp off the catheter and disconnect the tubing.

6. Open the catheter and drain all of the bladder contents into a collecting vessel.

7. Measure the fluid drained from the bladder and record as "bladder capacity." The value should check closely with the measured inflow.

In the ambulatory patient without catheter, the amount of urine voided after maximum voluntary inhibition of emptying reflex gives a fair indication of bladder capacity.

In the patient with indwelling catheter, the amount of urine voided after the catheter has been clamped off to point of tolerance is also an indication of bladder capacity. This test should not be undertaken without close medical supervision in the case of an atonic bladder.

Management of the Neurogenic Bladder

The means of dealing with areflexic and spastic bladders have been indicated above. The following is an outline summary:

A. Routine management of flaccid bladder

    1. Indwelling catheter on continuous drainage or

    2. Catheterization every 8 hours, minimally twice daily

B. Routine management of automatic bladder

    1. In men: external urinal

    2. In women: diapers and plastic panties or indwelling catheter

C. Residual urine. Catheterize at least twice daily.

D. Urinary tract infection

    1. Eliminate indwelling catheter if possible.

    2. Catheterize to remove residual urine (see above).

3. Use acidifying agents (ammonium chloride in gelatin capsules, *not* enteric coated; calcium mandelate) in sufficiently large doses to maintain urine pH below 6.0, testing all urine specimens for pH.

4. Use specific antibiotics to treat acute episodes of urinary tract infection (fever, chills, etc.) after identifying and determining drug sensitivity of organisms.

E. Ureteral reflux

1. Maintain indwelling catheter to assure bladder emptying.

2. Transform spastic bladder into flaccid bladder by surgical interruption of motoneural pathways.

Some surgical procedures such as the use of a suprapubic catheter or an ileal bladder are used by some in the management of neurogenic bladders. In our opinion they are rarely indicated.

INCONTINENCE IN THE ELDERLY AND THE CHRONICALLY ILL, NOT DUE TO NEUROLOGIC IMPAIRMENT OF THE BLADDER AND THE BOWEL

Differential Diagnosis and Evaluation

While this section is concerned with disorders causing organic involvement of visceral innervation of the bladder and the bowel, it is important to interject a brief discussion of problems often mistakenly attributed to neurologic impairment. Functional disorder of the bladder and the bowel is much more frequent than organic disorder. Loss of urinary control, constipation, impaction and bowel incontinence are often preoccupations of nursing staff in chronic illness hospitals and institutions for the elderly. Sometimes, these problems are inevitable in the mentally impaired, but they occur much more frequently as a result of mismanagement based on inadequate understanding of the physiology of elimination.

Therefore, it is important to differentiate between incontinence due to atonic or spastic bladder or loss of voluntary control of bladder and bowel due to sensory defect, and incontinence that is induced by circumstances having little to do with the nervous system or the viscera as such. The wet and soiled bed that is still too often the stigma of the chronic illness ward is due to habituation of patients to a way of life that is either a manifestation of neglect or a lack of interest due to boredom and frustration. The *most common cause* for this type of incontinence among the bedfast *is delay in responding to their calls for the bedpan or urinal.* Antedating this cause are the many factors that may lead to unnecessary bed rest, including failure of instruction in and stimulation of self-care. Routine ward care, especially scheduled bedpan service aimed at efficiency rather than satisfying patient needs, is often the direct cause of incontinence. In some institutions it has led to the use of a linen changing routine with what amounts to overt encouragement of incontinence. Repeated delay or disregard of patient calls for bedpan or commode are contributory causes of general deterioration. The ultimate consequences of dejection and depersonalization due to neglect are indistinguishable from the passivity, hostility or infantilism of patients with organic brain damage.

In order to differentiate between organic disorders of bladder and bowel function and those induced by poor or negligent care, it is essential to know the basic physiology of these organs as outlined at the beginning of this section. Patients with hemiplegia, arthritis, hip fracture, lower extremity amputations, cardiopulmonary disabilities and many other chronic non-neurologic disorders who comprise the great majority of patients in nursing homes and chronic illness hospitals do *not* have sensory or motor defects of the bladder and the bowel. They may have impairments of memory, orientation or perceptive acuity due to cerebral arteriosclerosis or other incidental causes, but the anatomic components for normal physiologic function of the bladder and the bowel are preserved. These are the all too frequently incontinent patients, many of them permanently dependent on indwelling catheters. Their fate can be changed sharply for the better by application of very simple methods once one understands the causes of their difficulties. Studies of rehabilitation potential among nursing home occupants have shown that it is not special measures of treatment that are necessary. All that is needed for many patients is opportunity to get out of bed, to be able to move about the institution and to have a chance to go to the toilet whenever it is necessary to do so.

Management of the Potentially Incontinent Disabled Patient

The following points merit special emphasis:

1. Adequacy of intake of fluid and bulk, to provide bowel content of sufficient quantity and proper consistency for evacuation, and for adequate urinary output.

2. Avoidance of preoccupation with elimination by discontinuing repeated inquiry about bowel movements. Busy patients and busy nurses can dispense with much of the discussion of elimination that is now often routine.

3. Stimulation of normal bowel action by exercise and activity.

4. Development of bowel habit by taking advantage of postprandial peristaltic activity, regularly at the same time of day, use of suppositories to initiate defecation during the early phase of bowel training, use of the commode instead of the bedpan and assurance of privacy during elimination.

5. Avoidance of delay. Delay is prevented most easily if the patient is independent of nursing assistance. If he can go to the toilet or commode, if he can reach his bedpan or urinal and cleanse himself, there is no opportunity for delay. The problem may merely be suitable arrangement of the patient's space and facilities. If the patient is not independent and if his mental status makes it impossible for him to signal adequately, he should be provided with the bedpan or urinal at frequent intervals. If he can signal, his request for service should be answered at once—not when it is convenient to do so.

6. Avoidance of conflict. The disgruntled patient, frustrated by his disability, irritated by disparaging remarks, subjected to casual and dependency-fostering nursing care and delay in service, often uses one of the few forms of aggression at his command to express his hostility. His repeated soiling of bed linen has an obvious connotation.

Management of the Convalescent Patient with an Indwelling Catheter
When the Catheter is Required

1. The catheter should be changed every 5 to 10 days according to the ease and effectiveness of irrigation in preventing sludge.

2. The bladder should be gently irrigated daily with 0.5 per cent acetic acid, normal saline or other prescribed sterile isotonic, preferably weakly acid solutions.

3. The urine should be examined periodically, and sediment smears should be stained to determine the bacterial flora present.

4. During acute illness, it may be necessary to use an indwelling catheter, sometimes solely for the purpose of accurate measurement of output. In the unconscious patient there may be temporary loss of reflex emptying, and good nursing care may require use of the catheter. This temporary resort to the catheter involves the calculated risk of infection.

Preparation for Removal of Catheter

1. Culture urine, determine bacterial invaders and their sensitivities to antimicrobial drugs.

2. Determine and record bladder capacity.

3. Remove catheter.

After Removal of Catheter
1. Record urine output and time of voiding.
2. Observe for signs of urinary retention and catheterize twice daily, if necessary, until spontaneous voiding resumes.
3. Test for residual urine; determine need for additional catheterization. (This decision is the responsibility of the physician.)
4. Help establish inhibition of emptying and incontinent urination by scheduled offer of bedpan, commode, urinal or visit to toilet. Expedite self-care and exercise program. Encourage ordinary dress. Often, patients are continent when wearing clothes but incontinent in hospital garments. Dignity, enhanced by accepted ways of dressing and relating to other persons, is a strong deterrent of infantile behavior such as wetting one's clothing.

SUMMARY

1. An understanding of normal physiology of the bladder and the bowel is essential to evaluation and management of neurologically impaired elimination.
2. Bowel training requires consistency and patient use of a well-planned, well-scheduled program.
3. The bladder must be managed according to the neurologic disturbance. Complications of bladder paralysis are stone formation and infection.
4. Incontinence that commonly occurs in the chronically ill and the disabled is often due to other than neurologic causes. This incontinence can be prevented and treated effectively when its pathogenesis is understood.

REFERENCES

1. Abramson, A. S.: "Exercise in Paraplegia," in Licht, S.: Therapeutic Exercise, 2nd Ed. New Haven: Elizabeth Licht, 1965.
2. Bors, E. and Comarr, A. E.: Neurological Urology. Baltimore: University Park Press, 1971.
3. Fitzpatrich, W. F.: "Sexual Function in the Paraplegic Patient." Arch. Phys. Med. & Rehab., 55:221, 1974.
4. Plum, F. and Posner, J. B.: The Diagnosis of Stupor and Coma, 2nd Ed. Philadelphia: F. A. Davis Co., 1972.
5. Souther, S. G., Carr, S. D. and Vistnes, L. M.: "Wheelchair Cushions to Reduce Pressure Under Bony Prominences." Arch. Phys. Med. & Rehab., 55:460, 1974.

16

Disabling Conditions Due to Musculoskeletal Impairment

Section A. Chronic Arthritis

Arthritis is defined as inflammation of a joint (or joints). If the inflammation persists or recurs over a prolonged period (years), the arthritis is chronic. Examples of chronic arthritis are rheumatoid arthritis, osteoarthritis and gouty arthritis.

STRUCTURE AND FUNCTION OF JOINTS

Joints are hinges that permit motion between two segments of bone (Fig. 16-1). To assure freedom of motion, the opposing bony surfaces are covered with a smooth but strong layer of cartilage, and they are bathed by a lubricant called synovial fluid. In order to contain the fluid the joint is surrounded by a fibrous capsule. The inner lining of the capsule is smooth synovial membrane that secretes the synovial fluid.

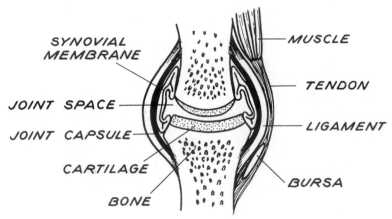

Fig. 16-1. Diagram of normal joint.

Stability of joints for weight-bearing and carrying loads is provided by the surrounding ligaments and by tendons inserted near the joint surfaces. Friction of tendons and ligaments is minimized by the smoothness of the tendons, some of which are surrounded by special sheaths filled with synovial fluid and also by interposition of flattened sacs or bursae containing synovial fluid. Often, these periarticular structures become involved in chronic arthritis. They may also be inflamed independently and cause interference with joint function.

In arthritis, the importance of joint mobility for overall function depends on the location of the involved joint. Immobility of the wrists and the ankles in good position is a relatively minor handicap. However, immobility of the hips interferes considerably with walking, and immobility of all fingers eliminates fine hand functions. By means of surgery it is sometimes possible to improve general function or relieve pain by immobilizing a joint by fusion of the two bony segments in a position that permits useful function. It is also possible at times to restore mobility to a joint that has become fused as a result of disease. This procedure is called arthroplasty.

TYPES OF CHRONIC JOINT INVOLVEMENT

The two most common types of chronic joint involvement are rheumatoid arthritis and osteoarthritis.

Rheumatoid Arthritis

Rheumatoid arthritis is by far the most disabling of all forms of chronic joint disease and therefore will be given special consideration in this chapter. Rheumatoid arthritis may occur from early childhood to old age. It may involve one, several or all joints, and the degree of joint involvement may vary from mild pain and swelling to complete destruction. The cause of the disease is not known, although many hypotheses as to its origin have been formulated.

Local Pathology.   For proper management and rehabilitation of patients with rheumatoid arthritis, it is necessary to visualize the condition of each joint. The pathologic process goes through several stages (Fig. 16-2). First, there is inflammation of the synovial membrane with or without secretion of excess fluid into the joint space. During the second stage, the synovial membrane proliferates and thickens. This thickening and the presence of fluid are responsible for swelling of the joint. During these two stages there is usually pain and frequently redness and heat of the joint tissues.

To this point the pathologic process is reversible, and the joint

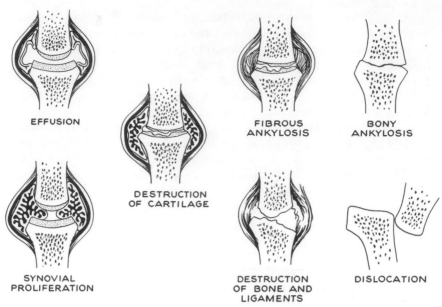

Fig. 16-2.   Pathologic changes in rheumatoid arthritis.

may become completely normal following remission. However, during the next stage the synovial membrane grows over the cartilaginous surfaces and destroys the cartilage. At this point, the x-ray picture may show narrowing of the joint space. Irreparable damage has been done to the joint, since the cartilage will not be replaced. Further progression causes destruction of the bony surfaces in contact with each other, leading to loosening of capsular and ligamentous structures. During the final stage, if the joint has been kept immobile, the bony surfaces may grow together, a process called ankylosis, or they may be separated from each other by muscular pull leading to dislocation.

When such anatomic damage has occurred, *use of the joint* can cause additional damage. The proliferated synovial membrane may be pinched, causing acute attacks of swelling and pain. Further erosion of the roughened joint surface by movement and crushing of softened bone by pressure adds to the destructive process. On the other hand, *lack of use* because of pain or immobilization leads to atrophy of the surrounding muscles, osteoporosis of the adjoining bones and limitation of joint range of motion by contracture.

An understanding of the pathologic process in rheumatoid arthritis leads to the conclusion that random immobilization and random exercise are equally detrimental in their effects. Activities of daily living without protection of involved joints are rarely good exercise for the arthritic. A specific management for each joint has to be considered according to its stage of involvement.

General Pathology. Rheumatoid arthritis is a disease with systemic manifestations, i.e., febrile episodes, elevated sedimentation rate, anemia and involvement of other organs such as the uveal coat of the eye, e.g., iritis, and rarely, the lungs and the valves of the heart. However, there is no known systemic medication that will arrest the disease. Systemic medications are symptomatic for pain relief or suppression of inflammation. Drugs may be valuable adjuncts in rehabilitation but cannot by themselves prevent disability.

The disease may follow a completely erratic course. It may involve one or many joints once or repeatedly without reaching the stage of cartilage destruction and may subside eventually without residual damage. One form of rheumatoid arthritis, namely, *rheumatoid spondylitis* or *Marie Strümpell disease,* may involve only the apophysial joints of the spine that eventually become fused completely. However, at times, bilateral hip and shoulder arthritis may occur in this disease. In the peripheral form, the limbs are involved while the spine and the hips are frequently spared. In the most severe form, both the spine and the extremities may be involved. Complete ankylosis of almost every joint, usually with marked deformity, is the final consequence of such severe disease.

Osteoarthritis (osteoarthrosis)

The pathogenesis of osteoarthritis is understood fairly well although some controversy still exists. Osteoarthritis is essentially a disorder of mechanical origin, and the pathologic changes that occur at the joint are reactions to the physical stress of weight-bearing and motions. While the intact normal joint can tolerate a considerable amount of movement and stress without producing any reaction in bone or cartilage, a slight alteration of joint structures due to a single trauma or to repeated minor injuries often leads to irritation and secondary reactions. Elderly persons, who have decreased elasticity of ligaments, muscles, joint capsules and intra-articular structures are very vulnerable to minor injury. Osteoarthritis occurs most commonly in the joints that are subject to repeated trauma and heavy loads. The cervical and lumbar vertebral joints and the knees are especially vulnerable because they are very mobile in most activities and subject to injury. Sometimes, a slight irregularity of the joint due to congenital defect or to injury may initiate changes that lead to osteoarthritis.

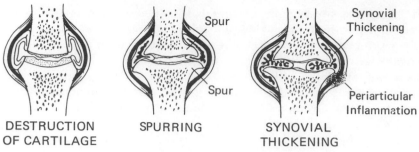

Fig. 16-3. Pathologic changes in osteoarthritis.

Frequently, this seems to be the case in osteoarthritis of the hip (malum coxae senilis). Since osteoarthritis is not primarily an inflammatory disease, the suffix -osis is sometimes used instead of -itis. Osteoarthritis of the spine has been called *spondylosis* and osteoarthritis of the hips, *coxarthrosis*. Osteoarthritis, unlike rheumatoid arthritis, is not a systemic disease.

The local pathology of osteoarthritis differs from that of rheumatoid arthritis (Fig. 16-3). The synovial membrane is not primarily involved, but the initial changes occur in the cartilage. There is erosion of cartilage and loosening of ligaments, leading to a slight degree of joint instability. This abnormal functional status leads secondarily to thickening and spurring of bone. In the third phase, the irritative effect of the moving spurs and of irregular motions in an unstable joint lead to irritation of the surrounding soft tissues. The inflammatory response to such irritation tends to subside when the joint is put at rest.

The initial pathologic changes in cartilage and ligaments in osteoarthritis are influenced by the following factors: (1) old age, because wear and tear has been of longer duration, and the structures are less elastic, (2) acute injury to the joint, causing alteration of the mechanical structure (the resulting osteoarthritis is then called traumatic arthritis) and (3) congenital defects in joint configuration that lead most commonly to osteoarthritis of the hips in late adult life.

The most disabling forms of osteoarthritis are those involving the hips, the knees and the spine. The latter, particularly in the cervical region, may also lead to neurologic disabilities (see Chap. 13). The traumatic arthritides that follow acute joint injury and the changes that develop in certain neurologic disorders causing sensory defect, e.g., Charcot joint of tabes dorsalis, are variants of osteoarthritis. Since pronounced mechanical derangements occur in rheumatoid arthritis, it is inevitable that osteoarthritic reactions will be found also in rheumatoid arthritis. Sometimes, the arthritis is designated as combined rheumatoid arthritis and osteoarthritis, although the joints may not show the typical spurring because of osteoporosis and inactivity of the parts. Older patients with rheumatoid arthritis also will show osteoarthritic changes in joints that were spared by the rheumatoid disease.

Other Types of Chronic Joint Involvement

All other forms of arthritis are overshadowed by rheumatoid arthritis and osteoarthritis as causes of morbidity and disability. *Chronic gouty arthritis* occurs in some patients, with the systemic disturbanace of uric acid metabolism called gout. Originally, the joint pathology consists of small deposits of urates in bone or soft tissue near the joint surface. These deposits may break through the cartilage and cause damage, which is then aggravated by joint activity.

A group of inflammatory diseases related to rheumatoid arthritis and called *collagen system diseases* also may cause chronic joint involvement. In disseminated lupus erythematosus, the joint manifestations are indistinguishable from early rheumatoid arthritis. Dermatomyositis is an acute collagen system disease with skin and subcutaneous tissue inflammation, muscle pain and joint manifestations. Scleroderma causes hardening and loss of elasticity of skin and other soft tissues and may lead to severe limitations of joint motion.

Some blood disorders such as hemophilia and leukemia may cause chronic joint disturbances. Finally, we should again mention the periarticular manifestations that are very common and frequently complicate chronic arthritis. These are periarthritis, bursitis, tendinitis and tenosynovitis.

DISABILITIES CAUSED BY CHRONIC JOINT INVOLVEMENT

The variety of disabilities caused by rheumatoid arthritis is so great it encompasses the whole spectrum of joint impairments of any cause. Therefore, it is possible to limit this discussion to the effects of rheumatoid arthritis. Other joint disorders may cause some but not all of the disabilities that can result from rheumatoid disease.

Widespread rheumatoid arthritis causes severe disability in all motor activities. Unlike progressive neurologic disorders and vascular disorders of the nervous system, rheumatoid arthritis does not cause organic mental or sensory impairment. Therefore, patients with the disease usually are responsive to and are able to participate in rehabilitative procedures. On the other hand, severe pain or wide-spread joint involvement may deprive them of the advantage of an uninvolved portion of the body, the principal resource in other disabilities. The principal disabilities of rheumatoid arthritis are *pain, muscular weakness* and *disturbances of joint function.*

Pain

Pain is the most common and most disabling complaint of patients with chronic arthritis. Pain may be present in or near the affected joints or it may be more generalized and difficult to relate to a particular joint. Pain may be experienced while the patient is at rest; it may be produced and aggravated by voluntary as well as passive motion. Even touch and pressure may cause pain in certain areas. Pain may be controlled to some extent by analgesic medications.

In rheumatoid arthritis it is often assumed that all of the pain is due to the rheumatoid process. However, the patient with longstanding rheumatoid arthritis may have pain produced by other causes, some of which may be secondary to the rheumatoid process. Pain may be due to the disease, to the secondary effects of treatment or to causes entirely unrelated to rheumatoid arthritis. In the list below, the causes of pain in rheumatoid and other chronic arthritides are classified according to the structure in which the pain is produced.

CAUSES OF PAIN IN CHRONIC ARTHRITIS

Articular pain
  Joint inflammation
    Rheumatoid arthritis
    Osteoarthritis
    Traumatic arthritis
  Mechanical joint disturbance
    Joint instability
    Irregularity of joint surfaces
Periarticular pain
  Bursitis
  Tendinitis
  Tenosynovitis
  Capsular tear

Bone pain
  Osteoporosis
  Compression fractures
Muscle pain
  Postural strain
  "Charley horse"
Skin pain
  Fibrositis or panniculitis
Nerve pain
  Root irritation (as in spondylitis or spondylosis

Muscular Weakness

Muscle weakness is a common disability of rheumatoid arthritis. It may have several causes, many or all of which may be active at the same time. True weakness and atrophy of muscle are produced by disuse (Chap. 3). Strong muscular contractions, essential to maintain strength, are inhibited by pain or joint derangements, and thus disuse atrophy of muscle results. At the same time, there is impairment of function greater than is accountable by muscle atrophy, because pain and joint disturbances also interfere with voluntary motion. The presence of this pseudoweakness explains the apparent recovery of strength after medication when actually only pain and stiffness have been relieved. True strengthening and rebuilding of atrophied muscles by exercise is not possible as long as motion is painful. For effective strengthening, exercise must therefore be prescribed concomitantly with physical or medical measures which relieve pain.

Disturbances of Joint Function

For good function, the joint must be moved easily through its normal range and must provide stability in each position. The disturbances caused by chronic arthritis are impairment of range of motion (ROM), impairment of ease of motion and impairment of joint stability.

Impairment of ROM.   This disturbance may be caused in several ways. In the initial state, painful motion associated with synovial proliferation and excess fluid tends to limit range. After a certain length of time, shortening of soft tissues (capsules, ligaments, tendons) leads to contractures. After destruction of the cartilage, the bony surfaces may fuse together, and bony ankylosis results. If mobility is maintained, subluxation and dislocation of joints may lead to mechanical blocks. While active exercise and passive motion may diminish contractures, such mobilization may cause further destruction if the limited ROM is due to a mechanical block.

Impairment of Ease of Motion.   This type of impairment is caused by synovial proliferation and by destruction of cartilage. Ease of motion is hampered also by dislocation of the joint and by joint instability. Frequently, the opposing joint surfaces are so uneven that a cogwheel effect is produced, with audible clicks as the joint moves. This leads to considerable slowing of the motion that often requires the patient to relax in the middle of a motion to permit the joint surfaces to pass by a rough area which blocks motion.

Joint Instability.   Joint instability is caused by damage to the supporting ligaments with or without subluxation or dislocation, by damage to the joint surfaces, or by both. It is most common in the finger and the knee joints. Instability of finger joints precludes a strong grip and thereby leads to apparent weakness. Instability of the knees leads to a gradually increasing valgus (knock-knee) deformity on weight-bearing. Exercise and use of an unstable joint lead to greater deterioration. Protection by splints and braces or surgical stabilization is the only means of achieving functional improvement.

MANAGEMENT OF DISABLED JOINTS

The Painful Joint

Articular Pain.   Articular pain may be due to inflammation of synovial membrane or to mechanical abnormalities in joints. In acute arthritis and recurrent attacks of swelling associated with pain, the inflammatory process is the major cause of pain. In chronic arthritis, pain results from disturbed joint function due to spurs or uneven joint surfaces. Regardless of the cause, the principal means of relief of pain, aside from analgesic drugs, are rest of the joint and intra-articular injection of adrenal corticosteroids.

Rest relieves pain in rheumatoid arthritis and may bring about remission of the disease. For this reason, treatment is often started with a prolonged period of bed rest. Of course, this is the way to give relative rest to all joints, and it is still favored by some physicians. However, bed rest involves the risk of interference with function and causes secondary disuse disability. Therefore, it must be weighed carefully as to its advantages and disadvantages.

Treatment of painful joints challenges the art of medicine to find a way to assure rest and immobility for one or several joints without interfering with the general activity of the patient. A certain number of joints can be immobilized and allowed to rest while the patient remains active. For example, the knees, the wrists and the ankles can

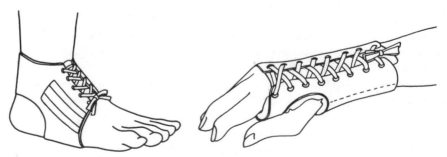

Fig. 16-4.   *(Left)* Leather anklet. *(Right)* Leather wristlet.

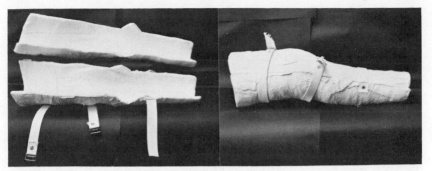

Fig. 16-5. Bivalved cast.

be immobilized without curtailing a person's ability to ambulate or perform daily activities. He is able to walk with stiff knees and stiff ankles by compensating for their motions through his hips and lumbar spine. He can compensate for wrist motions by use of the shoulders, the elbows and fingers. However, if the hips, the shoulders and the fingers are involved, immobilization would interfere greatly with function. In this case, intra-articular injection of corticosteroids becomes the method of choice.

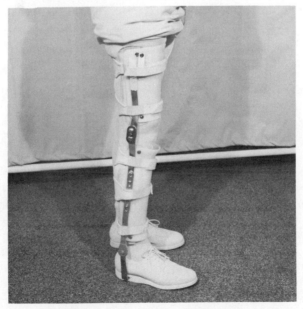

Fig. 16-6. Knee stabilization brace.

Disabling Conditions Due to Musculoskeletal Impairment 335

At times, restriction of motion by bandaging may be helpful. The bandage used should be of the Ace type, but it should not contain elastic fibers. Elasticity should result solely from the weave. Usually, the proper bandage is labeled "cotton elastic." Somewhat more restrictive supports that are applied easily and quickly are the leather anklet and wristlet (Fig. 16-4). Usually, these appliances can be slipped on and laced tightly by the patient himself. For effective immobilization of the knee joint, either a leather molded splint or a bivalved plaster cast (Fig. 16-5) is used.

Since a stiff knee is a rather severe disability, functional bracing of the knee may be used. Either a double bar functional long leg brace with thigh and leg lacers or a single lateral bar long leg brace with thigh and leg cuffs may be used (Fig. 16-6).

Whenever immobilization methods are used, it is essential to carry out ROM exercises twice daily, preferably in a warm bath, to prevent contractures of the immobilized joints. If the disease is advanced and prognosis for recovery of joint function is poor, permanent immobility in the knees, the ankles or the wrists may be considered desirable. Only in such circumstances should ankylosis or contracture be permitted. The prolonged use of plaster of Paris casts may then be appropriate.

Intra-articular injection of hydrocortisone or related compounds tends to diminish inflammatory joint reaction—whatever its cause. Therefore, it will afford pain relief for a certain length of time. Sometimes, the anti-inflammatory effect of the corticosteroids seems to favor some smoothing of the joint surfaces, and a more permanent beneficial effect may be achieved. However, a danger of this medication is the possibility of damage from pain-free joint activity without mechanical protection.

Periarticular Pain. Periarticular pain is caused by bursitis, tendinitis, tenosynovitis, ligamentous sprains and capsular tears. All these conditions are very responsive to local injections of corticosteroids into the affected areas. However, one must be sure to inject the inflamed or injured structure. The area to be injected is recognized by tenderness to pressure. Pain, as distinguished from tenderness, is often perceived remote from the site of disorder. Injecting vague painful areas leads to disappointing results. It is very important to determine whether the pain is of articular or periarticular origin since intra-articular injection of steroids and immobilization will not relieve periarticular pain. In fact, in the case of periarticular pain, it is important to attain maximum ROM for successful management. Limited ROM indicates that the periarticular structures are short and tight. Pain will persist until there has been full restoration of motion. Physical therapy, including gradually increased passive and active ROM exercises, must be used to supplement the local treatment.

The Contracted Joint

Limitation of joint ROM and joint deformity are very common features of rheumatoid arthritis. The most frequent disorders are flexion contractures of the hips, the knees and the elbows; limitation of shoulder motion in flexion and abduction; and limitation of finger flexion. This means that the hips, the knees and the elbows cannot be fully extended, while shoulders and fingers cannot be fully flexed. In the early stages of rheumatoid arthritis while all joint disabilities are still reversible, rehabilitation should aim toward restoration of joint integrity. At this phase, the functional goal is normal joint ROM everywhere. However, when there is disabling arthritis, when the patient has multiple joint involvement and severe articular damage, the goal of treatment may be merely to attain a more favorable position of certain contracted joints. Limitations of ROM that do not greatly impede functional activities in the partially disabled person may have to be tolerated. In other words, corrective measures should be undertaken to improve the particular joints in which useful and significant improvement of function can be anticipated.

Active and Passive Mobilization. The simplest and most widely accepted methods of increasing ROM of contracted joints are active and passive mobilization. There are a number of dangers inherent in these methods. The periarticular structures may have been so weakened by inflammation that they can be torn and disrupted by a vigorous muscle contraction. Furthermore, since the bone in the vicinity of inflamed joints is very osteoporotic, pressure exerted on joint surfaces at the fulcrum of the motion may easily result in small compression fractures. Finger joints are most vulnerable. The distal ends of phalanges are easily fractured not only by passive stretch but also by active motion. Therefore, restoration of joint ROM by active or passive mobilization must be carried out cautiously and gradually. The techniques are most applicable to joints with early rheumatoid changes where the inflammatory process has not gone beyond the synovial membrane and where osteoporosis is minimal. Passive mobilization is indicated also for use at the hip and shoulder joints and may be done safely if a certain amount of traction is exerted so that the femoral and humeral heads are not used as fulcra.

Active mobilization is carried out by having the patient move his joint forcefully through the maximum ROM. For example, in cases of finger extension contracture, the patient is requested to attempt to close his fist as hard as he can and repeat this 4 or 5 times. Two or three daily exercise periods should be prescribed.

Passive mobilization may be carried out by someone else or by the patient himself. For increasing ROM in fingers, the patient would be instructed to grasp the affected fingers with the other hand and to assist them in motion. However, he must be instructed exactly in which direction and how hard to push and also to exert a slight pull in order to avoid injuring the joints. For more proximal joints, such as the shoulder or the hip, passive mobilization is done preferably by another person.

Prior to active or passive mobilization, it is desirable to prepare the affected joints by means of hot packs or hot baths. Heat, especially moist heat, diminishes pain and decreases muscular spasm. Most patients with rheumatoid arthritis have to struggle constantly to maintain useful ROM of the involved joints.

Casting. When pronounced contractures are of long standing, neither active nor passive mobilization by manual means is likely to restore mobility. Very powerful structures such as the ligaments posterior to the knee joint become shortened, and flexion contracture appears irreversible. Under such circumstances, a series of plaster-of-Paris casts are used, each with slightly increased extension of the joint. For treatment of a flexion contracture of the knee, a cylindrical cast is applied that immobilizes the knee in the maximum degree of extension attainable without injury. Then, the patient is allowed to use the leg either by walking on it or by carrying out exercises involving muscles of the thigh and the leg. If the cast is removed after 1 week or is cut across at the level of the knee so that the knee can be extended further, one will find that a small increase of extension will have been gained. This has been achieved by the muscular pull exerted on the posterior structures of the knee. Supported by the cast at the point of maximum possible extension the muscles within the cast are allowed to loosen and lengthen themselves by their own pull. If this maneuver is repeated several times, the knee may be straightened to nearly complete extension and become functionally sufficient for walking. Usually, serial increments of extension are achieved by inserting a wedge into the posterior portion of the transected cast followed by application of additional plaster bandage.

The Unstable Joint

There are two principal categories of unstable joints: (1) the joint that maintains normal alignment and contact of articulating surfaces throughout its motion but is loose or unstable because supporting structures have been stretched abnormally; (2) the joint in which the articulating surfaces are no longer in contact or normal relationship. Such joints are subluxated or dislocated.

Instability. Slight degrees of instability or minor subluxation may not interfere greatly with joint motions. However, there is a degree of insecurity from wobbliness that occurs when forceful muscle pull is exerted. This wobbliness leads to irritation and pain and eventually to deformities such as ulnar deviation of the hand and the fingers and valgus deformity of the knee. Instability of the weight-bearing joints, particularly the knees and the ankles, should be counteracted as early as possible by an appropriate support, such as a bivalved plaster cast, a leather molded splint or a long leg brace.

Dislocation. Sometimes, stability of a joint has been so completely disrupted that the joint surfaces no longer have contact at any angle of motion. A new fulcrum is established, either at a point of bony contact or entirely in soft tissues. In one case, ROM may be severely limited by a bony block. In the other, the fulcrum would have no strength because of the elasticity of soft tissues. Active and passive mobilization will neither increase strength nor ROM; such exercises will only increase joint disruption and cause greater damage. Dislocated joints either have to be used within the range and strength that they may have, or they must be treated surgically. Dislocated finger joints may pose no serious problem. Dislocated major joints may require either fusion or arthroplasty.

Surgical Procedures

Tenotomy. The surgical treatment for contractures is tenotomy, which consists of cutting shortened tendons and other structures in or near a contracted joint. Tenotomy is indicated for severe contractures of strong tendons like the achilles and the hamstring tendons. Since postsurgical immobilization of the joint, and to some extent of the patient himself, is necessary this procedure must be used wisely in severely disabled patients with multiple joint involvement.

Arthrodesis. Arthrodesis is the surgical fusion of joints in functional position. If successful, this assures relief from pain and instability. Since joint motion is sacrificed in arthrodesis, fusion gives best functional results in wrists, ankles and spine where stability is more important than motion. In hips and knees, fusion is now being replaced by the use of prosthetic joints.[8]

Arthroplasty. Arthroplasty is a surgical reconstruction or alteration of a joint. Placement of a smooth vitallium cup over an arthritic femoral head is called a cup arthroplasty. Partial or complete prosthetic replacement of joints has been very successful so far only with hip and finger joints. In the hip the femoral head may be replaced by a metal head. The acetabulum is replaced by a plastic prosthesis to form a new socket (see Sect. B, Hip Disabilities). Finger joints may be replaced as a means of overcoming a severe disability of rheumatoid arthritis. The joints themselves are replaced by a long spindle of silicone rubber (silastic), the two ends of which insert into the adjoining bones and the expanded center of which constitutes the joint.

Synovectomy.   In rheumatoid arthritis where the synovial proliferation causes pain, destruction and mechanical interference with motion, surgical removal of the proliferating synovial tissue, called synovectomy, may not only relieve pain and stiffness but may also arrest the progress of the disease in the involved joint.

MANAGEMENT OF THE PATIENT WITH CHRONIC ARTHRITIS

While it is essential to know how to manage arthritic joints in order to rehabilitate patients with chronic arthritis, such knowledge by itself does not lead to rehabilitation. The arthritic patient's disability depends only in part on the degree of joint involvement and the number and location of the joints involved. Also, it is determined by his general health status and by possible associated impairments. The goals of rehabilitation for patients with chronic arthritis are: (1) specific medications, (2) relief of pain, (3) achievement of locomotion and self-care and (4) psychosocial adjustment.

Specific (Curative) Medications for the Treatment of Arthritis
Rheumatoid Arthritis
Two remedies used for the treatment of rheumatoid arthritis are gold therapy and chloroquine.

Gold Therapy.   In this form of treatment the patient is given weekly intramuscular injections of gold salts until a maximum dose has been achieved. The patient usually responds to gold therapy within 3 or 4 months. If his arthritic symptoms are greatly reduced, the period between injections may be extended to 2 weeks, at first, and then to 3 weeks.

If gold is administered, the patient must have weekly urinanalysis and blood counts prior to treatment. If there is albuminuria, gold should be stopped. If the white count falls significantly, it is necessary to stop treatment. This is particularly necessary if the granulocytes or the platelets are depressed. The sedimentation rate is a valuable aid in determining what the course of the disease may be under gold therapy. The worst complication of gold therapy is exfoliative dermatitis; the occurrence of a typical watery exudative skin eruption is indication that gold injections be stopped immediately.

Chloroquine.   The other drug fairly widely used is chloroquine, an anti-malarial agent which may produce a remission after 6 months. It has been used in varying dosages but 250 mg. twice daily represents the maximum acceptable now. Patients receiving chloroquine should be closely observed by an ophthalmologist in order to determine accurate visual fields. If any indentation of the field occurs, the drug should be stopped, particularly since ocular damage continues to occur even after cessation of the drug.

Gout

Another form of arthritis is gout, which can be treated with colchicine. Colchicine is very useful not only in aborting acute attacks but also in combating chronic gouty arthritis. In such treatment, a tolerable dose is administered for long periods of time. Diarrhea is the guide to the level of drug which is effective. This side effect should be prevented by giving colchicine up to a dose which is almost productive of diarrhea. Other drugs may also be used in the treatment of gout. Phenylbutazone (Butazolidin) may be used for a brief period of time to suppress an acute attack, indomethacin (Indocin) is effective. Probenecid (Benemid) increases the excretion of urate from the blood and is helpful, while allopurinol (Zyloprim) is effective in reducing the level of the uric acid in the blood by suppressing the chemical processes leading to synthesis of uric acid. The latter two drugs, probenecid and allopurinol, are effective in reducing tophaceous deposits in tophaceous gout.

Pain Relief

The General Approach to the Patient with Arthritic Pain.   It is not uncommon to find a bedridden patient with rheumatoid arthritis who will scream even before he has been touched. This degree of fear is the consequence of careless and thoughtless management to which such patients have been subjected in the course of treatment, often during institutional care. Not only overt carelessness, but such thoughtless gestures as a friendly handshake or a cordial slap on the back may cause unanticipated suffering. Personnel involved in patient care, from ambulance crew to nursing staff, may cause needless pain in transporting, moving or bathing patients unless made aware of the special precautions necessary to handle inflamed and damaged joints. It would be well to have signs over the beds of arthritic and other vulnerable patients, indicating that they must not be handled or moved except according to specified directions.

Since it is impossible for anyone to know which motion or pressure will be painful on any particular day, the patient should always have his say about how he should be moved. Turning and moving should be carried out very slowly, giving the patient a chance to call a halt before severe pain has been caused. Turning and transfer should be discussed with the patient, not only to prepare him for the act but also to plan how it can be carried out with the least amount of pain. The patient himself is best able to avoid painful motions, and therefore he should be set up in such a way that he can carry out most of his positioning and transfer unassisted or with only minor assistance. Knowledge of which joints are involved and the use of protective splinting for these joints are also helpful in preventing pain while moving or otherwise assisting the patient.

Physical Measures for Pain Relief.   Texts on arthritis emphasize the importance of physical therapy. However, physical therapy is of value only if the proper measure is applied for its specific indication. Frequently, pain caused by fibrositis or panniculosis is relieved by fibrositis massage or skin rolling. The pain of periarticular involvement responds not only to local injections of anesthetic agents plus corticosteroids but also to active and passive ROM exercises. Temporary relief from pain can be achieved by all forms of heat. For the severely involved patient, full immersion in a Hubbard tank or bathtub may be the only means of applying heat and also allowing some degree of active and passive mobilization of his joints. Moist hot packs may be applied to individual painful joints before strengthening or ROM exercises (See management of painful joints, p. 334). Both the value and the limitations of physical therapy must be understood. Many methods that have been recommended for pain relief have failed to meet the test of time.

Splints and braces have already been described (p. 336). Instruction and exercises for posture control and correction may also be useful. In general, the prescription for physical therapy and supportive devices requires expert technical knowledge.

Medications for Pain Relief.   The two most effective medications are aspirin and corticosteroids. Aspirin may be given in very high doses for relief. If it is inadequate to relieve pain, consideration has to be given to the use of other drugs, including corticosteroids which are almost always effective in relieving pain. Other medications include indomethacin (Indocin) and phenylbutazone (Butazolidin). Cortico-steroids and adrenocorticoprophic hormone (which has to be given by injection) relieve pain by suppressing inflammation and sometimes dramatically improve the ability of the patient to be active. Because of the numerous and serious side effects of these medications, long-term use requires both careful and judicious supervision.

In treating the arthritic it is essential to be aware of different causes of pain. If pain is due to peripheral neuropathy very little can be done. If pain is caused by osteoarthritis or by a postural defect these conditions must be relieved and corrected if possible. Whenever a new complaint occurs its cause must be investigated and whenever possible specific treatment should be instituted.

Special Measures to Relieve Pain in Osteoarthritis of the Hip (Coxarthrosis or Malum Coxae). (See also, Sec. B, Hip Disabilities). This condition may occur in one or both hips as an end result of congenital anomaly or trauma. Hip pain radiating to the leg and increasing limitation of ROM leads eventually to adduction contracture.

Conservative treatment by intra-articular injection of cortico-steroids and ROM exercises is helpful. In advanced disorder, hip fusion or prosthetic replacement may be indicated.

Special Measures for Relief of Pain Due to Cervical Osteoarthritis (Cervical Spondylosis). In persons over 40 years of age, abnormalities of the cervical vertebrae commonly are noted in roentgenograms of the neck. Narrowing of intervertebral foramina, spur formation and disk flattening are found most frequently betwen C-5 and C-6 vertebrae. There may be no clinical evidence of disorder. Sometimes, pressure on cervical nerve roots or soft-tissue injury causes pain in the neck, shoulder or arm. Root or cervical spinal cord compression may result from severe derangement of intervertebral disks, vertebral osteoarthritis or injury to ligamentous structures about the cervical spine.

Treatment consists of immobilizing the neck with a collar and using neck traction and graduated ROM exercises.

Locomotion

Ambulation is handicapped by arthritic involvement of any joint in either lower extremity. Rheumatoid arthritis of a small joint of the foot may cause disability that interferes with walking. Generalized disease of the knees, the ankles and the feet presents one of the most formidable challenges in rehabilitative practice. If the disability cannot be overcome or circumvented, the arthritic faces the possibility of

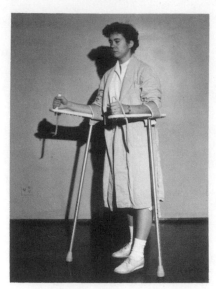

Fig. 16-7.   Platform crutch.

being confined to a wheelchair or bed for life, and, in either case, threatened with the array of secondary effects that has been emphasized throughout this book. Great effort should be made to maintain ambulation by using every protective device and technique available. Avoidance of the wheelchair is more important for the arthritic than the paraplegic since often the former is lacking in upper extremity function and strength and cannot maintain mobility by the use of his hands and his arm muscles.

The ambulatory arthritic should be kept ambulatory by precautionary use of protective devices and by careful supervision of care. The chronic arthritic who is bedridden or bound to a wheelchair must be approached with the same evaluative methods used for all severely disabled persons. A search must be made for uninvolved parts of the body that may be exploited to substitute somewhat for the disabled parts. For example, consider the patient with unstable and somewhat deformed knees and ankles whose arthritis is quiescent enough to permit weight-bearing and whose hips and spine are not involved by the disease. Potential for ambulation that is inherent in normal hips and spine can be realized by stabilizing the knees and the ankles in functional position. Assuming that the shoulders are normal or retain some degree of function, this patient can learn how to transfer from bed to standing position and from chair to standing, and he can succeed in ambulating if some or all of the following rehabilitative measures are carried out:

1. Use of a molded inlay in well-fitted or special shoes to provide a stable, pain-free, weight-bearing surface when feet are painful and deformed.

2. Use of laced leather anklets if the ankles are painful and lack stability.

3. Use of wedge casts and exercises to overcome contractures if the knees are limited in extension but permit some weight-bearing.

4. Use of long leg braces, bivalved plaster shells or cylindrical casts if the knees are painful and unstable.

If any or all of these supportive devices and related exercises are required, the patient will be able to walk with a stiff-legged gait, swinging his lower extremities from the hips and rotating the trunk with each step. Because rigid lower extremities limit stability, it may be necessary to use crutches for safe ambulation. If the wrists and the fingers are arthritic and conventional crutches cannot be used, a special platform crutch (Fig. 16-7) should be provided. This crutch is useful also for the arthritic with flexion contracture of the elbow whose ambulation depends on upper extremity assistance.

Once the problems of support and stabilization of arthritic joints have been dealt with satisfactorily, the patient with lower extremity arthritis must develop new methods of transfer. To get out of bed when fully braced, the patient should be instructed to turn face down and slide his legs over the edge of the bed. As his feet reach the floor, he stabilizes himself on his elbows and then stands erect by extending his hips. A similar technique is used for standing up from a chair. A second armchair is placed adjacent to his. With his hands or elbows on the arms of the adjacent chair he rolls to the face-down position, supports himself on both arms and stands by extending his hips and spine.

Obviously, if in addition to arthritis of the knees, the ankles and the feet, there is also involvement of one or both hips, the prognosis for ambulation and transfer is affected adversely. Under such circumstances, it is mandatory to maintain hip joint mobility in order to succeed. Here, the use of all the measures described for treatment of the painful joint may be required, namely, heat, cautious exercise and intra-articular injection of corticosteroids.

Self-Care

Self-care is handicapped especially by arthritis of the upper extremities. Often, the fingers cannot grasp ordinary objects because of limitation of flexion. At times, wrist pain makes the simplest acts of self-care intolerable. Shoulder and elbow motion may be so restricted in range that the patient cannot reach his mouth for feeding or his body and legs for bathing and dressing. If ROM cannot be restored, the self-care handicaps of the arthritic can be overcome in varying degree by the use of assistive devices and adapted equipment. At times, new devices must be invented to meet individual problems, but there is available a large battery of gadgetry that has arisen out of the needs of the handicapped and the fertile imaginations of physical and occupational therapists. A few examples of readily available devices are the following:

A large dowel or sponge rubber padded handle for eating utensils for the arthritic hand with limited grasp.

Long-handled utensils—toothbrush, comb and hairbrush—when elbow and shoulder flexion are limited.

Wire stocking holders or tapes with garter clasps to help place and pull up stockings when spine or hip motion is limited.

Long-handled shoehorn and fixed elastic laced shoes when dressing and lacing of shoes are difficult (Chap. 7, Fig. 7-3).

Psychosocial Adjustment

Much study has been devoted to the question of possible correlations betwen somatotype and personality and organic disease. Rheumatoid arthritis has been of special interest in this regard, and data have been presented to support the view that individuals with this disease tend to be dependent, to suppress anger and to present a bland type of psychological reaction to their environment while suffering severe consequences in the form of somatic deterioration. These views are of interest but they do not offer much immediate assistance in dealing with the manifest problems of the arthritic.

The spectrum of personalities among patients with this disease seems to be broader than that which is suggested by reported psychosomatic correlations. The characteristics that rheumatoid patients have in common are their helplessness, which often seems out of proportion to the extent of disease, and their vulnerability to pain. One cannot but inquire whether their psychological, social and somatic problems do not arise out of the highly disabling and poorly understood disease from which they suffer rather than from genetic determinants.

Pain and weakness are not adequately appreciated by the observer who, lacking empathy, often blames the arthritic for failure to exert enough effort in attempts to restore motion or function. Often, measures are prescribed and carried out that are potentially harmful because they are not based on full understanding of the need to protect diseased joints. Recognition of the gravity of symptoms is essential in order to plan the activity programs of the arthritic. When eating meals is agony because of painful motion of the elbow, it is not unreasonable for the arthritic to prefer to be fed. If weight-bearing causes great pain, it is not easy to relinquish the comfort of the bed.

In general, the rheumatoid patient seems as well motivated toward recovery as any other handicapped person. To assist in his rehabilitation, it is essential for family members and therapeutic personnel to recognize the nature and the degree of disability, to bring to bear all the methods possible for restoration of function and self-care ability and also to offer that degree of personal assistance that is needed to prevent undue suffering.

SUMMARY

1. The most common types of disabling chronic arthritis are osteoarthritis and rheumatoid arthritis. The latter causes more severe and more widespread joint involvement.

2. The disabilities of chronic arthritis are pain, muscular weakness and mechanical joint disturbances.

3. Rehabilitation of the arthritic involves consideration of each affected joint as well as of the over-all function of the individual. It must be planned with due concern for avoidance of painful and potentially damaging effects on involved joints.

Section B. Hip Disabilities

CAUSES OF HIP DISABILITIES

The two most common causes of hip disabilities are osteoarthritis of the hip and fractures of the hip.

Osteoarthritis of the Hip (Coxarthrosis, Malum Coxae Senilis)

This disability usually appears in middle aged persons and is frequently the result of minor congenital anomalies of the hip. Less frequently it develops as a result of severe injury to the hip joint, although sometimes the cause is unknown. The pathology is typical of osteoarthritis consisting of thinning of the cartilage and formation of spurs. The major disability is caused by pain. Secondary disabilities such as muscle spasm and loss of range of motion occur later on and may eventually interfere with ambulation.

Rehabilitation in the early phase consists of medical management. When the disability is severe the management of choice is total hip replacement.

Fractures of the Hip

Hip fractures constitute a serious cause of disability among the elderly. However with improved techniques of surgical care, the functional prognosis of hip fractures has been very favorably influenced. While walking ability is usually restored, a prolonged period of convalescence is frequently necessary. In the patient with additional disabilities, such as neurologic or organic mental impairment, the immobilization required for the treatment of a fracture often leads to secondary disabilities. The rehabilitation procedures discussed in this section will be especially oriented toward the hip fracture patient with multiple disabilities.

Just as the young amputee offers only a minor problem of rehabilitation, so does the otherwise physically fit, relatively young patient with a hip fracture. However, as soon as this disability is combined with other musculoskeletal, neurologic or mental impairments, rehabilitation following hip fracture requires skillful management.

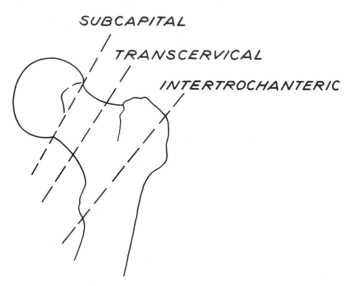

Fig. 16-8. Types of hip fractures.

Unfortunately, hip fractures frequently occur in the elderly patient who has neurologic or musculoskeletal impairment and is more likely to fall and fracture his hip.

The most frequently encountered types of hip fracture are fractures of the femoral neck and the trochanters. The upper or proximal femur consists of the greater and the lesser trochanters, the femoral neck and the head of the femur. The fracture line may pass through the trochanter or through the femoral neck (Fig. 16-8).

There are three possible approaches to hip fracture management:

1. Conservative treatment may be used in treating an *impacted fracture*. If the two fragments are held together because one is wedged into the other, it may be advisable to keep hands off and accept the minor deformity that may result.

2. Usually, internal fixation of the hip is carried out for *intertrochanteric fractures* by opening the skin over the greater trochanter and forcing a nail through the trochanter and the femoral neck into the femoral head. This is done after manipulation and alignment of fragments under x-ray guidance.

3. Prosthetic replacement of the femoral head is the method of choice for *subcapital and transcervical fractures*. In this method, which involves more extensive surgical intervention, the fractured portion of the femoral head and neck is removed and replaced by a metal femoral head and neck that is inserted by a long stem into the medullary canal of the femur. The Austin-Moore prosthesis is widely used for this procedure.

The method of rehabilitation and the time required for return of normal walking ability depend on the choice of surgical procedure. In conservative treatment of impacted fracture and in internal fixation, weight-bearing on the fractured hip must be postponed until the bone has healed. This takes from 3 to 8 months, sometimes longer. In fact, at times healing never occurs. During this prolonged period, the patient's mobility is restricted greatly, and if he walks at all he will have to use either a walker or crutches. If a prosthetic femoral head is inserted, the patient may bear weight very soon after surgery.

REHABILITATION OF HIP DISABILITIES

Conservative Management of Coxarthrosis

The major recommendation for conservative management of coxarthrosis is to reduce weight-bearing motion in the hip joint. This is achieved at first by restriction in weight-bearing activity in general. The necessary ambulation should be carried out with the assistance of a cane or crutches. For long distances the use of a wheelchair is advisable even if ambulation is possible. The patient may use a pedometer to monitor the total distance walked during the day.

Another important measure is the maintenance of hip range of motion by physical therapy. If a marked loss of range of motion has occurred and if passive hip motion is painful, physical therapy may be assisted by the use of medications. Indomethacin (Indocin) in doses as low as 25 mg. a day may be helpful. In cases of acute hip pain an intra-articular injection of xylocaine and a corticosteroid is also useful for pain relief. However, the patient must be instructed to be particularly meticulous in the restriction of weight-bearing during the period of freedom from pain caused by the corticoids.

REHABILITATION OF THE PATIENT WITH INTERNAL FIXATION OF THE HIP

Like the hemiplegic, the hip fracture patient goes through a bed phase, a unilateral weight-bearing phase and a bilateral weight-bearing phase. The unilateral weight-bearing that is on the uninvolved side includes stand-up exercises from the edge of the bed, stand-up exercises from the chair and walking with unilateral weight-bearing.

Bed Phase
Positioning of Patient after Internal Fixation
1. Place a small pillow under the popliteal space to prevent hyperextension of the knee and external rotation of the leg.
2. Place a sandbag or trochanter roll along the lateral side of the thigh and the leg. A sandbag gutter is preferable.
3. Elevate the backrest every 2 hours out of 4 hours for 2 hours.
4. Keep the bed completely flat for the intervening 2 hours. Be sure that the involved hip is fully extended. The patient may be in a back-lying or side-lying position; face-lying should first be allowed 3 weeks after intertrochanteric fracture and only after 3 or 4 months following a subcapital fracture. While the patient is turned on the side, pillows should be placed between the two legs. When the patient is lying on the side, the uppermost leg should be flexed at the knee. The feet should be supported against a footrest.

Sitting on Edge of Bed
The patient rolls over on the side of the uninvolved leg. The good hip and knee are flexed at right angles, and the operated hip (and

knee) are flexed as far as possible without pain. The legs are brought over the edge of the bed, and the patient swivels into a sitting position. He should sit on the edge of the bed from 3 to 5 minutes at a time several times a day. Special precautions are necessary:

1. If the patient is greatly overweight, he should be assisted by two persons. A very strict reducing regimen should be instituted immediately.

2. If the patient gets dizzy and faints, he may be suffering from orthostatic hypotension. Use of an abdominal binder or corset may be indicated. If there is a tendency for the feet to swell, the patient should be provided immediately with elastic stockings.

Unilateral Weight-bearing Phase

One-Legged Stand-up Exercises

1. Initially, stand-up exercises can be performed from the edge of the bed. The back of a heavy armchair or a high walkerette should be placed in front of the patient. He should be instructed to bear all his weight on the uninvolved leg and place the foot on the involved side flat on the floor beside the weight-bearing foot. The bed height should be 50 per cent greater than the distance from the floor to the patient's knee so that he can stand up with ease. He should carry out up to 10 stand-ups as tolerated for each session. There should be several sessions each day.

2. After a few days, the patient may transfer to a chair. This will be a one-legged weight-bearing transfer with a slight pivot on the weight-bearing leg. From this point on, the stand-up exercise can be done from the chair according to the method described for the hemiplegic patient (Chap. 14). While standing, the patient should practice straightening his involved knee and hip joint without weight bearing on that side.

The patient may be up in the chair 3 times daily for meals and do stand-up exercises 6 times daily, before and after each meal. He should not be in the chair for more than 1 hour at a time without standing or lying flat to prevent hip and knee flexion contractures.

3. Standing posture. Both feet should be flat on the floor, and both knees should be straight. The patient must stand completely erect with hips extended. The weight should be on the uninvolved leg, with only enough weight on the affected leg to keep the foot flat and the knee straight. This prevents contracture of the knee and the hip. It puts no undue stress on the injured limb but gives the patient a sense of balance. He must learn good standing posture before he can learn to walk in a walker or on crutches. He should not be allowed to

flex his hips and compensate by hyperextending the back, and he should not try to stand on one foot and hold the other off the floor.

4. The problem patient. A number of patients with hip fracture have various communication disabilities, such as hearing loss, aphasia or organic mental syndrome that may make it difficult to convey directions or ideas to them. In such instances, the technique must be modified slightly. The patient may be provided with only one shoe to be worn on the uninvolved side that will keep the involved leg off the ground. The fact that the foot on the involved side is bare will help to remind him not to put weight on this leg.

Walking With Unilateral Weight-Bearing
Ambulation With a Walker. The walkerette is most suitable for this purpose, since it is easy to lift and its four crutch-tipped legs provide stable support. The heavier walkers with casters are not sufficiently stable for unilateral weight-bearing. The patient must have enough strength in his arms to push himself up as he steps forward with the uninvolved leg. Then he puts his weight on the uninvolved leg and advances the walker. If the patient has difficulty comprehending the

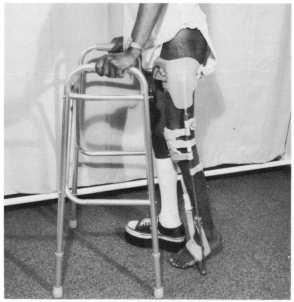

Fig. 16-9. Ischial weight-bearing orthosis.

method, it may be advisable to have him wear a shoe with a 1-inch wooden lift on the uninvolved leg so that his involved leg is kept suspended well off the ground.

Crutch-Walking. The patient walks with an amputee 3-point gait (Sect. D, p. 386).

Ambulation With an Ischial Weight-bearing Brace. One-legged walking requires considerable arm strength and balance which is frequently not available in the elderly patient. For this reason the introduction of an effective ischial weight-bearing brace has been helpful in permitting early ambulation in patients with hip fractures and also with fractures of the femur or the leg.[12] This appliance consists of an ischial weight-bearing quadrilateral socket (similiar to the one used for amputees) attached to two bars which unite into a walking tip 2 inches (5 cm.) below the foot (Fig. 16-9). The patient wears a 2 inch (5 cm.) rise under the opposite shoe and he may use crutches or a cane in the hand which is opposite to the arthrosis.

Bilateral Weight-bearing Phase

Bilateral weight-bearing must be introduced gradually in the stand-up exercise and while the patient is using a walker and crutches. Weight-bearing on the fractured side may begin 8 weeks after intertrochanteric fracture and 8 months after subcapital fracture. However, the specific decision to permit weight-bearing and the degree of weight-bearing has to be based on review of serial roentgenograms of the fracture site. Weight-bearing must be ordered specifically by the physician.

A simple method of introducing gradual weight-bearing on a lower extremity is to have the patient stand in parallel bars with the normal leg on a 2-inch (5-cm.) wood block and the involved leg on a bathroom scale. The patient is then requested to put 10 pounds (5 kg.) of pressure on the scale for a certain number of repetitions. The amount of weight-bearing can be increased gradually every week until the patient is able to support his body weight. If the patient's vision is not good enough to read the bathroom scale, the therapist will have to read it for him.

During the weight-bearing phase, the patient continues stand-up, and crutch-walking exercises. As soon as 50 per cent of the weight can be borne on the involved leg, the patient may start to walk with one crutch and soon thereafter with one cane. At this point, the patient may begin stair climbing with the use of a rail, at first leading with the good leg and later leading with the affected leg.

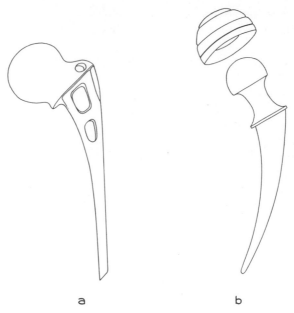

a   b

Fig. 16-10. (a) Austin Moor prosthesis; (b) Charnley total hip prosthesis.

REHABILITATION OF THE PATIENT WITH PROSTHETIC HIP REPLACEMENT

Partial hip replacement by a prosthetic femoral head is commonly used in transcervical or subcapital hip fractures. The Austin-Moore prosthesis is most commonly used for this purpose (Fig. 16-10a). Previously the Austin-Moore prosthesis was also used in the treatment of coxarthrosis but has now been largely replaced by a total hip prosthesis.[5,10]

The total hip prosthesis (Fig. 16-10b) consists of a plastic acetabular prosthesis and a metal femoral head prosthesis.

Postoperative Care After Prosthetic Hip Replacement[6,9]

The postoperative care of the patient with an Austin-Moore prosthesis or a total hip replacement is very similar. In both instances early weight-bearing is possible since no bone healing is required. Postoperative healing of the soft tissues, however, is necessary to prevent dislocation of the prosthesis, and for this reason precautions have to be taken during the early management. Adduction and rotation are to

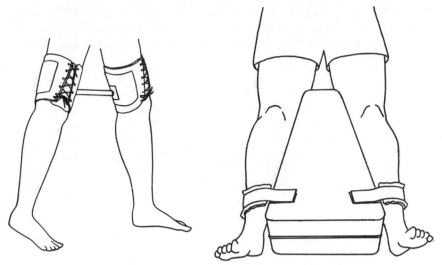

Fig. 16-11, *left,* hip-abduction brace; *right,* hip-abduction wedge.

be avoided in the early phase—external rotation for total hip replacement and internal rotation for the Austin-Moore prosthesis. These motions can be avoided by keeping the lower extremities in a hip abduction splint for the first few days. Two examples of hip abduction devices are presented in Figure 16-11.

The detailed prescription of postoperative care is the function of the surgeon who operated on the patient and may vary from surgeon to surgeon and sometimes from case to case. We shall describe an example of an average regimen.

Bed Phase (about 1 week)

Following surgery a hip abduction splint is applied. Elevation of the head part of the bed should be limited to 40 degrees to avoid hip flexion. The bed should have a foam rubber mattress and an overhead trapeze. The patient should be turned regularly, changing from back to operated side to abdomen, to nonoperated side. On the first day he will receive only breathing and coughing exercises. On the second and third postoperative day, ankle and quadriceps exercises may be started. On the third day he may be placed on a Nelson bed so that he can have two periods of partial weight-bearing a day. If no Nelson bed is available the weight-bearing can be initiated on a tilt table (p. 275). On the fourth day the patient may be started on active assisted hip and knee flexion exercises and straight leg raising exercises. During the exercise the hip abduction splint is removed. On the fifth or sixth day the patient may be started on ambulation but the use of the hip abduction brace in bed should be continued for a period of 2 weeks.

Ambulatory Phase

The ambulatory phase starts in the second week. If hip flexion is still limited the patient must transfer from the lying position to the standing position without assuming a sitting position. During the transfer the hip abduction brace should remain in place. To prevent his hips from being forced into flexion, the patient may use an elevated seat such as the edge of the bed or a raised toilet seat. Ambulation is started with a walkerette. The hip abduction brace is removed

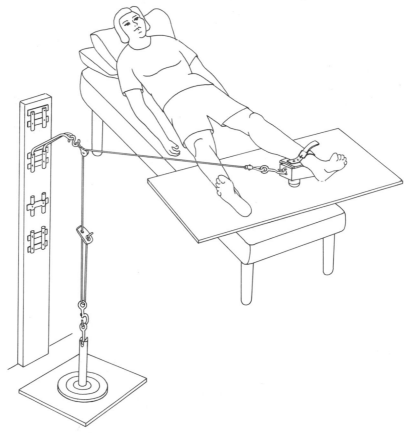

Fig. 16-12. Hip-abduction pulley exercise.

for ambulation and the patient is advised to put about 10 per cent of his weight on the operated leg initially. By the end of the second week the patient should be able to transfer from lying to standing position and to walk well with a walker. If desirable he may then be instructed in crutch-walking prior to discharge from the hospital. Two weeks postoperatively the patient may be discharged. In the third postoperative week he should be started on active and resistive hip abduction exercises and stair-climbing. After 6 weeks to 2 months he may drive a car.

Stair-climbing Phase

The stair-climbing phase starts 3 weeks postoperatively and includes stair-climbing exercises and resistive hip abduction exercises. The stair-climbing exercises are similar to those in the hemiplegia program. The patient should start with 2-inch (5-cm.) steps and increase gradually to 6-inch or 8-inch (15- or 20-cm.) steps. Initially he should lead with the operated leg which is to be strengthened and improved in range of motion. Later on he may lead alternately with each leg.

Strengthening of the hip abductors is best performed by the pulley exercise with the patient in supine position and the exercised leg supported on a skate or a powder board (Fig. 16-12). If the cuff is applied at the ankle an abduction strength of 15 to 20 pounds (7 to 9 kg.) should be achieved. If the cuff is applied above the knee, double the weight is needed to achieve identical strength.

SUMMARY

1. Hip fractures occur either in the region of the femoral trochanter or at various parts of the femoral neck. The former tend to heal faster and better than the latter.

2. Hip fractures may be managed conservatively (in selected impacted fractures) or surgically either by internal fixation (nailing) or by substitution of a femoral head and neck prosthesis (Austin-Moore prosthesis).

3. Rehabilitation of the patient with an impacted fracture or a nailed intertrochanteric hip fracture permits at best only unilateral weight-bearing on ambulation for a prolonged period (at least 3 months). Rehabilitation may be difficult to carry to a successful conclusion in elderly patients with multiple disabilities in addition to hip fracture, if ambulation is long delayed.

4. Patients with coxarthrosis with minor disability should be man-

aged conservatively. Major disability is best treated surgically by total hip replacement.

5. While insertion of a prosthetic femoral head and total hip replacement are complicated and prolonged surgical procedures, satisfactory ambulation is soon possible postoperatively, and the rehabilitation technique is simple.

Section C. Low Back Disabilities

INTRODUCTION

Disease and injuries of the low back may cause *paralysis, stiffness* or *pain.* Paralysis is discussed under neurologic disabilities (p. 211).

Permanent stiffness of the back occurs in ankylosing spondylitis and surgical fusion of the spine. Temporary stiffness is associated with pain syndromes of the low back. While stiffness of the spine without pain represents a disability which interferes with some occupations and creates minor problems with activities of daily living, it never leads to the severe disability seen in the chronic and acute pain syndromes of the low back. This chapter will be concerned only with low back disability resulting from low back pain.

Low back pain may cause different degrees of disability:

1. When pain is severe and continuous, never relieved but only dulled by large doses of narcotics, the patient may be bedridden most of the time and require assistance in activities of daily living.

2. When pain is moderate or mild but becomes severe as a result of any kind of physical exertion the patient may be severely restricted in activities for fear of causing an attack and may be totally disabled for work.

3. When pain occurs intermittently in acute attacks, as it does in a group of patients who are temporarily disabled, the restriction of activity is brief, and the pain subsides completely after a few days or weeks of rest.

CAUSES OF LOW BACK PAIN

The causes of low back pain can be divided into two groups:

1. Backache due to specific generally recognized pathology.

2. Backache, the pathogenesis of which is a matter of debate. The specific origins of the backache can be visceral, vascular, muscular, skeletal or neurologic. Some important causes of specific backache are listed in Table 16-1, but there are many others.

TABLE 16-1. Low Back Pain Due to Specific Pathology

A. PATHOLOGY OF THE NERVOUS SYSTEM
 1. Infections: Epidural abscess
                 Meningitis
                 Arachnoiditis
                 Herpes Zoster
 2. Neuropathies
 3. Neoplasms: Meningioma
                Ependymoma
                Glioma
                Neurofibroma
 4. Polymyositis
B. PATHOLOGY OF THE SKELETAL SYSTEM
 1. Infections: Osteomyelitis
                 Tuberculosis
                 Brucellosis
                 Coccidioidomycosis
                 Disc space infections
 2. Neoplastic bone disease: Multiple myeloma
                              Leukemia
                              Hodgkin's disease
                              Osteosarcoma of the pelvis
                              Metastatic disease
 3. Metabolic Bone Disease: Osteoporosis
                             Osteomalacia
                             Paget's disease
 4. Fractures and dislocations
 5. Arthritis: Marie Strumpell disease
                Scheuermann's disease
                Sacroiliac arthritis:
                  Rheumatoid
                  Ulcerative colitis
                  Reiter Syndrome
                  Psoriatic arthritis
C. VISCERAL PATHOLOGY
 1. Abdominal Pathology:
    Pancreas—Pancreatitis Tumor
    Stomach or duodenum—Peptic ulcer or tumor
 2. Pelvic Pathology: Uterus & ovaries
                       Tumor of the colon
                       Iliopsoas abscess
                       Prostatic tumor
 3. Retroperitoneal Pathology:
    Kidneys—Stone—Hydronephrosis
    Abscess or tumor—lymphoma
                       sarcoma
                       carcinoma
    Retroperitoneal sclerosis
D. VASCULAR PATHOLOGY:
 1. Intermittent claudication
 2. Aortic aneurysm

Nonspecific low back pain may be *organic* or *psychogenic*. The organic low back pain which is not due to specific causes is assumed to originate from stresses and strains imposed on the structures of the low back either by normal activities or by excessive activities or even by injuries. It has, therefore, been called "mechanical" backache. The mechanical "failure" has been attributed to a number of causes which are listed in Table 16-2.

TABLE 16-2. POSTULATED CAUSES OF MECHANICAL LOW BACK PAIN

A. DEFECTS IN BONE STRUCTURE
   1. Congenital: Spina bifida occulta
                  Spondylolysis (split pedicle)
                  Transitional L-5, S-1 vertebrae (lumbarization
                    sacralization)
   2. Degenerative: Lumbar spondylosis
   3. Spondylolisthesis
B. JOINT DYSFUNCTION (FACET SYNDROME)
C. SOFT TISSUE LESIONS
   1. Lumbar Disc lesions
   2. Low back sprain: Iliolumbar
                        Sacroiliac
                        Interspinous
   3. Postural low back pain

Psychogenic back pain comprises a heterogenous group of clinical entities such as tension syndrome, hysteria, malingering and traumatic neurosis.

In our opinion defects in bone structure, with the exception of severe spondylolisthesis, play no role in severe low back disability. The existence of joint dysfunction is questionable. Most specialists discount low back sprain and postural low back pain as causes of severe disability. There is general agreement, however, at this time, that lumbar disc lesions can cause severe low back disability, particularly by nerve root compression. We shall therefore limit this chapter to the rehabilitation of disabilities caused by lumbar disc lesion.

DISABILITIES CAUSED BY LUMBAR DISC LESIONS

The intervertebral disc is a fibrous structure located between two vertebral bodies. It is composed of an outer shell, the annulus fibrosus, and a gelatinous inner core called the nucleus pulposus. If as a result of excessive pressure a tear occurs in the annulus, material of the core herniates through the opening. Disc herniations in the posterolateral area of the disc may compress and irritate the nerve root causing pain and paralysis.

Frequently disability starts as the result of lifting a heavy load. The patient experiences sudden acute low back pain and has to stay in bed for several days before he is able to walk again. From then on he may have such attacks once or twice a year following an effort or without any apparent reason. Finally he may develop sciatic pain in one lower extremity which does not subside with bed rest. He may be hospitalized for pelvic traction for 2 to 3 weeks, see a chiropractor or acupuncturists and finally end up with disc surgery which may or may not give complete relief. In addition to pain, a disc lesion may lead to paralysis of one or several lower extremity muscles and in severe cases to complete paraplegia.

MANAGEMENT OF LUMBAR DISC LESION

The management of a lumbar disc lesion can be surgical or conservative. The most common surgical procedure is a laminectomy following by removal of the herniated nucleus pulposus. Some surgeons then fuse the lumbar spine. Another still experimental method is the injection of an enzyme into the nucleus pulposus. The enzyme "digests" the nuclear material.

There are numerous conservative measures including pelvic traction, exercise, manipulation, physical therapy and injection of corticosteroids. We shall describe in this chapter a comprehensive program of conservative management which has been very successful with patients who are willing and able to carry it out.

It is commonly accepted that a patient suffering from symptoms of a herniated nucleus pulposus (lumbar disc lesion) should be given a trial of conservative management prior to surgery.[1,3,10] The reasons for this view are the danger of surgical complications, the certain damage to the stability of the spine and the possible failure of surgery to relieve symptoms. Follow-up study of conservatively managed lumbar disc lesions in Britain has shown a respectable percentage of good results.[10]

While the value of conservative management appears to be accepted, the methods commonly used in the "conservative trial" are frequently inadequate. Thus, a much larger number of patients fail the "conservative trial" and come to surgery than would be the case with more adequate conservative management.

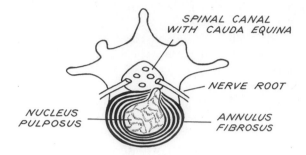

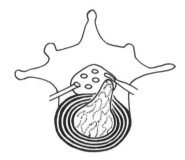

a. INITIAL PROTRUSION

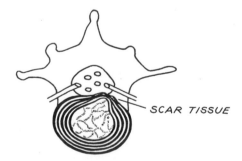

b. NERVE ROOT COMPRESSION

c. HEALING WITH SCAR FORMATION

Fig. 16-13. Evolution of lumbar disc lesion.

Rationale for Conservative Management

The Evolution of a Lumbar Disc Lesion[1]

In recent years the evolution of a lumbar disc lesion has become better known from animal studies, postmortem studies, and the study of surgically removed human disc specimens. The disc lesion goes through three phases: (1) intradiscal changes, (2) herniation or expulsion of the disc material and (3) fibrosis and healing (Fig. 16-13).

Intradiscal Changes. The intradiscal changes which start in the teenager are chemical in nature and gradually lead to fragmentation of the nucleus pulposus and weakening of the posterior portion of the annulus fibrosus. This stage is probably asymptomatic.

Herniation. Herniation of disc material through the weakened annulus fibrosus is a result of mechanical pressures exerted on the disc. The protruded disc material first distends the posterior spinal ligament which may cause low back pain. Later, it may progress laterally and compress and irritate the facet joint or the nerve root. At this point acute low back pain or sciatica results. Anterior herniations as well as protrusion upward and downward into bone may occur—but cause no symptoms.

Fibrosis and Healing. Under favorable circumstances, the protruded portion of the nucleus pulposus shrinks by dehydration, and pain disappears. Fibrosis consolidates the posterior wall of the annulus fibrosus over a period of months and complete recovery results. However, if excessive pressure on the disc occurs before healing of the annulus fibrosus is completed, there will be recurrence of the tear with expulsion of additional disc material which causes aggravation and prolongation of symptoms.

The present rationale of conservative management is to keep the intradiscal pressure low enough, long enough to permit adequate healing of the annulus fibrosus.

Studies of Intradiscal Pressure

Measurement of the intradiscal pressure in vivo has shown that intradiscal pressure is lowest when the subject is lying supine with hips flexed.[8,9] It increases progressively in side-lying, standing and sitting positions and with forward bending and lifting (Fig. 16-14). It is also increased by straining, coughing and sneezing. Strong compression of the abdomen by a tight corset decreases the load on the disc up to 50 per cent in a standing and sitting position.[2,7,8]

These studies of intradiscal pressure explain the empirical fact that bed rest and a tight corset relieve the pain of lumbar disc lesions. The protruded disc is most vulnerable to increased intradiscal pres-

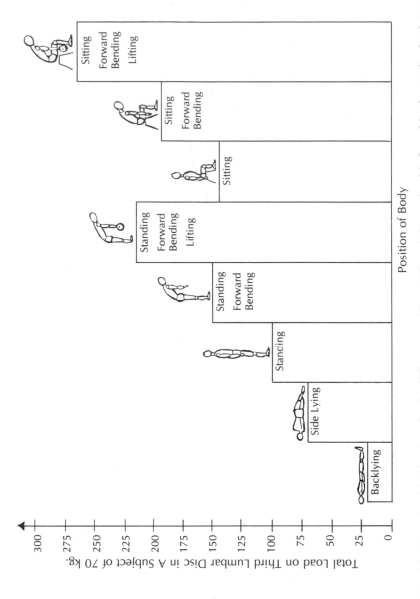

Fig. 16-14. Total load on the third lumbar disc in different positions. The minimum load is found in the supine horizontal position and increases in the standing and sitting positions and with forward bending and lifting. (Hirschberg, G.: "Treating Lumbar Disc Lesion by Prolonged Continuous Reduction of Intraducal Pressure, Texas Med., Vol. 70, No. 12. Dec., 1974.)

Position of Body

Total Load on Third Lumbar Disc in A Subject of 70 kg.

0 25 50 75 100 125 150 175 200 225 250 275 300

Backlying

Side Lying

Stancing

Standing Forward Bending

Standing Forward Bending Lifting

Sitting

Sitting Forward Bending

Sitting Forward Bending Lifting

sure immediately following a protrusion. Therefore, treatment consists of complete bed rest for 2 weeks. After this period the disc can tolerate moderate pressure. Therefore standing, sitting and walking with a corset or body jacket may be permitted. The corset may be required for 6 months to a year or longer for lifting and other heavy duty activities to protect against a new disc protrusion.

MANAGEMENT OF THE PATIENT ON CONTINUOUS COMPLETE BED REST

If the patient is in horizontal position the weight of the body does not affect the disc. Nevertheless, intradiscal pressure can be increased by pain and muscle spasm, voluntary activities, and involuntary muscular contractions. Therefore, these three factors must be controlled.

Control of Pain and Muscle Spasm

Control of pain and muscle spasm is attempted by positioning the patient in bed and by prescribing medication. Pain relief is defined here as the complete disappearance of severe root pain to the point that the patient can lie comfortably and relaxed. Paresthesia, fleeting pains and minor aches and pains in the low back may be disregarded for this purpose.

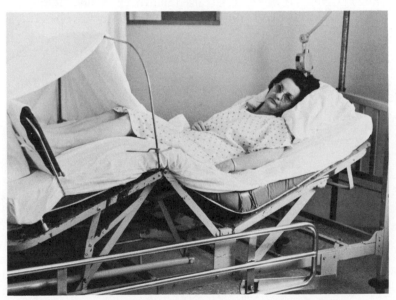

Fig. 16-15.   Bed treatment of lumbar disc lesions.

The patients can be divided into three groups according to their response: Group 1. Pain relief is achieved by positioning in bed alone. Group 2. Pain relief is achieved after 3 or 4 days of bed rest and administration of narcotics. Group 3. No pain relief is obtained in 3 or 4 days.

The Pain is Relieved by Positioning Alone

Methods of Positioning. The crucial position for maximum decrease of intradiscal pressure and for pain relief is the so-called semi-Fowler's position in which the patient lies on his back with head and knees slightly elevated (Fig. 16-15).

The bed should be equipped with a 4-inch (10-cm.) foam rubber mattress over a slatted or folding bedboard which permits the mattress to adapt to the contour of the bed frame. The overhead trapeze should be removed from the bed frame so that the patient will not be tempted to pull himself up. There should be a cradle over the knees in order to allow free movement of the legs and a footboard for support. It may be advisable to have lamb's wool or a foam rubber pad under the sacral area to minimize discomfort.

It is preferable to have a hospital bed with electrically controlled adjustment of position. Initially the head of the bed is raised 12 inches (30 cm.) above the level of the hips. Under no circumstances should the head portion of the bed be raised above 12 inches (30 cm.). The portion under the knees, usually marked "feet" or "seat" on the electric adjustment is raised to the maximum. From this position the bed can be lowered at the head or foot in order to achieve maximum comfort.

During the first week the adjustment of the bed should not be changed. The patient should remain in this semi-Fowler's position day and night for the first 2 to 3 days of the bed phase. He may be moved passively into side-lying position for brief periods only for examination or use of the bedpan.

After 3 days the side-lying position may be assumed for longer periods alternating with the supine semi-Fowler's position. The elevation of the bed keeps the hips and knees flexed when the patient is in a side-lying position. However, the patient should still be moved to his side passively.

After 1 week the bed position may be altered from the semi-Fowler's position to a completely flat bed if desired and the patient may roll actively to his side by using his arms to pull himself onto his side by grasping the side rail. Under no circumstances should the patient assume a prone position during the bed phase.

Supportive Medication. To maintain proper positioning some patients may require two kinds of medication. Minor analgesics such as aspirin, Empirin, and Bufferin may be administered for relief of aches and pains resulting from lying in one position. Furthermore, tranquilizers may be given to facilitate tolerance of the enforced immobility. According to the patient's temperament and interest, one may choose between sleep-inducing tranquilizers such as diazepam (Valium) and meprobamate and those causing less or no sleep such as prochlorperazine (Compazine) and trifluoperazine (Stelazine).

The Pain is Not Relieved by Positioning Alone

If positioning alone does not relieve the pain, it is important to use medications to keep the patient completely pain free so that he can relax in semi-Fowler's position and avoid turning and twisting from discomfort. Analgesics are usually inadequate to accomplish this goal at the initial stage and narcotics must be used. The choice of narcotic is determined by the tolerance of the patient and the effectiveness of the drug. Frequently, a dose of ½ grain to 1 grain of codeine in the form of Empirin with Codeine administered orally is adequate for pain relief. Sometimes meperidine (Demerol) or morphine is needed. It is best to give the medication every 3 or 4 hours around the clock during the first 3 days. When medications are administered on demand, patients frequently wait until their pain is severe before they request them. It may then take a half-hour to an hour before the drug is actually administered and another half-hour before pain relief actually starts. This may prolong the patient's pain for periods up to 2 hours.

If the patient is not completely pain free and relaxed with the administration of narcotics around the clock, it is necessary to add a muscle relaxant, for instance meprobamate in adequate dose, to relax the patient even to the point of keeping him asleep most of the time.

After 3 days, the narcotic is given only when requested by the patient. The patient must be instructed to request the medication immediately at the onset of pain and the nurses must be instructed to give it promptly upon request. Rarely is a patient completely pain free after the first 3 days of narcotic administration but he will usually require medication less often than every 3 or 4 hours and in subsequent days this demand will diminish. Some patients may still require medication following the use of the bedpan. Others may wake up in the middle of the night with sciatic pain. If narcotic requirement has decreased to one or two doses a day the patient may be given the choice between Empirin and Codeine or Bufferin. At the end of 1 week most patients are pain free. The positioning program may then be relaxed similar to that of Group 1 but complete bed rest must continue until 2 weeks are completed.

The Pain is Not Relieved by Positioning and Narcotics

If after 3 days the demand for narcotics continues to be for doses every 3 or 4 hours, one should first ascertain that the patient has actually followed the complete bed rest program diligently. If that is the case it would be advisable to use anti-inflammatory medication such as prednisone provided that there are no serious contraindications to its use.

The rationale of the use of prednisone is to reduce the inflammatory swelling of the nerve root and thereby accelerate pain relief. About 15 to 20 mg. of prednisone a day for a week or two are usually given. If effective pain relief generally starts within a few days the patient should be kept on complete bed rest for another week after pain relief is complete. This may prolong the bed phase up to 3 weeks. This is the maximum time we have had to use in the treatment of sciatica. If pain relief is not obtained in 3 weeks, surgery may be indicated.

A word must be said about two commonly used physical methods for the relief of pain and muscle spasm in lumbar disc lesions, namely, hot packs and traction. Pelvic traction is most widely used. It helps to keep the patient quiet in a semi-Fowler's position.[6] Unfortunately it has to be removed for the use of the bedpan and it is frequently removed for the patient's bath. At times, the patient takes it off himself and puts it on again. This additional motion, in our opinion, outweighs the usefulness of the traction.

A similar argument may be cited against the use of hot packs. Hot packs are an excellent means of providing pain relief and relaxation of muscle spasm if applied expertly. In practice, however, we have found that the movement of the patient during the application and removal of the hot pack has frequently aggravated pain and proven more harmful than helpful. If one chooses to make use of hot packs or traction, care must be taken that the patient is moved as little and as carefully as possible.

Control of Voluntary Activity

The restrictions of voluntary activity are defined in the term "continuous complete bed rest."

Bed Rest Must be Continuous

In accordance with the rationale to prevent any increase of intradiscal pressure, the bed rest must be continuous. A single brief instance of sitting up or getting out of bed may produce protrusion of disc material and start a new attack. It is very difficult to convince the patient, the nurses and physicians of this fact. The patient must not be raised for meals beyond the 12-inch (30-cm.) limit despite the difficulty of eating in the horizontal position. He cannot have bathroom privileges, though it may be true, as is often pointed out, that placing the patient on a bedpan is more damaging than the use of a bedside commode.[3,10] However, there are methods of using a bedpan which are safer for the patient than using the commode.[5]

To carry out all activities of daily living in bed requires skilled nursing. One may have to use all of one's ingenuity to keep the patient continuously horizontal for the required period if the patient is hospitalized. However, it is possible to carry out this program at home.

If a hospitalized patient has to be transferred from his bed for diagnostic purposes, he must remain in horizontal position. Any procedures requiring sitting or standing must be postponed until the patient is ready for the corset phase.

Bed Rest Must be Complete

Complete bed rest is defined as bed rest with assistance in eating, changing body position, using the bedpan and other activities.[4] It is commonly used for patients with recent myocardial infarction to avoid exertion. In the management of disc patients exertion per se need not be totally avoided. However, any motion which increases intradiscal pressure must be avoided or minimized, and many harmful activities can be completely avoided. Other activities such as eating and elimination cannot be avoided for a prolonged period and the patient must be assisted.

Activities to be Avoided. The patient should be told not to raise his head, to turn, to reach for any distant object or to lift himself by pulling on any part of the bed. All necessary equipment should be within easy reach, including the call light, T.V. switch, telephone, etc. He should be instructed to call the nurse for any items not within easy reach. For reading he should have a reading rack and prism glasses which enable him to read in supine position without moving his head.

Activities to be Assisted. *Eating.* Most patients are able to eat without assistance in semi-Fowler's position provided the food is cut up and positioned properly. Fluids can be taken through straws. If patients have great difficulty feeding themselves in supine position and are pain free, they may be allowed to feed themselves in a side-lying position. However, patients with severe sciatic syndrome who are aware that the slightest body motion causes aggravation have to be fed until they become pain free.

Bathing. Patients may be allowed to wash their hands and face. In patients with severe pain this is all that is permissible during the first few days. A bed bath involving the body should be postponed for a few days. After the patient is pain free a bed bath may be given by the nurse. The patient must be passively rolled on his side and returned into supine position. Great care should be observed that the patient remain relaxed during the rolling and does not participate in the effort. At no time should the patient be requested to wash his own trunk or lower extremities during the bed phase.

Bowel Program. Evacuation of the bowels seems to be a great stumbling block in the conservative management of lumbar disc lesions. It puts the patient in double jeopardy, because the straining which is involved in evacuation of the bowel increases intradiscal pressure, as does the use of a bedside commode or a regular bedpan.

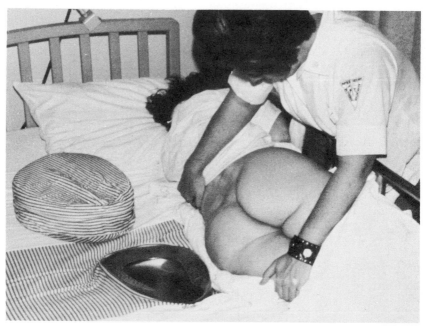

Fig. 16-16. Sunken bedpan. (Arch. Phys. Med. Rehab. 53:192-193, 1972.)

For over 10 years we have used a sunken bedpan as a successful method of defecation in the supine position.[4] A hole the exact size and contour of a regular bedpan is cut into a 4-inch (10-cm.) foam rubber mattress at the appropriate place. The cut out section and the edges of the hole are covered with mattress ticking. For use of the bedpan the patient is rolled to one side of the bed, the plug is removed, the bedpan is put into the hole (Fig. 16-16) and the patient is rolled onto his back. This involves no activity by the patient.

Though the described procedure reduces considerably the danger of disc damage during defecation, it is still advisable to limit the bowel evacuation as much as possible and to assure evacuation without strain. During the first few days while the patient still has sciatic pain, bowel evacuation is avoided entirely. If narcotics are used for pain relief they assist in this endeavor by their constipating action. Then the patient is placed on a bowel softener such as dioctyl sodium sulfosuccinate (Doxinate), 240 mg., two to three times a day and a bowel movement induced every second or third day by a Fleet enema. The patient must be encouraged not to strain during the bowel movement.

Bladder Program. The activity of daily living which tends most frequently to interfere with complete bed rest is the emptying of the bladder. In male patients this can be managed with a urinal without a change in the semi-Fowler's position. For women the sunken bedpan is used.

Quite frequently patients have difficulty voiding in supine position. Measures to induce emptying of the bladder are the sound of running water, hot packs to the suprapubic region, or medications such as bethanecholchloride (Urecholine) and neostigmine bromide (Prostigmin). If the patient still cannot void, he should be catheterized. Frequently, patients become able to void in supine position after one catheterization. However, if this is not the case and the patient has to be catheterized repeatedly, the use of an indwelling catheter is advisable. This decision should be made within the first 24 hours. In women with severe sciatica, an indwelling catheter may be used from the outset in order to avoid the bedpan procedure.

Recommended Activities

In the endeavor to avoid disuse phenomena as much as possible the patient should be encouraged to carry out activities which do not involve contraction of the trunk muscles. These are activities of the upper and lower extremities.

The upper extremities are usually exercised adequately by use during the patient's daily activities—eating, washing his hands, reading, writing, and using the telephone. If the patient needs additional activities to be fully occupied, crafts may be considered. In all these activities it is always important to warn the patient not to raise his head.

Activity in the lower extremities is even more important, not only for the prevention of disuse but also for the prevention of thrombotic phenomena. The markedly immobilized patient at bed rest is in danger of pelvic thrombosis and possible pulmonary emboli. The recommended leg exercise consists of simultaneous flexion of hip and knee while the heel of the foot is gliding along the mattress. The hip and knee may be flexed until the foot rests on the crest of the raised portion of the bed. The patient should be encouraged to perform approximately five such motions with each leg every 2 to 3 hours.

Other thrombosis preventing measures may also be taken. Women should always be taken off birth control pills. The patients may wear elastic stockings up to the knee. Heparin may be administered daily. Aspirin 1 Gm. three times a day, may be added.

Suppression of Involuntary Muscular Contractions

Coughing. If the patient is given morphine derivatives, cough will be controlled during the first 2 or 3 days. Later on, if the patient has a tendency to cough he should be given medication every 3 to 4 hours around the clock. Empirin with Codeine could be used for this purpose.

Sneezing. If the patient is known to be allergic and is likely to sneeze because of a cold, a systematic program of antihistaminic medication should be instituted.

Vomiting. To avoid drug-induced vomiting it is important to inquire which narcotics the patient tolerates best. In case of nausea and vomiting, antiemetic medication such as atropine or prochlorperazine (Compazine) should be given promptly.

PATIENT MANAGEMENT DURING THE AMBULATORY PHASE

Choice and Application of Corset or Body Jacket

Many types of corsets, braces and plaster jackets have been recommended for the management of lumbar disc lesions. In order to effectively decrease intradiscal pressure they must put considerable pressure on the abdomen and restrict the mobility of the trunk, particularly forward flexion. Two appliances which satisfy these conditions are the Hoke Corset and the Raney Flexion Jacket.

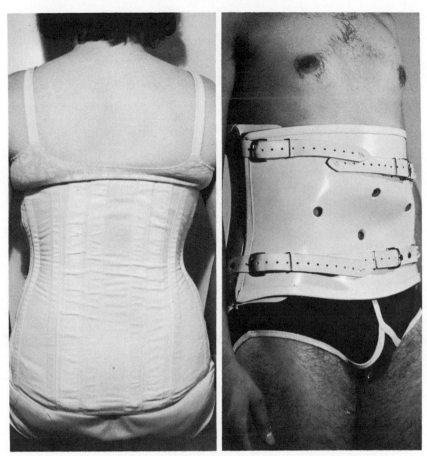

Fig. 16-17. *(Left)* Modified Hoke corset. *(Right)* Plastic dorso-lumbar flexion jacket.

The Hoke Corset.   The Hoke corset (Fig. 16-17) is a canvas cylinder which surrounds the trunk of the patient from the pubis to the sternum in front and from the sacrum to the middle of the shoulder blades in the back. It is closed in front by straps and buckles and has paravertebral pockets in the back for the insertion of steel stays. The corset must be fitted and shaped to the figure of the patient. It is particularly important to have a marked narrowing in the waist. This prevents the corset from sliding up and when properly adjusted exerts considerable abdominal pressure. The stays should be bent in such a way as to minimize the lumbar lordosis.

The paravertebral stays should be located to either side of the protruding spinous processes. The corset must be applied while the patient is in supine position. The lowest strap of the corset should be at the upper border of the pubic bone. The lower straps which tighten the corset around the pelvis should be snug. The middle straps at the waist should be as tight as possible and should exert noticeable abdominal pressure. The uppermost strap which should be at the lower portion of the sternum can be loosened to allow epigastric expansion during breathing.

The Raney Royalite Flexion Jacket. The Raney Royalite Flexion Jacket (Fig. 16-17), like the Hoke corset, surrounds the trunk completely and reaches, in front, from the pubis to the sternum and, in the back, from the sacrum to the middle of the shoulder blades.[11] It is made of Royalite and, therefore, is light and comfortable. The Raney Jacket is divided into an anterior and posterior shell hinged by leather straps in the axillary line. It is designed with a deep indentation anteriorly between the pubis and the sternum. This anterior indentation serves the double purpose of keeping the lumbar spine in flexion and of exerting pressure on the abdomen. The indentation also prevents the corset from sliding upward or from rotating. It should be applied to the patient in supine position. The anterior lower border of the jacket should be at the superior edge of the pubic bone.

The manufacture of the Raney Flexion Jacket presents one problem. Initially a plaster mold is made with the patient in sitting position. This may produce a recurrence of lumbar disc herniation even after a patient has been at bed rest for 2 weeks. To prevent this complication we have given each patient a Hoke Corset first which can be measured, fitted and applied in lying position. The plaster mold for the Raney Jacket was then applied over the Hoke corset which protected the patient while in sitting position.

Both appliances have drawbacks and advantages. The Raney Jacket if properly tightened stays in place without motion. It probably produces a greater and more constant abdominal pressure than the Hoke Corset whose straps tend to loosen. The Raney Jacket does not deteriorate while the canvas corset, of course, after a while tends to tear, and the straps have to be replaced. As far as comfort is concerned, some patients prefer the jacket and others the corset.

The First Three Months Following the Bed Phase

While many patients accept the very exacting bed phase as a necessary evil possibly because they are aware of the fact that it is the bed rest which has relieved the pain, they are greatly puzzled by the strict corset regimen which follows the bed phase for a period of 3 months. It is very important to repeatedly explain the mechanism of the disc herniation, the effect of the load on the disc and the role the corset or jacket plays in diminishing it to the patient. For the first 3 months following the bed phase the patient should wear a corset or jacket at all times unless he is in horizontal position in bed. This in itself imposes some restrictions in activity. All restrictions in activity must be clearly outlined for the patient. The average patient needs to be seen by the physician approximately four times during the first 3 months, 2 weeks after the discharge from the hospital and then again at the end of the first, second and third months. Usually there will be some problems with the design or the application of the corset that will need to be altered. The patient also needs psychological support in order to persevere in the restrictions of activity.

Bath and Shower Restrictions

If the patient cannot leave the horizontal position without a corset or body jacket he needs to alter his usual routine for cleanliness. It is simplest to forgo baths and showers altogether and have the patient take a sponge bath while wearing the corset. The corseted area of the body can be cleaned with a sponge bath in bed or a visiting nurse can perform this procedure. However, if the patient insists that he must take a shower, the following procedures are possible:

  a. The patient can cover his corset with a plastic sheet while taking a shower to prevent it from getting wet.
  b. The patient may have two corsets, one of which will get wet during the shower. He will then have to lie down on a bath towel on the bed, remove the wet corset, dry his body with some assistance and apply a dry corset.
  c. The patient using a Raney Flexion Jacket may have a second unlined jacket which is used only for showers. After the shower, he will then have to switch jackets while lying in the horizontal position.

Regardless of which method the patient chooses to take a shower, the area under the corset will still have to be cleaned by a sponge bath while the patient is in a horizontal position.

Restrictions on Sexual Activity

Studies of intradiscal pressure during sexual activity are not available at present. From clinical experience it is known that sexual activity is a frequent cause of recurrent symptoms when carried out early in the recovery phase. We recommend the following routine:

a. For 2 weeks after the bed phase, no sexual activity whatsoever.
b. From 2 weeks to 2 months sexual relations only while wearing the corset or body jacket. The patient should be supine during sexual intercourse with his hips and knees flexed and should restrict trunk activity to a minimum.
c. From 2 to 3 months after the bed phase, sexual activity without corset may be permitted but the same rules for position and avoidance of violent motions should be observed.

Restrictions in Activities of Daily Living

During the first 3 months following the bed phase activities which increase intradiscal pressure should be avoided. The most common activities which need to be regulated are sitting and lifting.

Sitting. For 2 to 3 weeks following bed rest sitting should be limited to periods of 30 minutes. The use of an elevated chair to a height of 22 to 24 inches (55 to 60 cm.) prevents the lower edge of the corset or jacket from pressing on the thigh. In addition, getting up from and sitting down on an elevated seat requires less effort and less forward bending. On the toilet the patient should use a 6-inch (10-cm.) raised toilet seat. Since driving a car is inevitably associated with sitting, it will have to be limited to short periods initially. The car seat should be as high as possible and the back of the seat should be slightly reclined. After 3 weeks sitting can be gradually increased to longer periods, and 2 months after bed rest the patient may sit for several hours, but still on an elevated chair.

Lifting. Nothing heavier than 10 pounds should be lifted. Picking up an object from the floor should be accomplished by bending at the knees and not by leaning forward. Heavy pushing and pulling, such as pushing a lawn mower or pulling weeds, also must be avoided.

For patients who need physical activity, walking is recommended. There is no medical indication for any exercise other than walking at this time and it is best to postpone any specific therapeutic exercise until after the third month.

Work Restrictions

The restrictions on activities of daily living give an indication of necessary restrictions in work. Many patients can resume work during the corset phase. The teacher who can prepare his lesson plans in a horizontal position and do his teaching in a standing position can go back to work shortly after the bed phase. So can salesmen, executives, and many other white collar workers. Patients whose occupations involve sitting for several hours, such as typists, can return to work after

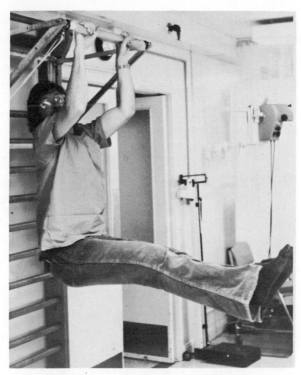

Fig. 16-18. Abdominal strengthening by chinning.

1 or 2 months following the bed phase provided they arrange to sit on an elevated chair. A housewife can do most of her chores, provided she avoids lifting and sitting.

Patient Management After the Third Month

If 3 months have passed since the bed phase and the patient has had no recurrence of disc symptomatology the conservative management can be considered successful. Nevertheless, the disc is not healed, treatment is not complete and further medical supervision is necessary. The goals of medical management after the third month are gradual elimination of the corset and restoration of normal trunk mobility and strength.

Gradual Elimination of the Corset

After wearing the corset or jacket for 3 months the patient has become adjusted to it, feels quite comfortable and is frequently reluctant to discard it.

Disabling Conditions Due to Musculoskeletal Impairment 377

Normally the contraction of trunk muscles protects the lumbar disc in cases of increased load. The patient has to become gradually conditioned to contract the trunk muscles during effort. For this reason the corset has to be eliminated gradually. It is best to start this process under controlled conditions, that is, at times of complete leisure, after work, on weekends or on days off.

Initially the corset will be worn approximately 75 per cent of the day, then after a week or two 50 per cent and finally 25 per cent. The corset should always be put on again for sitting, driving, any heavy activity and any sports activity. At the 6-month point the corset may, in most cases, be discarded.

Trunk Strengthening

Always conscious of the fact that the injured disc still has not competely healed and is still vulnerable to excessive loads, we have

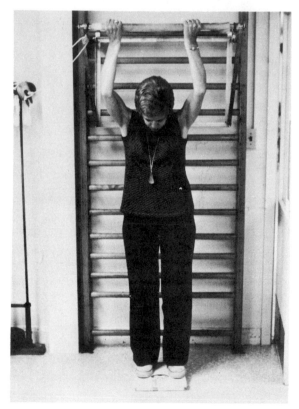

Fig. 16-19. Chinning exercise on a bathroom scale.

looked for a method of trunk strengthening which puts a minimal load on the disc. For this reason we prefer exercises in suspended position.

If the patient is able to chin himself at a horizontal bar this will be the exercise of choice. The patient will start chinning while flexing trunk, hips and knees. This flexor synergy facilitates strengthening of the abdominal muscles. Later on the patient should chin while flexing trunk and hips but keeping the knees extended (Fig. 16-18). This places a greater load on the abdominal muscles. Eventually he can add a weight to his ankles in the form of a sand bag weighing from 2 to 10 pounds. It is agreed that strengthening of the abdominal muscles generally is the crucial exercise for trunk stability and disc protection. If a patient is unable to chin he may push himself up on a parallel bar and carry out the same program—first, trunk flexion with hip and knee flexion and later trunk and hip flexion with knees extended and finally the same exercise with an additional weight at the ankle.

If the patient is unable to chin himself he may start out with a graded chinning exercise. In this exercise the patient stands on a bathroom scale under a chinning bar which is located about 6 inches (10 cm.) above his head (Fig. 16-19). After checking his weight on the scale the patient grasps the chinning bar with a supinated grip and pulls himself up. He then reads on the scale by how many pounds he has diminished his body weight. By doing 10 chinning exercises daily he will gradually improve to the point where he can lift his whole body weight. Then he may begin regular chinning exercises.

Other very good trunk exercises are swimming, jogging and walking up hill. All these activities are permissible after the third or fourth month. Jogging, however, should still be performed with a corset or body jacket.

Restoration of Trunk Mobility

When the patient is examined for the first time without his corset at the 3 months check-up, there is usually limitation of trunk mobility, particularly forward flexion. The fact that trunk flexion has been avoided for over 3 months has led to contracture or shortening of the lumbar fascia and the tendons of the hip and back extensors. On his first attempt at forward bending the patient's extended fingertips are frequently from 15 to 20 inches (40 to 50 cm.) from the floor. Restoration of normal range can be accomplished in many ways. We have chosen a simple exercise which the patient can carry out himself under the shower. Standing with knees extended and legs slightly spread, the patient bends forward passively as far as the weight of his trunk will pull him without any additional muscular effort and without any momentum. He stays completely relaxed in this position and allows very hot water from the shower to run over his lumbar, sacral, and gluteal region. The patient then straightens up slowly and repeats this maneuver two more times. This exercise places a greater load on the disc than it has had in the preceding months and for this reason has to be done with great care. Usually the patient's trunk flexion becomes normal after 1 month of these forward bending exercises.

By the sixth month the patient should have adequate trunk strength and mobility. At this point most patients can go without the corset and carry out all their regular daily activities. However, since they have shown by their original disc lesion that they have vulnerable intervertebral discs they are advised to use the corset for heavy duty. This term needs to be explained since it may mean different things for different patients.

The person who is not usually involved in heavy lifting should put his corset or jacket on before he moves furniture or undertakes a repair job in the house which involves some carrying of medium loads. For the mechanic or any person involved in his ordinary life in lifting loads up to 50 pounds the corset will be needed when he is confronted with a task involving an extra heavy load. It probably would be advisable for a person having suffered a lumbar disc lesion not to lift anything heavier than 50 pounds for the rest of his life wherever this is possible. In the case of a laborer whose very livelihood depends on being able to lift heavy loads the question arises whether or not he should ever be allowed to go back to work. In a younger person the occurrence of a lumbar disc lesion should not be a condemnation to retirement. It would be advisable for this person to return to work wearing a corset or body jacket. Unfortunately, it is most unlikely that an employer is willing to employ a worker having the medical order to wear a corset. As far as laborers over 40 and 50 are concerned, it would be more reasonable to consider either retirement or, if feasible, vocational rehabilitation.

Section D. Amputations of Lower Extremities

GENERAL PRINCIPLES

As a result of the experience with war casualties and recent progress in limb manufacture, it is now relatively easy to solve the problem of mere ambulation for the young, able-bodied amputee who has lost a lower extremity. For this patient, the principal remaining objectives are a normal-appearing gait and the ability to dance, ski and possibly roller skate with an artificial limb. However, for the elderly amputee the outlook is by no means so favorable. Because he often has either additional disease or disability, he is frequently declared unsuitable for a prosthesis. Advanced age, arteriosclerosis, heart disease or a poor amputation stump may be the reasons for an unfavorable prognosis. Although it has been shown that crutch-walking is more strenuous for the leg amputee than the use of a prosthesis, the elderly amputee is frequently sent home from the hospital with only crutches or a wheelchair.

As a rule, the elderly and sick patient adjusts more slowly and has more difficulty with prostheses than the young healthy person. This is due to a variety of causes.

Motivation. Some elderly people are satisfied to restrict their activities to the extent that an artificial limb is a nuisance rather than a help. Others would use a limb if it were a mere matter of fitting and walking with ease, but they are not willing to work through the training and adjustment period. Introduction of the prosthesis must be planned carefully, and training should be carried out slowly to avoid frustration.

Costs. The use of a prosthesis may be short-lived because of the likelihood of additional morbidity or disability, even death, within a few months. Under such circumstances, the cost of artificial limbs is often considered to be too high.

Danger to Health. Damage to a poorly vascularized stump may occur from an ill-fitted socket, and injuries may occur due to falls. Overexertion during the training period may precipitate cardiac decompensation or other medical complications.

Poor Planning. Since it is frequently assumed that the elderly patient is not a candidate for a prosthesis, the surgeon may not plan the amputation with future use of an artificial limb in mind. Other manifestations of poor planning may be evidenced by unsatisfactory care of the stump or by delay in referral to a rehabilitation service. Frequently, patients whose limbs are amputated have long been bedridden and severely debilitated before amputation.

While there may be valid objections to prescription of an artificial limb for some, it is usually possible to provide an elderly person with a prosthesis without being thwarted by the difficulties listed above. Following are rules of management which may obviate some or all of the obstacles to a prosthesis:

The surgeon should consider each amputee as a candidate for some kind of appliance. He should treat the stump accordingly and refer the patient to a rehabilitation service immediately after amputation. When possible, the patient should have consultative rehabilitation guidance prior to amputation.

Conditions and procedures must be provided for optimal stump healing and prevention of disuse during the healing period.

As soon as the stump is healed, the patient should be provided with a temporary prosthesis with a plaster socket and should be trained in ambulation with this pylon. The socket may need to be changed after shrinkage of the stump.

If after several months of use of the temporary prosthesis, the patient has shown no harmful effects, walks well and is satisfied with the pylon, he may then be fitted with a permanent artificial limb.

The quality of gait expected in the elderly amputee is less than perfect. The patient may need a cane, crutches or a walker but this does not contraindicate the use of a prosthesis.

METHODS OF REHABILITATION

Discussion will be limited to the two most frequent types of lower extremity amputation, namely, the below-knee (BK) amputation and the above-knee (AK) amputation at the level of mid-thigh or higher.

At present three general approaches to the above-knee and below-knee amputee are used: (1) delayed fitting with a permanent prosthesis; (2) early fitting with a temporary prosthesis; and (3) immediate postoperative fitting with a temporary prosthesis.

Delayed Fitting with Permanent Prosthesis

After amputation and wound healing, the patient undergoes a long-range physical therapy program designed to prepare his stump for a prosthesis. This preparation includes shrinking, toughening, strengthening and maintaining or increasing range of motion. Shrinkage is accomplished by bandaging or by elastic shrinkers, toughening by massage and strengthening by weight and pulley exercises. When he is ready, the patient is fitted with a prosthesis and trained in its use.

It is difficult to achieve complete shrinkage by this method and after some time the patient will usually require a new socket for his prosthesis because of additional shrinkage.

Early Fitting with a Temporary Prosthesis

After amputation and wound-healing, the patient is provided with a temporary prosthesis which in its simplest form is a pylon with a plaster of Paris socket. He then starts walking and weight-bearing

immediately. Toughening, shrinkage, strengthening and maintenance of range of motion are achieved by walking and weight-bearing.
The plaster socket is replaced by a smaller one from time to time as
the stump shrinks. When shrinkage is complete and the patient has
proven that he is able to handle the pylon, a prosthesis is prescribed.
This method seems to us most suitable for the elderly amputee and is
also the most economic. Therefore it will be described in detail on
pages 383-395.

Immediate Postoperative Fitting with a Temporary Prosthesis

In this method the stump is wrapped with a rigid plaster of Paris
dressing immediately after amputation. This cast is used as a socket,
and weight-bearing on a temporary prosthesis is started even before
wound-healing has occurred. This method has the advantage of faster
rehabilitation and sometimes better wound-healing. For success this
method requires very skillful surgery and an exacting procedure to
apply the immediate postoperative cast. For this reason its use is not
widespread and mostly confined to amputee centers.

REHABILITATION BY EARLY FITTING OF A TEMPORARY PROSTHESIS

Rehabilitation progresses through three successive phases: the
wound-healing phase, the phase of temporary prosthesis and the
prosthetic phase.

Wound-Healing Phase

This phase starts immediately after surgery and lasts until satisfactory healing of the stump wound has occurred. The rehabilitative
measures during the wound-healing phase are: skin traction, positioning and general activities.

Skin Traction

Skin traction is to be applied to the stump immediately after
surgery and should be maintained continuously until complete closure of the stump has occurred.

Purpose. Traction on the skin of the stump protects the wound in
several ways. Above all, it prevents retraction of soft tissue and pre-
serves a cushion between bone and skin. It also protects the wound
against injury since the traction strips form a protective cuff around
the stump. Furthermore, traction maintains the knee joint and the hip
joint in extended position and prevents flexion contractures. Finally,
it affords resistance to all movements of the stump and thereby pre-

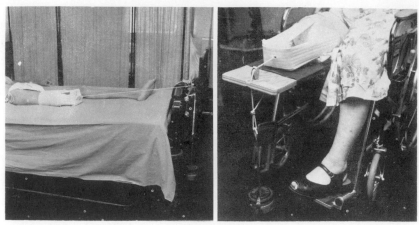

Fig. 16-20. *(Left)* Skin traction for AK amputee in bed. *(Right)* Skin traction for AK amputee in chair.

vents disuse atrophy. In a way, it replaces the weight of the missing limb. The traction device can be used in a chair as well as in bed.

Method. Unless there is known allergy to tincture of benzoin, the stump to be placed in traction may be sprayed with it for better adhesion of the traction strips.

Two traction strips, 3 inches (18 cm.) wide, are placed, one from the anterior to the posterior aspect of the stump and one from the medial to the lateral aspect. They must be long enough to allow the loops to clear the end of the stump by about 2 inches (5 cm.). The strips are held in place by a cotton elastic bandage (Fig. 16-20, *left*).

A block of wood, covered with moleskin, is placed inside of these strips at the point where they cross, to act as a spreader. A rope is knotted and put through the block and then through the strips and over a pulley at the end of the bed. Then, a weight hanger with 3 to 5 pounds (about 2 kg.) of weight is attached (Fig. 16-20).

Traction can also be kept on when the patient is in a chair by using a seat board with a pulley designed for this purpose (Fig. 16-20, *right*).

Positioning

Positioning is essential to prevent flexion contractures at the hip and the knee (in the BK amputee). Proper positioning supplements the preventive effect of traction. The patient should be placed in face-lying position without pillows under the hips at least 4 times daily for 1 hour. Preferably, the patient should sleep the greater part of the night in the face-lying position. Flexion of the hip should be avoided.

Pillows should not be placed under the knee since this will cause flexion at the knee and the hip. Prolonged sitting is also detrimental to the lower extremity amputee since the hip and the knee are flexed at 90 degrees in this position. The chair should be used as little as possible until the wound-healing is complete. Then, a vigorous exercise program can be carried out to counteract the tendency to form contractures.

Activities

The postoperative stump of the arteriosclerotic BK and AK amputee is very vulnerable. For this reason, it is wise to limit the patient's activities during early phase care. Often, elderly patients are very awkward and weak, and during a simple transfer from bed to chair or while sitting in a wheelchair they may strike the stump against the bed or the chair. This may cause the wound to split open or may result in bleeding into the stump. Therefore, it is recommended that the patient remain at bed rest until most of the skin and subcutaneous tissue have grown together. During this stage, bed exercises should be performed. Toward the latter part of the wound-healing phase, chair exercises, stand-up exercises and hopping exercises may be added. Finally, the patient is trained in amputee crutch gaits.

Bed Exercises. *Trunk Flexion.* Trunk flexion strengthens the trunk in preparation for crutch-walking.

1. While lying on back, lift head and shoulders forward as high as possible without coming to a sitting position. Relax.

2. Repeat 5 or 6 times, several sessions daily.

Face-lying Push-ups. Push-ups are used to strengthen the arms and shoulders.

1. While lying face down, bend elbows and place hands flat on bed under shoulders.

2. Extend arms and push trunk off the bed. Keep the pelvis and stump flat on the bed.

3. Slowly return to starting position.

4. Repeat 10 times, several sessions daily.

Chair Exercises. Seated push-ups are also helpful in strengthening the arms and shoulders.

1. Place hands on chair arms forward of trunk.

2. Push down gradually straightening the arms.

3. Lift body off the chair as high as possible.

4. Slowly let body down into the chair.

5. Repeat push-ups 5 or 6 times, several sessions daily. Gradually increase the number of push-ups done at each exercise period.

Stand-up Exercises.   During the later part of this phase, one-legged stand-up exercises are carried out from the edge of the bed. During all these activities skin traction should be maintained. For the stand-up exercise a 1-lb. (½ kg.) weight can be suspended directly from the traction cuff.

Hopping Exercises.   Hopping exercises are for strengthening the remaining leg. Hopping may also be used by an amputee without a prosthesis as a means of propelling himself for short distances at a fairly rapid rate if necessary. Variations of hopping exercises are:

Hopping in Place
1. Stand up. With one hand hold on to a firm support.
2. Hop up and down in place as tolerated.
3. Sit down. Repeat.

Progressive Hopping
1. Stand up. Place one hand on bar forward of body.
2. Hop one step forward.
3. Move hand forward.
4. Repeat, hopping one step forward and moving hand forward.

Hopping with a Walker
1. Stand up with walker in front with both hands on walker.
2. Lift and move walker forward one step.
3. Hop forward one step.
4. Repeat, moving walker forward and hopping forward.

Amputee Crutch Gaits.   *Stance.*   Stand against the bed or a wall. Place crutches under arms with the crutch tips about 4 inches (10 cm.) in front and 4 inches (10 cm.) to each side of the normal foot position, forming a wide base. Hold head up. Stand tall with pelvis over the feet.

Gait No. 1.   The Tripod Alternate Crutch Gait
1. Move right crutch forward.
2. Move left crutch forward.
3. Drag body and leg forward.

Gait No. 2.   The Tripod Simultaneous Gait
1. Move both crutches forward.
2. Drag body and leg forward.

Gait No. 3.   The Swing-To Gait
1. Move both crutches forward
2. Lift and swing body and leg up to crutches.

Gait No. 4.   The Swing-Through Gait
1. Move both crutches forward.
2. Lift and swing body and leg beyond crutches.

Wound Care

The stump wound is not only vulnerable to mechanical trauma but is also subject to infection. For this reason, frequent changes of dressing should be avoided. If the postoperative course is satisfactory, i.e., uncomplicated by fever, pain or bleeding, the original dressing may be left in place until the 10th day. Then, the wound should be inspected to see whether it is sufficiently healed for removal of sutures. Initially, it is best to remove only every other suture and to anchor the skin in the area by means of an eleastic adhesive tape butterfly bandage. The remaining sutures may be removed within a few days if the wound is healed. The butterfly bandages should be left on for another week or 2 and should then be removed very carefully. One should not hesitate to delay removal of sutures if healing of the tissues has not occurred.

If there is any sign of infection of the wound, cultures should be taken, and the patient should be placed immediately on broad spectrum antibiotics. When bacteriologic studies are completed, specific antibiotics should be prescribed and continued for 2 weeks. If granulation tissue protrudes beyond the skin in certain areas of the wound margin, it should be touched with silver nitrate every other day until the proliferating portion has disappeared.

THE TEMPORARY PROSTHESIS

The completely healed stump is not yet ready for use of an artificial limb. Usually, it is very tender and the skin of the thigh has to be prepared to tolerate the pressure and friction to which it will be subjected inside the socket of a prosthesis. The measures used to alleviate the sensitivity and vulnerability of the skin of the stump are known as *stump-conditioning*. The freshly healed stump is swollen, and if subjected to the pressure of weight-bearing, it will shrink. Thus, an objective of stump care is maximal shrinkage of the swollen tissues. Finally, the stump must be strong to be able to move the prosthesis and to stabilize the body when weight is borne on it.

Before a permanent prosthesis is prescribed, shrinking, strengthening and conditioning of the stump should be completed. This can best be accomplished by the use of a temporary prosthesis. This seems to be the method of choice for the elderly patient for several reasons. Motivation is an important factor. The elderly patient is likely to accept an exercise that allows him to stand immediately and to walk fairly soon after amputation. This can be done with the temporary prosthesis. He is less likely to cooperate in doing pulley exercises, and he may be intolerant of tedious, complicated bandaging of the stump. Furthermore, the temporary prosthesis accomplishes all three objectives of conditioning, shrinking and strengthening without requiring additional measures.

The services of a prosthetist are needed for preparation of the temporary prosthesis and manufacture of the permanent artificial limb.

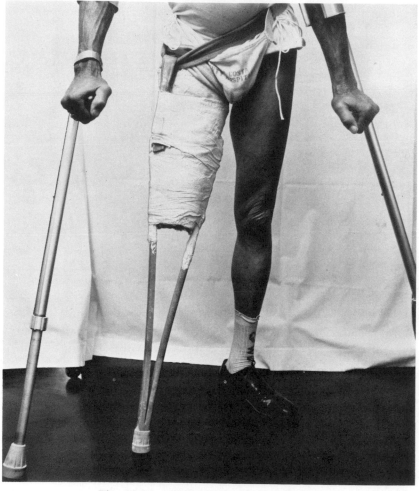

Fig. 16-21.   Temporary AK prosthesis.

The Pylon

The temporary lower extremity prosthesis or pylon is a "peg leg" and consists of three parts—a bucket or socket that fits over the stump, a stick or peg attached to the socket that bears weight on the ground and a strap or belt that holds the socket in place on the stump. Often, the stick is made from the lower portion of a crutch, and it is covered with a rubber crutch tip. The socket is made of plaster of Paris.

1. The socket for AK amputations has a quadrilateral opening and is conical in shape. Its upper rim is flattened in the posterior portion to provide an ischial seat. Usually, it is open at the bottom unless some end-bearing of the stump is desired. The socket is attached to the patient by means of a belt (Fig. 16-21).

TECHNIQUE FOR MANUFACTURE OF PLASTER PYLONS

The BK Pylon

1. Fit a wide strip of ¼-inch (½ cm.) felt snugly around the entire BK stump.

2. Wrap 2-inch (5-cm.) adhesive tape around the felt in spiral fashion from the patella to the lower third of the stump. Apply this adhesive tape as tightly as possible. The lower third of the stump must remain untaped.

3. Apply plaster of Paris to the stump. Use two 4-inch (10-cm.) rolls. Mold it around the condyles of the femur. Go up as high as the middle of the patella and depress the plaster below the patella.

4. When the plaster has set (after a half hour), trim the posterior portion of plaster down to the level of the depression in front.

5. Fix suspension buttons to either side of the socket, ¾-inch (2 cm.) below the brim at the junction of the posterior and lateral surfaces, using plaster of Paris.

6. Apply the wooden crutch part to the socket by winding the plaster in figure-8 fashion around the bars of the crutch and the socket.

The AK Pylon

1. Fit medium weight cardboard around the AK stump from the crotch to 2 inches (5 cm.) below the stump. On the outside of the thigh this cardboard should cover the trochanter.

Disabling Conditions Due to Musculoskeletal Impairment **389**

2. Take a piece of ½-inch (1 cm.) felt 4 inches (10 cm.) wide and fold it over the upper rim of the cardboard and glue it in place.

3. Place the cardboard snugly around the stump with the seam to the outside. Hold it in place with three strips of 2-inch (5-cm.) adhesive tape and mark the line of overlap with a pencil.

4. Remove the cardboard from the stump and advance the overlap a half inch to diminish the circumference.

5. Wrap two 6-inch (14 cm.) plaster bandages around the cardboard molding the upper rim into a quadrilateral shape. Maintain an anteroposterior distance equal to the crotch measurement from the ischial tuberosity to the adductor tendon.

6. After the plaster has set apply the wooden crutch portion to the socket with additional plaster bandage after shaving down the wooden bars for better fit.

7. Rivet the strap to the socket at the area of the trochanter in such a way that the buckle is in front of the socket.

An alternate for the crutch portion is a piece of 1-inch (2-3 cm.) dowel attached to a circular plate of ¾-inch (2 cm.) plywood that fits into the lower portion of the socket.

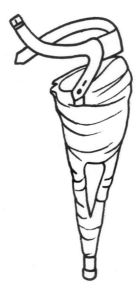

Fig. 16-22. Temporary BK prosthesis.

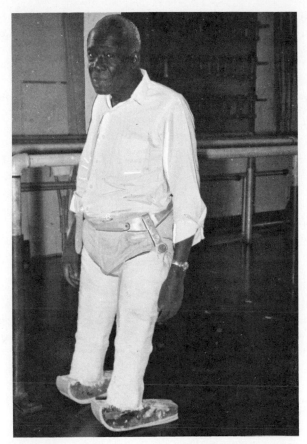

Fig. 16-23. Temporary prosthesis for bilateral AK amputee.

2. The socket for a BK amputation has the shape of a rounded cup. In front and on the sides it reaches to the level of the middle of the patella. It is lower in the back to permit flexion of the knee. A strap is attached on each side of the socket. These straps are buckled above the knee to hold the socket in place (Fig. 16-22).

The plaster sockets described resemble the wooden socket of the AK prosthesis and the soft patella-bearing socket of the BK prosthesis. A woolen stump sock is worn in all temporary prostheses.

3. For a bilateral lower extremity amputee the sockets are not attached to pegs but to flat, curved, wooden blocks that extend posteriorly like feet that have been turned 180 degrees (Fig. 16-23). These

Disabling Conditions Due to Musculoskeletal Impairment 391

blocks provide the standing stability that the bilateral amputee needs. The bottom of each block is covered with crepe rubber and is rounded in order to facilitate walking.

Exercises With the Temporary Prosthesis

The purpose in performing the exercises is stump-conditioning and shrinkage, strengthening and development of balance on the prosthesis. Initially, weight-bearing and use of the prosthesis will be limited to short periods, from 15 minutes to a half hour. These exercise periods should be frequent, at least 3 or 4 times a day. Later, the periods will be lengthened, and finally, the patient will wear the temporary prosthesis all day long and walk with it. The exercises are begun in the parallel bars; the patient then progresses to cane-walking with the prosthesis and finally, to walking without a cane, if this is feasible. Some very unstable patients may need to use a walker for a time, and some may always have to rely on a walker if balance is impaired by other disabilities.

During the parallel bar phase, the patient is at first allowed to use both hands on the bars and to bear weight gradually on the affected limb. Usually, a certain amount of hip-flexion contracture has occurred in the AK amputee, and an important exercise is to stabilize the prosthesis by pressing it down on the ground and hyperextending the hip. Another early exercise is the shifting of weight from the good leg to the stump and back to the good leg.

A second step is balancing on the prosthesis with both hands still on the bars. This is done by placing the good leg forward and backward and maintaining the hip of the amputation side hyperextended during this motion. Finally, the patient may start walking in the parallel bars. He should be encouraged to take very small steps with the prosthesis and very long steps with the uninvolved leg, hyperextending the hip on the amputated side with each step. After the patient can carry out these exercises with both hands on the parallel bars, he is led through the same exercise program with only one hand on a bar, that is, the hand opposite the amputation side. When he is capable of one-handed walking in the parallel bars, he starts on the same exercise routine with a cane and eventually without a cane. The procedure is the same for the AK and BK amputee, but usually the BK amputee progresses more rapidly and has less difficulty.

The exercise program for the double AK amputee differs somewhat from that of the unilateral amputee. He also starts out in low parallel bars; his weight-bearing will have to be accomplished at first by taking most of his weight on his arms and gradually letting himself

---

SUMMARY OF PYLON EXERCISES FOR THE UNILATERAL
LOWER EXTREMITY AMPUTEE

Practice for Standing Balance

1. Stand between parallel bars with body in good postural alignment. Place both hands on bars. Body weight should be supported equally on both legs.

2. Shift weight from side to side. As control of balance increases use only one hand on the bar, later balance without holding bar.

Practice Training in Ambulation

1. "Step-to" gait: Stand between parallel bars. Assistance by holding bars with hands is allowed at first, if necessary. Step forward one step with the normal leg; bring the prosthesis up to it. Repeat.

2. "Step-out" gait: Stand between bars. Step forward one step with normal leg. Step forward one step with prosthesis beyond normal leg. Take another step with normal leg. Repeat.

After practicing in parallel bars for stability, the patient does a series of "step outs" that constitute walking. With adequate balance, he begins cane-walking. Equal length of steps is stressed.

---

down into the sockets. Thus, the initial exercise is a push-up and relaxation for weight-bearing. Once he tolerates weight-bearing on both leg stumps, he starts to walk with a waddling gait and small steps, holding on to the bars with both hands. He may progress from there to walking with two short crutches and eventually with two short canes or without support. Since the use of this type of prosthesis (called a "stubbie") reduces the height of the patient considerably, he may have difficulty getting into the wheelchair or into bed. While it is at first easiest for him to control the stubbies if they are as short as possible, it may be advisable to lengthen the sockets gradually until the patient has reached the height from which he can transfer with ease to his bed and his wheelchair. Walking with stubbies is strenuous and very slow. Most elderly AK amputees thus prefer to forego prostheses and use only a wheelchair. For younger and athletic bilateral AK amputees it is also possible to progress to the use of regular AK prostheses.

Disabling Conditions Due to Musculoskeletal Impairment　　**393**

Stump-Conditioning. While the very gradual use of a temporary prosthesis may accomplish the stump-conditioning automatically, additional measures may be required for certain stumps. If the patient cannot tolerate the socket at all because of excessive stump sensitivity, the skin may be desensitized gradually by gentle massage and tapping. If there are some very painful spots within the stump, these may be due to the formation of neuromata, small knots of nerve fibers that may develop at the end of nerves. These can be treated with ultrasound, and the patient will be pain-free after four or five treatments. (The usual dosage is 2 watts for 5 minutes.)

Stump Shrinkage. During the wound-healing phase, swelling of the stump should be prevented by fairly snug bandaging. Further shrinkage will occur during the walking exercises with the temporary prosthesis. Shrinkage must be maintained when the socket is off. Traditionally, this is done by bandaging with a cotton elastic bandage. Since application of this bandage requires considerable skill and has to be done repeatedly during the day, it is preferable to use an elastic stump sock called a shrinker. This must be fitted properly to the size of the stump and have enough elastic power to compress it but not to interfere with circulation. Since shrinkers have a conical shape like the stump, they tend to slip off unless supported by garters. As the stump shrinks the patient must use additional stump socks during his walking exercises. If the shrinkage is considerable, it may be necessary to make a new plaster socket that will fit the shrunken stump.

Strengthening. Strengthening the patient's arms, trunk and stump begins during the wound-healing phase by means of the bed-exercise program, the stump-traction program and the one-legged stand-up program. Further strengthening of the stump and the patient in general occurs during the gait-training program in the parallel bars and with a cane. If additional exercises of the stump are needed, for example, because of weak hip extensors, it is easiest and best to carry them out with the temporary prosthesis by attaching a weight to the tip of it.

Special Problems. The principal complications that may interfere with the gait-training program are a painful stump and skin irritation or ulceration. The management of pain due to initial hypersensitivity and to neuroma was previously discussed. The only other likely cause of stump pain on weight-bearing is an ill-fitting socket. Usually, this is not the case initially since the socket has been molded to the stump, but it may occur after shrinkage. In this case, a new plaster socket should be made, or a soft liner may be added. When skin irritation or

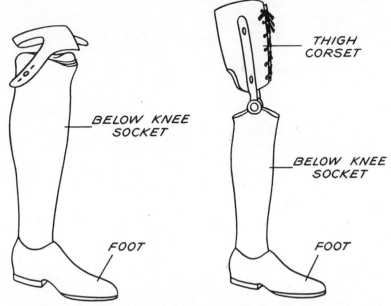

Fig. 16-24. *(Left)* Patella-bearing BK prosthesis. *(Right)* Standard BK prosthesis.

ulceration occurs, one must also look first for an ill-fitting socket. Other causes are excessive exercising before the skin is properly conditioned, or wrinkles in the stump sock.

PHASE OF PERMANENT PROSTHESIS

Artificial Limbs

Many types of artificial limbs are manufactured, and there is constant change and improvement of design. A few of the commonly used models will be described briefly.

Below-Knee Prosthesis

Patella-bearing Prosthesis.   This prosthesis has a soft socket for the BK stump. It is held in place by straps buckled above the knee (Fig. 16-24, *left*). The relative position of the foot and the ankle must be adjusted carefully to permit proper balance with only a small area of contact between the stump and the limb.

Standard BK Prosthesis.   This older type of appliance has a knee joint and a thigh corset which provides greater stability and control (Fig. 16-24, *right*).

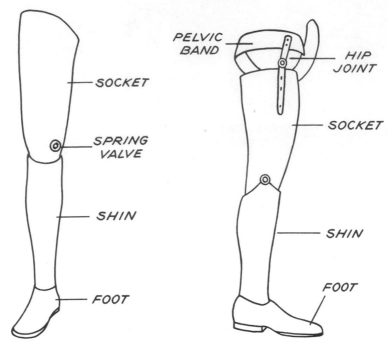

Fig. 16-25. *(Left)* Suction socket AK prosthesis. *(Right)* Conventional AK prosthesis.

Above-Knee Prosthesis

Suction Socket (Fig. 16-25, *left*).   The suction socket is held in place by negative pressure. After the stump has been introduced into the socket, a valve at the lower end is closed. Because of the snug fit no air enters the socket from above.

Conventional Socket (Fig. 16-25, *right*).   The conventional socket has a looser fit and is held in place by a pelvic band with hip joint.

Knee Joints.   The AK prosthesis has a knee joint that bends when the patient sits down and when he flexes his hip during walking. To bring his leg forward when walking, he has to flex the hip forcefully and quickly to obtain extension at the knee. A friction mechanism inside the joint regulates the speed with which the leg extends and diminishes the shock of full extension. The conventional knee joint will buckle when weight is borne on it while it is slightly flexed.

The Bock Knee is provided with a safety stop that prevents knee buckling. This knee flexes easily when no weight is borne but when weight is put on the slightly flexed knee (approximately to 25 de-

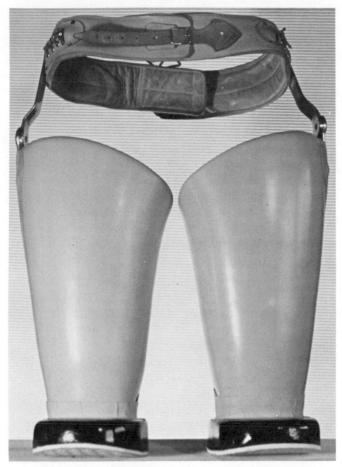

Fig. 16-26. "Stubbies" for bilateral AK amputee.

grees), the lock operates to prevent buckling. This is particularly advantageous for the elderly patient.

Prostheses for Bilateral AK Amputees

Stubbies (Fig. 16-26). These rather costly appliances are infrequently used because of their unnatural appearance and limited
functional usefulness.

Bilateral Conventional AK Prostheses. These prostheses afford
normal height and appearance and movable knee joints. However,
only athletic, highly motivated people master their use.

Disabling Conditions Due to Musculoskeletal Impairment   **397**

After his experience with the temporary prosthesis, the BK amputee will need only to become accustomed to the greater weight of the permanent prosthesis. Since there is no substantial difference in gait pattern, he will need no further instruction.

The AK amputee has a new problem to face. His temporary prosthesis has no knee joint; with the permanent limb he will have to learn how to handle the knee, i.e., he will need to gauge the force with which he propels the leg and to prevent the knee from buckling when bearing weight. He will have to lock a standard knee by striking the ground with the heel and pulling the knee back. In a Bock Knee the locking occurs on weight-bearing in slightly bent position. He must put full weight rather suddenly on the knee to prevent buckling.

SUMMARY

1. Frequently, the elderly amputee is not provided with an artificial limb and must use crutches or a wheelchair for locomotion. More elderly amputees can benefit from prostheses if they have an adequate stump and have demonstrated their ability to handle a temporary prosthesis (pylon).

2. An adequate stump is obtained by prompt use of postoperative rehabilitative measures such as skin traction, positioning, restricted activity and proper wound care.

3. A temporary prosthesis or pylon is used as soon as the stump is healed. It provides stump-conditioning, shrinkage and strengthening. It prepares the patient for use of a permanent prosthesis and also tests his ability to use it.

Section E. Amputations of Upper Extremities

CAUSES

Most upper extremity amputations are due to injuries, while a small number result from malignant tumors or birth defects. Thus the majority of upper extremity amputees are young.

DISABILITY

If only one upper extremity is involved the disability for activities of daily living is minimal since one functional hand is adequate. There is, of course, a vocational restriction. Children born without both arms can usually learn to substitute a foot for a hand for the purpose of eating, dressing, writing and most other needed activities. This was the only method of rehabilitation available prior to the development of modern prostheses. The severity of disability is proportional to the amount of upper extremity loss, i.e., the site of amputation: This can be disarticulation of the shoulder, amputation between elbow and shoulder or below the elbow.

REHABILITATION AND TRAINING

Upper Extremity Prostheses

The most important part of the upper extremity is the hand with its primary function of prehension. Mobility in shoulder, elbow and wrist enable the hand to be placed in the proper position to accomplish desired activities.

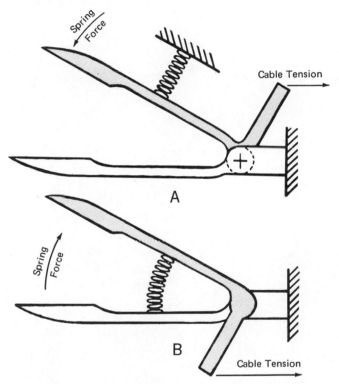

Fig. 16-27. *a.* Voluntary-opening and *b.* voluntary-closing terminal devices. (Based on Klopsteg, P. E., and Wilson, P. D.: Human Limbs and Their Substitutes. New York, Hafner Press, 1969.)

Disabling Conditions Due to Musculoskeletal Impairment **399**

The Terminal Device

The part of an artificial arm which replaces the hand is called the terminal device. If function of the upper extremity is the major concern the terminal device takes the form of a hook. If cosmetic appearance is the major concern, the terminal device will be a hand.

The Prosthetic Hook. A hook attached to an upper extremity stump is probably the oldest known prosthesis for the loss of a hand just as the pylon is the oldest known replacement for a leg. A simple hook can be functionally helpful and permit an amputee to carry heavy loads and manipulate certain machines.

In order to facilitate prehension, a split hook is now used most commonly (Fig. 16-29, 30). The two prongs of this device may be held together tightly by a rubberband or a spring. In this case the amputee activates a cable to open the hook (Fig. 16-27a) then grasps the object and releases the cable. The object is then held by the power of the elastic force. This method of voluntary opening does not allow the

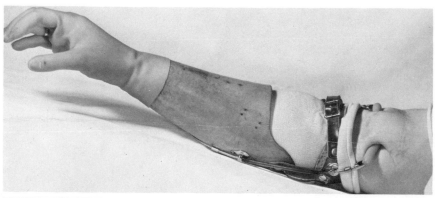

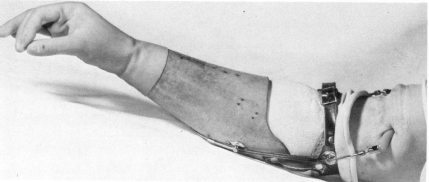

Fig. 16-28. Cineplasty with a cosmetic hand. (The American Limb Co.)

amputee to control the pressure exerted on the object held in the grasp.

Another variety of prosthetic hook is held open by an elastic force and the amputee activates a cable which closes the hook for grasping (Fig. 16-27b). With a simple voluntary closing hook, he will have to continue tensing the cable until he wants to release the object. In the APRL voluntary closing hook, a rather complex device, the pull which closes the hook also locks it. A second pull is needed to release the cable and allow the hook to open.

The hook most commonly used by our patients is the Dorrance hook with voluntary opening. The closing is done by a rubberband, the strength of which the amputee may choose according to the task he wishes to accomplish.

The Cosmetic Hand. To many amputees a cosmetic hand without any function may be acceptable. The terminal device can be readily exchanged so that the patient can use the prosthetic hook at work and the cosmetic hand for social occasions. Of course, grasping function can also be built into a cosmetic hand.

In this case the thumb replaces one prong of the split hook and the second and third fingers the other (Fig. 16-28). A pull on the cable can open the hand or close it according to the mechanism chosen. It must be kept in mind, however, that even an activated cosmetic hand cannot give the amputee the variety of functions that are possible with the prosthetic hook.

The Cable Control System. The most commonly used method to control the cable which activates the terminal device is a figure-of-8 harness around both shoulders (Fig. 16-29). The cable is relaxed

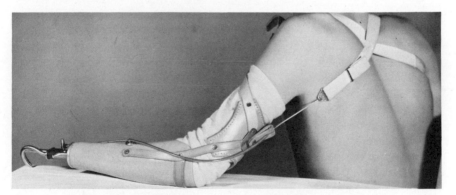

Fig. 16-29. Below-elbow figure-of-8 harness. (Institute of Rehabilitation Medicine, New York University Medical Center, New York, N.Y.)

Disabling Conditions Due to Musculoskeletal Impairment **401**

when the patient stands straight. It is shortened when he pushes one or both shoulders forward. There is adequate strength and excursion in this motion to cause a wide opening or a strong compression of the terminal device.

A rather ingenious method of plastic surgery called cineplasty is sometimes used for enabling the patient to activate the cable. In this procedure a tunnel is made through a strong muscle, for instance the biceps, and covered with skin. A pin is placed through the tunnel and the cable is attached to it (Fig. 16-28). When the patient contracts this

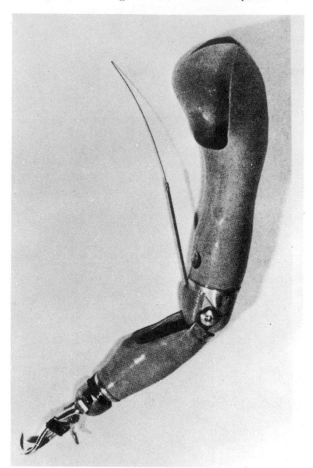

Fig. 16-30. Standard above-elbow prosthesis with wrist flexion unit, voluntary opening hook. (Institute of Rehabilitation Medicine, New York University Medical Center, New York, N.Y.)

muscle the shortening pulls on the cable and activates the terminal device. The advantage of this method is the elimination of the harness and the freeing of the opposite shoulder from participation in the process of prehension. A drawback is the fact that the excursion and strength of the cable motion is much less than that of the harness.

In recent years attempts have been made to use the action potential of a contracting muscle to control the cable either by activating an electric motor or by amplifying the action potential to the point that it can power the motor by itself.

The Joints

Wrist Units. The terminal device is attached to the remainder of the prosthesis by a wrist unit (Fig. 16-30). The wrist unit permits the terminal device to be manually rotated into pronation or supination. This position is maintained by friction. Some wrist units may also permit manual flexion or extension of the wrist.

The Prosthetic Elbow. The prosthetic elbow (Fig. 16-30) consists of a joint which can be locked in various positions. Usually the cable which activates the terminal device also flexes the elbow. A lever activated by the opposite hand of the amputee locks the elbow in the desired position. Once the elbow is locked the cable opens the terminal device.

Shoulder Units. The shoulder unit (Fig. 16-30) is primarily a device to attach the prosthesis to the torso in a stable fashion. The shoulder joint has no active motion though manually controlled passive motion is feasible.

Sockets. The prosthesis is attached to the stump by means of the socket (Fig. 16-30). This is usually made of plastic. In the below-elbow prosthesis, the socket fits the forearm stump and in the above-elbow prosthesis, it fits the arm stump.

Training

While the lower extremity amputee requires considerable preparation of the stump such as shrinkage and strengthening prior to the use of a prosthesis, and gait training with the prosthesis, the upper extremity amputee usually requires only instruction in the use of the prosthesis. Since the upper extremity amputee is ambulatory his rehabilitation can usually be carried out on an outpatient basis.

The majority of the upper extremity amputees are unilateral arm amputees with function in the opposite upper extremity. In these patients the purpose is to train the patient to use his prosthesis as a helper in two-handed activities. He must learn how to put on and take off his prosthesis *and* how to adjust the harness. It is advisable that he wear a T-shirt under the harness to protect the skin. Once the amputee has been shown how to operate the controls, terminal device, wrist unit, forearm, elbow lock, etc., he practices approach, grasp and release. Most of his skill eventually comes from practice. Finally, he must also be instructed in the proper care and maintenance of his prosthesis.

REFERENCES

1. Anderson, M. H.: Upper Extremities Orthotics. Springfield, Ill.: Charles C Thomas, 1970.
2. Armstrong, J. R.: Lumbar Disc Lesions, 3rd Ed. Baltimore: The Williams and Wilkins Co., 1965.
3. Bartelink, D. L.: "The Role of Abdominal Pressure in Relieving the Pressure on the Lumbar Intervertebral Discs." J. Bone & Joint Surg., 39B:718, 1957.
4. Bianco, A. J.: "Low Back Pain and Sciatica: Diagnosis and Indications for Treatment." J. Bone & Joint Surg., 50A:170, 1968.
5. Burgess, E. M., Romano, R. L. and Zettl, J. H.: "The Management of Lower Extremity Amputations." Prosthetics Research Study. Washington, DC: U.S. Government Printing Office.
6. Charnley, J.: "Low Friction Arthoplasty of the Hip Joint." J. Bone & Joint Surg., 53B:149, 1971.
7. Charnley, J.: "Total Prosthetic Replacement of the Hip in Relation to Physiotherapy." Physiotherapy, 54:406, 1968.
8. Chatton, M. J., Margen, S. and Brainerd, H.: Handbook of Medical Treatment, 14th Ed., Lost Altos, Ca.: Lange Medical Publications, 1974.
9. Coventry, M. B.: "Probable Place of Total Hip Arthoplasty in Rheumatoid Arthritis Involving the Hip." Orth. Clin. N. Amer., 2:697, 1971.
10. Eftekhar, N. S., Bush, D. C., Freeman, A. and Stinchfield, F. E.: "Perioperative Management of Total Hip Replacement." Orth. Rev., 3:17, 1974.
11. Eftekhar, N. S. and Stinchfield, F. E.: "Total Replacement of the Hip by Low Friction Arthoplasty." Orth. Clin. N. Amer., 4:2, 1973.
12. Friedman, L. W.: "The Prosthesis—Immediate or Delayed Fitting." Angiology, 23:518, 1972.
13. Grynbaum, B. B., Sokolow, J. and Lehneis, R.: "Adjustable Ischial Weight-Bearing Brace—Preliminary Report." Arch. Phys. Med. & Rehab., 50:460, 1969.
14. Hirschberg, G. G. and Robertson, K. B.: "Mattress Designed to Accommodate Sunken Bedpan for Patients with Lumbar Disc Protrusion." Arch. Phys. Med. & Rehab., 53:192, 1972.

15. Judovich, B. D. and Mobel, G. R.: "Traction Therapy; A Study of Resistance Forces." Amer. J. Surg., 93:108, 1957.
16. Klopsteg, P. E. and Wilson, P. D.: Human Limbs and Their Substitutes. New York: Hafner Publishing Co., 1969.
17. Morris. J. M., Lucas, D. B. and Bresler, M. S.: "Role of the Trunk in Stability of the Spine." J. Bone & Joint Surg., 43A:327, 1961.
18. Nachemson, A. and Morris, J. M.: "In Vivo Measurements of Intradiscal Pressure." J. Bone & Joint Surg., 46A:1077, 1964.
19. Nachemson, A. and Elfstrom, G.: "Intravital Dynamic Pressure Measurements in Lumbar Discs—A Study of Common Movements, Maneuvers and Exercises." Scand. J. Rehab. Med., Suppl. 1, 1970.
20. Pearce, J. and Moll, J. M. H.: "Conservative Treatment and Natural History of Lumbar Disc Lesions." J. Neurol. Neurosurg. & Psychiat., 30:13, 1967.
21. Raney, F. L.: "The Royalite Flexion Jacket in Spinal Orthotics." Washington, DC: Committee on Prosthetic Research and Development, National Research Council, 1969.
22. Santschi, W. R.: Manual of Upper Extremity Prosthetics, 2nd Ed. Los Angeles: UCLA, Department of Engineering, 1958.
23. Sullivan, R. A. and Tucker, J.: "Amputee Management Using a Fitted Temporary Prosthesis; A Preliminary Report." Arch. Phys. Med. & Rehab., 55:409, 1974.

CHAPTER
17

Disabling Conditions Due to Respiratory Impairment

THE FUNCTION OF RESPIRATION

The purpose of respiration is to bring oxygen to the blood, which is then distributed to the tissues via the general circulation, and to remove carbon dioxide from the blood. The exchange of oxygen and carbon dioxide between the air and the blood occurs in the alveoli of the lung by *diffusion* of these two gases through the alveolar epithelium (Fig. 17-1). A continuing exchange of gases is maintained by the *pulmonary circulation,* which assures continuous blood flow, and by *pulmonary ventilation* or the pumping of air through the alveoli of the lung, which assures the constant renewal of the alveolar air.

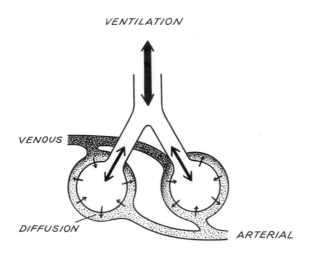

VENTILATION

VENOUS

DIFFUSION

ARTERIAL

(AFTER COMROE)

Fig. 17-1. Schematic Diagram of Ventilation, Diffusion and Circulation.

406

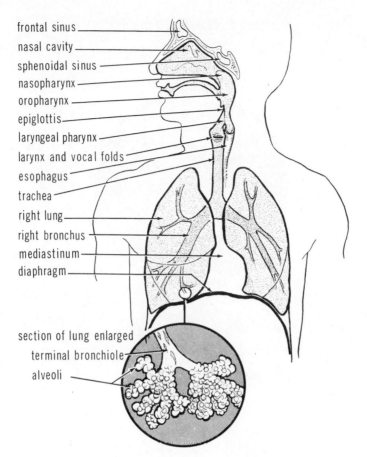

frontal sinus
nasal cavity
sphenoidal sinus
nasopharynx
oropharynx
epiglottis
laryngeal pharynx
larynx and vocal folds
esophagus
trachea
right lung
right bronchus
mediastinum
diaphragm

section of lung enlarged
terminal bronchiole
alveoli

Fig. 17-2. The respiratory tract. (From Memmler, R.: The Human Body in Health and Disease, 2nd ed. Philadelphia, J. B. Lippincott Co., 1970.)

Pulmonary Ventilation

Ventilation is a cyclic process of inspiration and expiration in which fresh air enters the lung and pulmonary gas is exhaled in order to maintain a homeostatic gas relationship in the lung. One likes to think of the lung as a bag into which fresh air is blown and from which used air is blown out rhythmically, but this is not strictly the case. The total surface of exchange is over 90 square meters. The lung consists of an enormous number of small bags or alveoli to which the air is evenly distributed by a network of branching tubes, starting with the trachea and branching to the bronchi and the bronchioli (Fig. 17-2).

Disabling Conditions Due to Respiratory Impairment   **407**

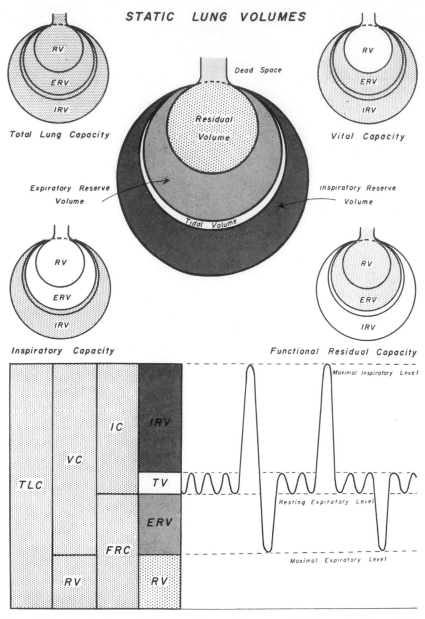

Fig. 17-3. Static Lung Volumes. (From Comroe, J. H., et al. (eds.): The Lung, 2nd ed. Chicago, Yearbook Medical Publishers, Inc., 1973. Used by permission.)

The pump consists of the chest and the diaphragm to which the lung is "attached" by a vacuum in the pleural space. Expansion of the chest expands the lung and sucks air into it. Contraction of the chest pushes air out of the lung. Chest expansion is produced by the action of the inspiratory muscles. Contraction of the chest is produced by the elasticity of the lungs during normal breathing. Forced expiration is accomplished by the action of the abdominal muscles, which are the principal expiratory muscles.

On its way to the alveoli, the air flows through the nose or mouth, the larynx, trachea, bronchi, and bronchioli. Since no exchange of gases occurs in the area of the airways, their volume is called "dead space." A certain amount of air which is pulled in towards the very end of inspiration and pumped out at the very beginning of expiration stays only in the dead space and never is available for respiratory exchange of gases. Under normal physiologic conditions this amount is about 150 ml. in the adult. In pathologic conditions, it may be increased. The amount can be calculated from samples of expired and alveolar air.[4]

Lung Volumes (Fig. 17-3)

The amount of air entering and leaving the lungs can be easily measured with a spirometer. During quiet breathing at rest, a person pumps a volume of 300 to 500 ml. in and out of the lungs with each breath. This is called *tidal volume* (TV). With a maximum inspiratory effort, an additional 1500 ml. can be breathed in. This quantity is the *inspiratory reserve volume* (IRV). If a forced expiration is made at the end of the normal expiration, another 1500 ml. can be breathed out. This quantity is the *expiratory reserve volume* (ERV). Some air remains in the lung which cannot be breathed out. This is the *residual volume* (RV). A combination of volumes has been given the following names:

TV plus IRV is called *inspiratory capacity* (IC).

ERV plus RV is called *functional residual capacity* (FRC).

TV plus IRV plus ERV is called *vital capacity* (VC).

VC plus RV is called *total lung capacity* (TLC).

The most commonly used measurement clinically is the vital capacity measurement, particularly as a physiologic measure of physical fitness.* In pathologic conditions, the determination of all lung volumes may be needed in order to evaluate ventilatory disability.

---

*Nomograms for the estimation of required tidal volume in tank respirators and also for estimation of vital capacity and forced expiratory volumes will be found in Chapt. 15 (pp. 307-308).

TABLE 17-1. PULMONARY FUNCTION TESTS MOST USEFUL TO THE CLINICIAN

TEST	CLINICAL SIGNIFICANCE	NORMAL VALUES
Vital capacity (VC) Maximum volume that can be expelled after a maximum inspiration. No time limit.	Repeated abnormal values (more or less than 20% of predicted) may be significant. Main value is in following course of cardiopulmonary or respiratory disease with serial tests.	Male: VC = $(27.3 - [0.112 \times$ age in years$]) \times$ height in cm. Female: VC = $(21.78 - [0.101 \times$ age in years$]) \times$ height in cm.
Forced expiratory volume (FEV) "Timed vital capacity." Maximum volume expelled in a timed interval, usually 1 or 3 seconds.	A reduced timed volume usually indicates obstructive bronchopulmonary disease. Improvement after a bronchodilator indicates some degree of reversibility.	FEV_1 sec = 83% of actual VC. FEV_3 sec = 97% of actual VC.
Maximal expiratory flow rate (MEFR) Measurement of maximal flow rate of a single expelled breath, expressed in liters/minute.	A reduced flow rate has the same significance as a reduced FEV. The test requires little effort, and several types of small, portable instruments are available. Suitable for screening tests.	Adult male = > 400 liters/minute. Adult female = > 300 liters/minute.
Maximal voluntary ventilation (MVV) "Maximal breathing capacity." Maximal volume expelled in 12–15 seconds of forced breathing, expressed in liters/minute.	Measures essentially the same function as FEV and MEFR. An additional confirmation test of FEV and MEFR. Requires sustained effort and cooperation of patient to a greater degree.	There is a wide variation of normal values depending upon age, size, and sex. The following formulas can be used as a guide for predicted values. Male = $(86.5 - [0.522 \times$ age in years$]) \times$ sq m body surface. Female = $(71.3 - [0.474 \times$ age in years$]) \times$ sq m body surface.
	When low values are obtained, the above tests should be repeated after administration of a bronchodilator.	
O_2 tension (arterial) (PaO_2)	Hypoxemia which is not apparent clinically can be detected. This and the determinations listed below are readily available in most hospital laboratories and are essential in the diagnosis of respiratory insufficiency and the management of oxygen and ventilation therapy.	Arterial O_2 tension (PaO_2) = 90–100 mm Hg
CO_2 tension (arterial) ($PaCO_2$) Plasma bicarbonate (HCO_3^-) pH of arterial blood	Important values in the diagnosis and management of respiratory acidosis due to CO_2 retention. (Now readily measured in arterial blood by the method of Astrup: Clin Chem 7:1, 1961.)	$PaCO_2$ 40 mm Hg Plasma HCO_3^- 24 mEq/liter pH 7.40

From: Krupp, M. and Chatton, M.: Current Medical Diagnosis and Treatment 1975. Lange Medical Publications, Los Altos, California, 1975.

Screening methods are available to determine most values in pulmonary function. Complete studies require a sophisticated pulmonary function laboratory.

Time Factors in Pulmonary Ventilation

Measurement of the lung volumes indicates how much air the lung can exchange per breath. It is important functionally, however, to know how much air the lung can exchange per minute (minute volume). The average frequency of breathing is about 11 to 14 breaths per minute under basal conditions. One can easily calculate the minute volume by multiplying the tidal volume by the frequency.

Common methods of measuring the efficiency of ventilation are shown in Table 17-1. Timed vital capacity or *forced expiratory volume* (FEV) measures how much air the patient can breathe out following a maximum inspiration within a ½ second, 1 second, 2 seconds and 3 seconds maximal. The time it takes to empty the lungs completely is an important determination. The fastest air flow of expiration, expressed in liters per minute, is the *maximal expiratory flow rate* (MEFR). A third test determines the patient's ventilatory efficiency over a period of time. The expired air is collected in a large bag (Douglas bag) or a spirometer, while the patient is trying to take as many deep breaths as he can over a period of 15 seconds. The amount of air, expressed in liters per minute, is his *maximum breathing capacity* (MBC), or *maximal voluntary ventilation* (MVV).

Alveolar Ventilation

Alveolar ventilation depends upon tidal volume, respiratory rate, and dead space: Alveolar ventilation per minute equals TV minus dead space times frequency. It may differ considerably from pulmonary ventilation even in normal subjects as seen in Figure 17-4. Average normal values of alveolar ventilation are approximately 2.0 to 2.5 liters per minute per square meter of body surface.

Hyperventilation.   Excessive ventilation has no effect on oxygen uptake which is limited by the oxygen saturation of blood; however, it leads to excessive loss of carbon dioxide with subsequent respiratory alkalosis.

Hypoventilation.   Insufficient ventilation has a double effect:

1. Retention of carbon dioxide with subsequent respiratory acidosis.

2. Inadequate oxygenation of the arterial blood (hypoxemia).

Uneven Ventilation.   Some degree of uneven ventilation occurs in everyone. One cannot expect that each alveolus of the lung will be equally ventilated. In the normal person, however, compensation occurs and the total expiratory gas exchange is what one would antici-

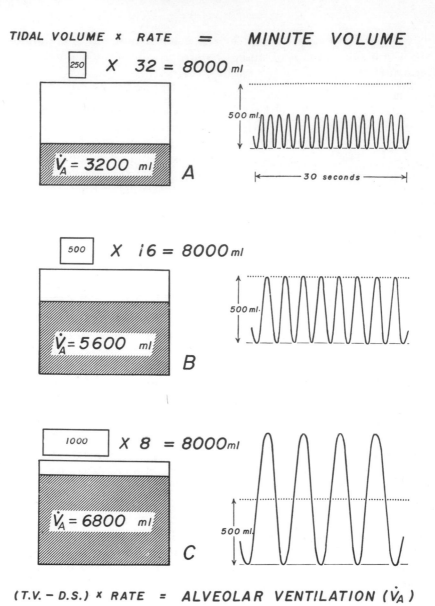

TIDAL VOLUME × RATE = MINUTE VOLUME

250 × 32 = 8000 ml

$\dot{V}_A$ = 3200 ml **A**

500 ml.

30 seconds

500 × 16 = 8000 ml

$\dot{V}_A$ = 5600 ml **B**

500 ml.

1000 × 8 = 8000 ml

$\dot{V}_A$ = 6800 ml **C**

500 ml.

(T.V. − D.S.) × RATE = ALVEOLAR VENTILATION ($\dot{V}_A$)

Fig. 17-4. Effect of Changes in Tidal Volume and Frequency on Alveolar Ventilation/Minute. (From Comroe, J. H., et al. (eds.): The Lung, 2nd ed. Chicago, Yearbook Medical Publications, Inc., 1973. Used by permission.)

CAUSES OF UNEVEN VENTILATION

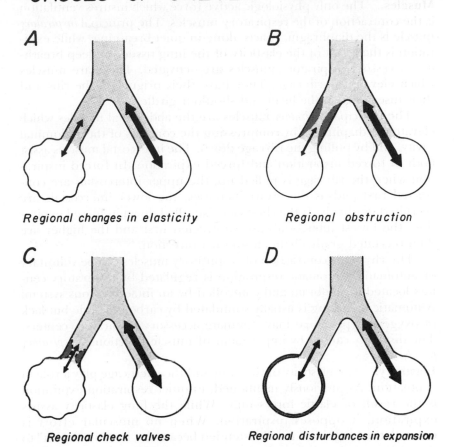

A
Regional changes in elasticity

B
Regional obstruction

C
Regional check valves

D
Regional disturbances in expansion

Fig. 17-5. Causes of Uneven Ventilation. Circular areas represent the alveoli. Wavy lines in *A* and *C* represent alveoli that have lost their elastic tissues. Thick line in *D* signifies alveoli that expand less than normally, although their elastic tissue is normal and there is no airway obstruction. Size of arrows indicates the volume of gas ventilating each region. (From Comroe, J. H., et al. (eds.): The Lung, 2nd ed. Chicago, Yearbook Medical Publishers, Inc., 1973. Used by permission.)

pate in even ventilation. Changes in elasticity and in expansion of the alveoli, as well as obstruction from mucus or other causes, can interfere with even ventilation (Fig. 17-5). When uneven ventilation becomes extreme, it is a significant cause of disturbed pulmonary ventilation.

Disabling Conditions Due to Respiratory Impairment **413**

Forces Involved in Ventilation

Muscles. The only physiologic active force which insures ventilation is the contraction of the respiratory muscles. The principal *inspiratory* muscle is the diaphragm. It acts alone in quiet breathing, while expiration is the result of the elasticity of the lung tissue. In deep breathing, accessory inspiratory muscles are activated. These are muscles which elevate the rib cage. They have their origins on the ribs and their insertions on the head and shoulder girdle.

The principal *expiratory* muscles are the abdominal muscles which elevate the diaphragm by compressing the contents of the abdominal cavity, and by pulling the rib cage down. The intercostal muscles assist both in forced inspiration and forced expiration. In forced inspiration when the rib cage is pulled up, the upper intercostals are contracted first and as the effort increases, the lower intercostals are recruited gradually. If the chest cage is pulled down in forced expiration, the lowest intercostals are contracted first and the higher are then recruited gradually in an upward direction.

The rhythmic contraction of respiratory muscles can be voluntary or automatic. Automatic respiration is regulated by respiratory centers located in the brain and controlled by an intact nervous system. Automatic breathing is usually stimulated by carbon dioxide but lack of oxygen (hypoxemia) may stimulate accessory respiratory centers. The disability caused by impairment of muscle function is *respiratory paralysis*.

Elasticity. The elasticity of the lung and the chest cage play a role in ventilation. As previously mentioned, in quiet respiration expiration is the result of elastic forces only. While the lung elasticity assists expiration, it opposes inspiration. When no muscular effort is exerted, the lung tissue is still distended because of its "attachment" to the pleura of the chest wall. In case of a pneumothorax, the lung collapses to a much smaller volume. On the other hand, the chest has a tendency to assume a resting position at a greater volume, so that the elasticity of the chest and the elasticity of the lung balance each other and produce the end expiratory position. The chest elasticity thus assists initial inspiration. On deep inspiration, however, the chest wall is also stressed and becomes an opposing force. The opposing elastic forces of lung and chest cage are expressed by a measurement which is the reverse of their resistance and which is called compliance. It is expressed in the number of ml. of air which can be forced into the lung by a pressure of 1 cm. of water. If the compliance is increased by pathologic conditions, the resulting deficit in pulmonary function is called a *restrictive disability*.

Gravity. The weight of the viscera attached to the diaphragm exerts a force dependent upon the position of the subject. In upright position, the weight of the viscera pulls the diaphragm down and thereby has an inspiratory effect. This is useful for patients with respiratory paralysis who have preserved their expiratory muscles or are using expiratory assistance. They can be sufficiently ventilated by expiratory breathing alone but only if they are in a near sitting or standing position. On the other hand, some patients with respiratory paralysis who have no functioning abdominal muscles may be able to breathe independently in horizontal position but lose this ability while in a sitting position or standing, because the weight of the viscera prevents the diaphragm from returning to its resting position. The rocking bed (Fig. 17-18) gives respiratory assistance by making use solely of gravity. The patient is brought alternately to head down (or flat) position where the weight of, or the thrust of, the viscera causes him to breathe out, and to foot down position where the weight of the viscera causes him to breathe in.

Friction. The friction between tissues resulting from ventilatory movements opposes ventilatory efforts. It increases with the rate and depth of respiration.

Airway Resistance. The movement of the air in and out of the lung through the airways also causes frictional resistance which is relatively small in quiet breathing. The resistance to air flow increases as breathing becomes deeper and more forceful. Under pathologic conditions, the resistance to air flow can be greatly increased and may cause an *obstructive disability*.

Diffusion

The transfer of oxygen (O_2) molecules from the alveolar air to the blood of the pulmonary capillaries and the transfer of carbon dioxide (CO_2) molecules from the capillary blood to the alveolar air is effected by the mechanism of diffusion. Diffusion is the spread of molecules from an area of higher concentration to an adjacent area of lower concentration until an even distribution is reached. Gas molecules like O_2 and CO_2 will diffuse in a gaseous atmosphere such as the ambient air and also in solution, as is the case in the fluids of human tissues.

In the lung, O_2 diffuses successively through the alveolar membrane where it is dissolved in tissue fluid, then through interstitial fluid, the capillary membrane, the plasma in the capillary and the membrane of the red cell. It then combines chemically with hemoglobin which permits the blood to transport considerably more O_2 than can be carried in solution by the plasma.

Disabling Conditions Due to Respiratory Impairment   415

On the other hand, CO_2 is dissolved in the plasma only and diffuses through the same media as O_2 only in the opposite direction. Emerging from the alveolar membrane, the dissolved CO_2 turns into gas and is carried away with the expired air in a quantity sufficient to leave the mixture in the lung at about 5 per cent CO_2 and 15 per cent O_2.

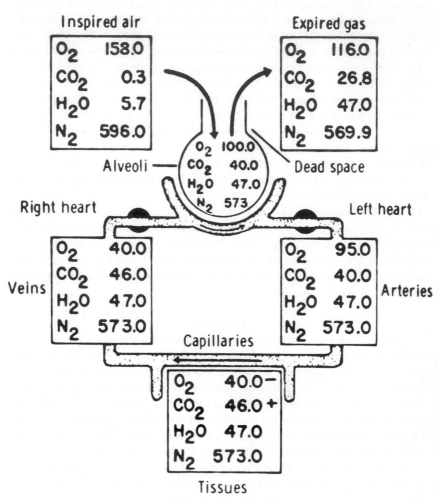

Fig. 17-6. Partial pressures of gases (mm Hg). (From Ganong, W. F.: Review of Medical Physiology, 7th ed. Los Altos, Lange Medical Publications, 1975. Values from Lambertsen in, Mountcastle, V. B., ed.: Medical Physiology, 13th ed. St. Louis, C. V. Mosby Co., 1974.)

Partial Pressure

The pressure of any one gas in a mixture of gases is called its *partial pressure*. It is equal to the total pressure times the percentage of the total amount of gas it represents. The composition of air is 21 per cent O_2 and approximately 79 per cent N_2. There are also small quantities of CO_2 (0.04%) and other gases (0.1%) present in the air. The basis for measuring partial pressure is the barometric pressure at sea level which is about 760 mm. of mercury. The partial pressure of O_2 in the ambient air is therefore 160 mm. Hg (or 21 per cent of the total pressure).

In the alveolar air, there is an additional gas in the form of water vapor which causes a reduction in the partial pressure of O_2 (pO_2) to 100 mm. Hg. The partial pressure of CO_2 (pCO_2) in the alveolar air is 40 mm. Hg. Therefore in *arterial* blood which has been exposed to gases at these partial pressures, pO_2 approximates 100 and pCO_2 approximates 40. However, in the blood of the *pulmonary capillaries,* which comes from the peripheral venous circulation, the pO_2 is reduced to 40 while the pCO_2 is elevated to 46 (Fig. 17-6. All p values are in mm. Hg).

Since gases diffuse from an area of high pressure to an area of low pressure, there is a constant flow of O_2 from the alveoli ($pO_2 = 100$) to the capillaries ($pO_2 = 40$) and of CO_2 from the capillaries ($pCO_2 = 46$) to the alveoli ($pCO_2 = 40$). The rate of diffusion depends upon the concentration gradient and the nature of the barrier between the two areas. The rate of diffusion between a gaseous and liquid area is also determined by the solubility of the particular gas in the liquid. For instance, CO_2 is about 24 times as soluble as O_2 in saline solution (the principal constituent of the membrane), and its diffusing capacity is 20 times as great as that of O_2, so that impairment of diffusion of CO_2 is rarely a clinical problem.

The diffusing capacity of the lungs is defined as the quantity of a gas transferred each minute for each millimeter of Hg difference in partial pressure of the gas across the alveolar capillary membranes. Its measurement requires complex laboratory equipment. In a normal person at rest, the diffusion capacity of O_2 is greater than 15 cc. It is increased during muscular exercise by an increase in capillary blood volume.

Impairment of Diffusion

When the *only* significant disturbance in pulmonary function is a decrease in diffusion capacity, the condition is called alveolar capillary block. This occurs in Boeck's sarcoid, berylliosis, asbestosis, pulmo-

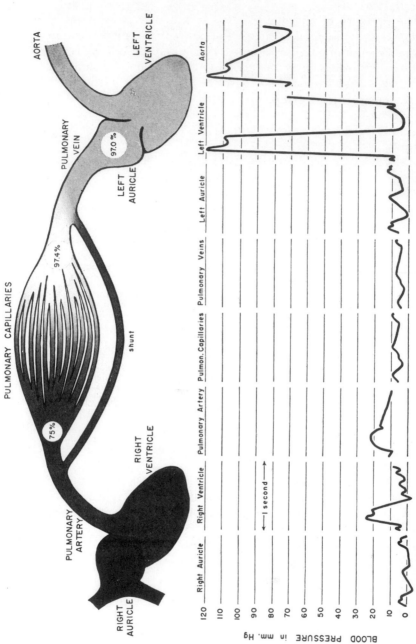

Fig. 17-7. The Pulmonary Circulation. (From Comroe, J. H., et al. (eds.): The Lung, 2nd ed. Chicago, Yearbook Medical Publishers, Inc., 1973. Used by permission.)

nary scleroderma, alveolar cell carcinoma and sulfur dioxide poisoning. In association with other respiratory disabilities, impairment of diffusion is found in many diseases of the lung.

Reasons for impaired diffusion are:
1. Reduction of surface by:
   a. A decrease in the number of patent capillaries.
   b. A decrease in the number of capillaries in contact with *functioning* alveoli (i.e., emphysema, pulmonary fibrosis).
2. Change of the alveolar capillary tissues.
   a. Intra-alveolar or interstitial pulmonary edema.
   b. Thickening of the alveolar or capillary membranes.

The only rehabilitative measure for improvement of diffusion capacity is to increase the oxygen content of the inspired air.

Pulmonary Circulation

Anatomically, the pulmonary circulation consists of the right auricle, right ventricle, pulmonary arteries, capillaries and pulmonary veins (Fig. 17-7). This unit is called the lesser circulation, and indeed it involves less territory than the left heart system, and the ventricular and auricular walls are less thick than the left. Pulmonary vascular pressures are much lower than systemic pressures. Right heart function is much less accessible for study; nevertheless, the right heart circulation is as vital to survival as the left circulation. The pathology of functional and anatomical disorders of this circulation are now recognized to be most important. The blood pressure values of the right circulation are shown in Figure 17-7. It will be noted that in comparison with left ventricular pressures of 110 or more, the right ventricle and pulmonary aorta have systolic pressures of only about 20.

"Wedge pressure" is determined by wedging a cardiac catheter as far as possible into the finest branch of the pulmonary arterial system, measuring pressure there. Wedge pressure is approximately the same as pulmonary venous pressure when there is no venular obstruction. Capillary pressure of the lung, while important, cannot be accurately measured.

Our concern with pulmonary circulation here is particularly in respect to ventilation and blood flow ratios. Under ordinary circumstances, relatively uniform blood flow occurs and accompanies uniform ventilation of the lungs. Under these conditions, the ratio of pulmonary blood flow to alveolar ventilation is 2.5 to 2.0, a ratio of 8 liters of blood to 10 liters of air. The normal ratio is expressed as 0.8. It can be achieved by various compensatory mechanisms within the

VENTILATION/BLOOD FLOW RATIOS

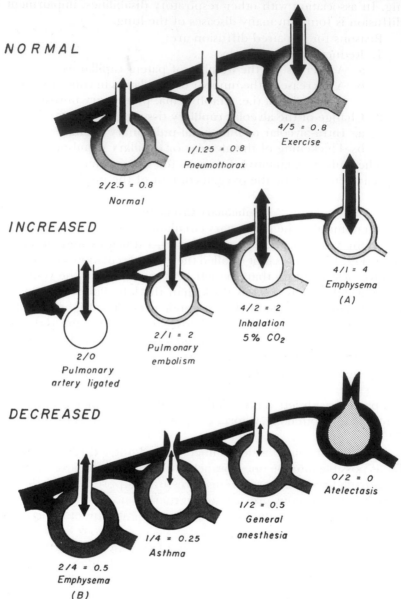

NORMAL

2/2.5 = 0.8
Normal

1/1.25 = 0.8
Pneumothorax

4/5 = 0.8
Exercise

INCREASED

2/0
Pulmonary
artery ligated

2/1 = 2
Pulmonary
embolism

4/2 = 2
Inhalation
5% CO₂

4/1 = 4
Emphysema
(A)

DECREASED

2/4 = 0.5
Emphysema
(B)

1/4 = 0.25
Asthma

1/2 = 0.5
General
anesthesia

0/2 = 0
Atelectasis

Fig. 17-8. Some Clinical Abnormalities in Ventilation/Blood Flow Ratios. (From Comroe, J. H. et al. (eds.): The Lung, 2nd ed. Chicago, Yearbook Medical Publishers, Inc., 1973. Used by permission.)

lungs if it is either uneven ventilation or circulation. However, if there is gross interference with blood flow, the ratio is increased and there may be much greater ventilation than circulation. With ligation of a pulmonary artery, the ratio is 2/0 (Fig. 17-8).

In the advanced pulmonary function laboratory, there are means of determining shunts and differences in ventilation-diffusion ratio by gas analysis.

Arterial Gas Analysis

Frequently the adequacy of ventilation, diffusion, and circulation cannot be measured clinically. In this case the overall efficiency of respiration can be determined by examining the arterial blood for O_2 and CO_2 content. Arterial samples are procured either by aspiration with a hypodermic needle from one of the available arteries in the arm, or the cannulization of the brachial, radial or femoral artery for interval samples. About 2 cc. of blood are aspirated in a heparinized glass syringe. Then the tip of the needle is immediately inserted into a rubber stopper to prevent contact with air. The syringe is then placed into an ice tray for refrigeration and taken to the laboratory.

The arterial blood normally has an O_2 saturation of 95 per cent and a pO_2 of 80 to 100 mm. Hg. The pO_2 is a more sensitive indicator of hypoxia than the O_2 saturation. If the pO_2 falls below 50 mm. Hg there is definite impairment of respiratory function.

The pCO_2 of the arterial blood is normally 40 mm. Hg. An increase is usually a sign that the patient is hypoventilated, while a decrease indicates that the patient is hyperventilated.

CO_2 dissolves in plasma to form carbonic acid. An excess of CO_2 due to hypoventilation therefore leads to respiratory acidosis while excessive loss of CO_2 by hyperventilation leads to respiratory alkalosis. Both are serious conditions and must be avoided or corrected. One can assess this condition by measuring the pH (concentration of H ions) of the blood which normally ranges from 7.35 to 7.45. The pH level will fall in acidosis and rise in alkalosis.

CAUSES OF RESPIRATORY DISABILITY

The causes of respiratory disability can be broadly classified under three headings: impaired ventilation, impaired diffusion and impaired ventilation-circulation ratio. We shall list the most common causes of respiratory disability, followed by a brief description of some of the most common disabling pulmonary diseases.

TABLE 17-2. COMMON CAUSES OF RESPIRATORY DISABILITY*

I. Impaired Ventilation
  A. Respiratory Paralysis
    1. Respiratory center damage or depression
      a. Cerebral trauma
      b. Cerebral, medullary or upper spinal cord disease: Infarction, tumor, abscess, virus diseases
      c. Toxic agents: Anesthetic, tranquilizers, barbiturates, narcotics
      d. High flow oxygen therapy (see p. 431)
    2. Upper motoneuron paralysis
      a. Brain or spinal cord injuries
      b. Multiple sclerosis
    3. Lower motoneuron or muscle paralysis
      a. Anterior horn cell disease: Poliomyelitis, progressive muscular atrophy, amyotrophic lateral sclerosis
      b. Root damage: Guillain-Barré syndrome
      c. Polyneuropathy
      d. Muscle involvement: Myasthenia gravis, muscular dystrophy, botulism, tetanus, curare
  B. Chronic Airway Obstruction
    1. Due to muscle spasm: Chronic bronchial asthma
    2. Due to bronchial collapse during exhalation: Emphysema
    3. Due to bronchial secretions: Chronic bronchitis, emphysema, asthma, respiratory paralysis
  C. Respiratory Restriction
    1. Decreased lung expansion
      a. Acute pneumothorax; pleural effusion
      b. Chronic fibrothorax, interstitial fibrosis
    2. Limited thorax expansion
      a. Acute: Multiple rib fractures; post-thoracic surgery
      b. Chronic: Kyphoscoliosis, rheumatoid spondylitis, respiratory paralysis
    3. Decreased diaphragmatic movement
      a. Acute: Abdominal surgery, peritonitis
      b. Chronic: Ascites, severe obesity; paralysis
II. Impaired Diffusion
  A. Pulmonary edema
  B. Pulmonary fibrosis
    1. The pneumoconioses
    2. Sarcoidosis
    3. Hamman-Rich syndrome
  C. Obliterative pulmonary vascular disease; pulmonary emboli
  D. Anatomic loss of functioning lung tissue
    1. Pneumonectomy, tumor, emphysema
III. Abnormal Ventilation-Circulation Ratio
  Emphysema, chronic bronchitis, bronchiolitis, atelectasis, pneumonia, thromboembolism, posttransfusion syndrome, respiratory distress syndromes

*Modified from: Petty, T. L.: Intensive and Rehabilitative Respiratory Care, 2nd Edition, Lea and Febiger, Philadelphia, 1974.

Common Causes of Respiratory Disability (Table 17-2)

While the following disabilities are classified according to their physiologic effect, it must be understood that in practically all respiratory disabilities, several disabling factors occur in combination. For example, in respiratory paralysis there is basically an impairment of ventilation because of muscular paralysis. In addition, however, these paralyzed patients have difficulty expelling bronchial secretions, thus having the added disability of chronic airway obstruction. In addition, the paralysis leads to contractures of the chest, adding a restrictive disability of impaired compliance. Some diseases, such as pulmonary fibrosis, lead simultaneously to impairment of diffusion and impairment of ventilation by restriction. For this reason, the same disease may be listed as the cause of several different disabilities.

Common Disorders of the Lungs Leading to Respiratory Disability

It is customary to divide the chronic lung disorders into obstructive and restrictive lung disease according to the major disability. Into the obstructive group fall chronic bronchitis, asthma, and emphysema. Restrictive lung diseases comprise two different groups of disabilities:

1. Those caused by chest cage restriction (e.g., severe kyphoscoliosis).

2. Those caused by lung pathology proper (e.g., pulmonary fibrosis).

Obstructive Pulmonary Disease

Chronic Bronchitis. In the United States this disorder is recognized as chronic inflammation of the bronchial mucosa. It is associated with production of secretion and cough. The presence of secretion within the bronchial tree seems to produce chronic obstructive pulmonary disease and eventually the manifestations of chronic pulmonary emphysema. Chronic bronchitis and emphysema are so similar that the term chronic bronchitis is used in Great Britain quite the same as we use the term pulmonary emphysema here.

Bronchial Asthma. Asthma is an intermittent disorder of the lungs and one in which obstructive phenomena are the result of spasm of bronchial and bronchiolar musculature. During the acute asthmatic episode, disability is very similar to that of pulmonary emphysema. The expiratory phase is prolonged, vital capacity is diminished and the cough is severe. After the episode has cleared, the lungs may or may not return to their normal status, depending upon the frequency of attacks, the occurrence of associated bronchitis and other factors.

TABLE 17-3. PNEUMOCONIOSES*

Disease and Occupation	Causative Particle and Pathology	Clinical Features	X-Ray Findings
Silicosis (mining, drilling, blasting, grinding, abrasive manufacture; various other processes exposing silica to high temperatures, such as iron moulding or ceramic manufacture)	Free silica, crystobalite, and tridymite (toxic isomers produced by exposure of silica to high temperatures) cause immunologic tissue reactions producing nodules, fibrosis, lymphatic blockage, emphysema, and hilar adenopathy.	Required exposure is 2–20 years. Dyspnea on exertion, dry cough. Frequent infections, especially tuberculosis. Pulmonary insufficiency, chronic cor pulmonale.	Hilar adenopathy; peripheral ("eggshell") calcification of hilar nodes; nodules (inner, midlung fields), overall increased radiolucency, fibrosis. Signs of associated tuberculosis.
Asbestosis (asbestos mining and processing)	Magnesium silicate (particle size 20–200 μm), rod-shaped bodies visible in tissue sections and sputum, causing obstruction of bronchioles, distal atelectasis, fibrosis (little nodulation).	Required exposure 2–8 years. Dyspnea early. Productive cough. Pulmonary insufficiency. "Corns" on skin of extremities (imbedded particles). Possible increased incidence of bronchogenic carcinoma and malignant mesothelioma.	Fine reticular markings in lower lung fields. Thickening of pleura ("ground glass" appearance), obliteration of costophrenic angles. Bilateral pleural calcifications.

Disease (source)	Pathology	Symptoms	X-ray findings
Berylliosis (beryllium production, manufacture of fluorescent powders)	Beryllium particles. Acute: Patchy infiltrations, resembling bronchial pneumonia. Chronic: Alveolar septal granuloma causing fine nodules. Fibrosis not prominent. Elastic tissue damaged, causing emphysema. No hilar adenopathy.	Acute: After a few weeks of exposure, upper respiratory symptoms; "bronchitis," "pneumonia" later. Chronic: Required exposure 6–18 months. Dyspnea, cough, weight loss, cyanosis, skin lesions, pulmonary insufficiency, cor pulmonale.	Acute: Clear at first, then patchy infiltrations. Chronic: Scattered minute ("sandpaper") nodules. Later, larger nodules, diffuse reticular markings. No hilar adenopathy.
Bauxite pneumoconiosis (Shaver's disease; aluminosis)	May be due to other toxic contaminants rather than aluminum dust per se, causing fibrosis, hilar adenopathy, atelectasis.	Required exposure is several months to 2 years. Dyspnea (marked pulmonary insufficiency). Attacks of spontaneous pneumothorax.	Hilar and mediastinal adenopathy, irregularity of diaphragms, fibrosis, emphysema.
Anthracosis (rarely dissociated from silicosis) (mining, city dwellers)	Coal dust, causing black discoloration of lungs, nodes, distant organs (nodules rare).	Progressive disease (fibrosis, emphysema) reported in Welsh soft-coal workers. Silica may be an important factor.	"Reticulation," fine nodules. Coal dust may produce large densities by deposition without fibrosis.
Siderosis (iron ore processing, metal drilling, electric arc welding)	Iron oxides, metallic iron, causing "red" (oxides) and "black" (metallic) discoloration of lung. "Red" type leads to fibrosis. "Black" type associated with silicosis.	Symptoms are those of associated silicosis.	Dependent mainly on associated silicosis.

*Actual exposure is rarely to one dust alone.
From: Krupp, M. A. and Chatton, M. J.: Current Medical Diagnosis and Treatment, 1975, Lange Medical Publications, Los Altos, California, 1975.

Pulmonary Emphysema. The most common form of respiratory impairment is that due to pulmonary emphysema or related disorders. In all forms of pulmonary emphysema, there is impairment of outflow of air. Without discussing all of the theories concerning the abnormal physiology of this disease, let us note that the important phenomenon is a difficulty emptying the lungs and a consequent increase of the residual volume of the lungs. Ordinarily, one can breathe out all but a relatively small portion of the total air content of the lungs. What is left (residual volume) usually measures between 1000 and 1500 ml. in the adult. In pulmonary emphysema and obstructive lung disease, residual volume tends to increase, and as it represents a pool of relatively immobile air, the amount of carbon dioxide in it tends to increase. Pathologically, the lung tends to lose its elasticity and to get larger. The diaphragm becomes flat, respiratory excursion is impaired, and there is not only accumulation of carbon dioxide but also diminution in the partial pressure of oxygen. Pulmonary emphysema occurs as a diffuse disorder of the lung, with enlargement of alveoli and loss of elastic tissue. It also occurs as a result of apparent central scarring with widening of the interspaces around centrilobular contractions. It is a phenomenon secondary to scarring in tuberculosis, silicosis, and other diseases. Eventually, some persons with advancing pulmonary emphysema may develop bullae, which are large bubble-like cysts in the lung, from which it is almost impossible to remove accumulated carbon dioxide. A bullous lung is very inefficient. Ultimately, the person with chronic obstructive pulmonary disease becomes more and more hypoxic. The CO_2 tends to rise higher and higher (hypercapnia), and the patient usually develops right-heart strain and right-heart failure and eventually dies.

Restrictive Pulmonary Disease

While the lungs of a person with obstructive pulmonary disease tend to enlarge and lose elasticity, the lungs of a person with restrictive lung disease, while also losing elasticity, tend to undergo fibrous contraction, resulting in a smaller lung volume. The patient does not have obstructive difficulty but he has difficulty getting enough air into the lungs and into contact with capillaries containing blood cells capable of carrying oxygen. The person with chronic fibrosis of the lungs from any cause, the person with severe tubercular scarring, and others with fibrous contraction of the lung space (Hammon-Rich syndrome) eventually have marked diminution of lung volume, inadequate oxygenation, low pO_2, chronic bronchitis, and eventually respiratory failure. They may also develop right-heart failure. Often, as stated above, the person with respiratory impairment suffers from a mixed obstructive-restrictive disorder.

Pulmonary fibrosis is caused commonly by the industrial diseases known as pneumoconioses (Table 17-3). An understanding of these disorders is complicated by the fact that many people who are exposed to harmful or nonharmful dust make claims under Workmen's Compensation insurance, thus tending to produce evidence one way or another which is not in fact substantiated. What we do know at present is that some particular chemicals are highly destructive to the pulmonary epithelium. Silicon dioxide in both its crystalline and amorphous forms (flint, finely powdered quartz, diatomaceous earth, etc.) is harmful. Particles of these minerals are phagocytosed by wandering cells and delivered to small lymphatic foci in the lungs where they produce inflammatory reactions, leading to scarring and marked secondary emphysema. In the course of time, silicosis may produce extreme destruction of the lung. Silicotic lesions are also susceptible to tuberculosis infection, and the often fatal combination is silicotuberculosis. Anthracite, or hard coal, can also produce severe lesions of the lung and so, it appears, can graphite and possibly soft coal as well. Clay can sometimes collect in enormous quantities in the lung and produce a condition known years ago as "potter's rot." New diseases came with World War II, e.g., berylliosis, a highly destructive inflammatory lesion of the lung.

Atelectasis

Atelectasis is the collapse of the alveoli of a section of the lung. This is usually due to bronchial obstruction. When no additional air enters the bronchial tree, the gases present in the alveoli diffuse into the bloodstream and the alveoli collapse. Atelectasis of a large area of the lung or of several small areas may constitute a severe respiratory disability because of the reduction in alveolar ventilation. Initially, the patient frequently becomes quite cyanotic and dyspneic because the continuing blood flow through the collapsed alveoli constitutes a shunt. After 24 to 48 hours, circulation in the collapsed alveoli usually decreases, and the patient tends to improve to some extent. Atelectasis is a common and serious complication of nearly all respiratory disabilities and diseases and a common result of immobility. It should be prevented if possible. This is done by all the measures used for elimination of bronchial secretions. Treatment of atelectasis calls for an increase in these measures: humidification, cupping and vibration, postural drainage and suctioning. The same measures should be applied with sufficient vigor as preventatives to avoid this disturbance.

Sometimes resistant bronchial obstruction must be unblocked by bronchoscopy or by careful aspiration via an open trachea tube.

Pulmonary Embolism

Until recently, pulmonary embolism was construed as a catastrophic phenomenon in which one of the large bronchial arteries became obstructed; the patient expectorated blood, became cyanotic, and frequently did not survive. With the introduction of the radiographic scan, or scintiphoto, it has become a well-known fact that pulmonary embolism is one of the most common disorders of persons at rest. A large number of persons who lie in bed develop thromboses in the veins of their lower extremities and these shed emboli which travel up the vena cava to the right heart and thus to the lungs. Pulmonary emboli may be multiple or single and of varying size; their management demands the cautious use of anticoagulant medication and frequent turning of the bedridden patient.

The method of administering anticoagulants is a subject of some controversy. Either partial heparinization or full anticoagulation with a warfarin product may be undertaken. If partial heparinization without prolongation of clotting time is truly effective, it is, of course, the method of choice in a rehabilitation facility where individuals may fall or become injured. There are, nevertheless, many advocates of anticoagulation with warfarin compounds.

TECHNIQUES OF RESPIRATORY REHABILITATION

As in neurologic and musculoskeletal disabilities, a few methods of rehabilitation are applicable to many respiratory diseases and disabilities. We shall describe the rehabilitation techniques under three headings: (1) Measures to improve oxygenation, (2) Measures to relieve airway obstruction and (3) Measures to improve ventilation.

Measures to Improve Oxygenation of the Arterial Blood (Oxygen Therapy)

Oxygen therapy is the administration of oxygen in concentrations greater than that found in the ambient atmosphere.

Indications of Oxygen Therapy

Oxygen therapy is indicated in hypoxia when the pO_2 falls below 50 mm. Hg, particularly if the hypoxemia is due to impairment of diffusion, abnormalities in the ventilation–circulation ratio, shunts and the loss of functional lung tissue. Impairment of diffusion may be caused by pulmonary edema, pneumonia, emphysema, pneumothorax and atelectasis. If hypoxia is due to ventilatory impairment or

TABLE 17-4. OXYGEN THERAPY EQUIPMENT AT AMBIENT PRESSURE*

EQUIPMENT	FLOW (LITERS/MIN)	APPROXIMATE O$_2$ CONCENTRATION DELIVERED (%)	REMARKS
Nasal cannula (prongs)	4–6	30–40	Nasal obstruction interferes.
Nasal catheter –	4–6	30–40	Misplaced catheter may cause gastric dilatation.
Mask (with exhalation valve)	6–8	35–45	May be difficult to fit and uncomfortable for prolonged use.
Mask (with bag)	8–12	45–65	
	6–8	40–60	
	8–12	60–90	
Venturi mask (Venti-Mask®)**	4–8	24, 28, 35†	Accurate concentrations delivered over wide range by Venturi principle. Light plastic mask.

*See also Table 17-5. Both types may be used for assisted ventilation (patient cycled) and controlled ventilation (machine cycled).
†Disposable mask for each concentration.
**These values also apply to the metered masks now available.

Modified from: Krupp, M. A. and Chatton, M. J., Current Medical Diagnosis and Treatment, 1975, Lange Medical Publications, Los Altos, California, 1975.

TABLE 17-5. Oxygen Therapy with Positive Pressure Units*

EQUIPMENT	APPROXIMATE O₂ CONCENTRATION DELIVERED (%)	REMARKS
Pressure controlled (Bennett, Bird, and others)	40–100 (when driven by oxygen).	"Air dilution" setting usually delivers more than 40% O_2 specified. Most commonly used. Not effective when airway resistance (mask pressure) exceeds 30 cm of water.
Volume controlled (Air Shields, Ohio, Bennett MA-1, Emerson, Engstrom, Ohio-560), Searle	21–100. (Newer models have more accurate O_2 concentration controls.)	Most effective for controlled ventilation. Can overcome high airway resistance. Newer models have positive end-expiratory pressure control.

*See also Table 17-4. Both types may be used for assisted ventilation (patient cycled) and controlled ventilation (machine cycled).

Modified from: Krupp, M. A. and Chatton, M. J., Current Medical Diagnosis and Treatment, 1975, Lange Medical Publications, Los Altos, California, 1975.

airway obstruction these disabilities must be treated adequately, but if this fails to relieve hypoxia, the addition of oxygen therapy can be helpful (i.e., severe asthma and bronchitis).

Dangers of Oxygen Therapy

1. A patient with long-standing chronic CO_2 retention, whose breathing center has become insensitive to CO_2 may have his breathing suppressed if oxygen is administered, because a high concentration of oxygen precludes the operation of secondary respiratory centers (carotid and aortic bodies) which are stimulated by low pO_2.

2. The administration of high percentage oxygen tends to increase the partial pressure of CO_2 in the lungs, because nitrogen is washed out and CO_2 takes its place. This may lead to respiratory acidosis, particularly if the patient is hypoventilated.

These dangers are minimal in patients who are mechanically ventilated and well monitored. In patients who breathe on their own power it is advisable to maintain the oxygen content of the inspired air below 40 per cent.

Methods of Administering Oxygen

The most common methods of administering oxygen are listed in Tables 17-4 and 17-5.

Oxygen Therapy at Ambient Pressure. Administration of O_2 is usually continuous throughout the hypoxic episode. A nasal catheter, nasal prongs or a mask is used for administration.

Nasal Prongs or Catheter. A loop or tubing with plastic prongs which extend about 1 cm. into each nostril is the most comfortable device. A nasal catheter (10-12 F urethral catheter) may be used. It should be lubricated and passed through one nostril until the tip (visualized through the mouth) just disappears in the hypopharynx. Humidification of the oxygen is essential. Nasal obstruction will interfere with oxygen delivery by this method.

Masks. A simple plastic nonrebreathing mask may be used in place of nasal prongs or catheter with similar effect, although a slightly higher flow rate is needed. One such mask, the Venti-Mask, is a disposable plastic mask which delivers measured oxygen concentrations by the Venturi mixing principle. An opening in the tube permits ambient air to enter the tube and mix with the oxygen. At a given rate of flow, the amount of air entering the tube depends upon the size of the opening. Thus a mixture with a fixed percentage of oxygen is achieved. Three separate masks (27 per cent, 30 per cent and 35 per cent) are available.

Disabling Conditions Due to Respiratory Impairment   **431**

There are also masks which have exchangeable color-coded rings which are inserted in the mask. Each ring permits air flow at a given speed and thus produces a known percentage of oxygen.

Oxygen Therapy with Volume Controlled Positive Pressure Units. This treatment is usually given to patients with severe respiratory failure. The equipment requires a closed circuit via tracheostomy with cuff tube (or cuffed endotracheal tube). Usually the patient also has severe ventilatory disability, and oxygen therapy is added if hypoxia cannot be relieved by ventilation alone. It must be continued until the pO_2 is adequate (60 to 80 mm. Hg) and then discontinued gradually.

Oxygen Therapy with Pressure Controlled Positive Pressure Units. For treatment of chronic pulmonary disorders, especially emphysema and bronchial asthma, pressure controlled intermittent positive pressure apparatus is usually preferred. This type of apparatus can be operated from an oxygen pressure source by an air compressor. Oxygen concentration can be varied from 20 to 100 per cent by various methods. The rate of breathing can usually be adjusted to 10 to 20 respirations per minute, and treatment is often applied at pressures of 10 to 20 cm. of water for about 15 to 20 minutes.

The percentage of oxygen delivered is only approximate. When the concentration must be carefully controlled, the gas delivered to the patient should be monitored with an oxygen meter.

Treatment of Upper Airway Obstruction
The larynx and pharynx may become obstructed in bulbar paralysis (see p. 303) and in some acute conditions such as diphtheria and edema of the glottis. In the emergency room, obstruction by injury or foreign body is often seen. Obstruction is relieved either by intubation or tracheostomy. Intubation is the insertion of an endotracheal tube through the larynx. Tracheostomy is the surgical insertion of a tracheal tube below the larynx. Both procedures are used not only to maintain an open airway but also to permit mechanical ventilation by positive pressure equipment and tracheobronchial suctioning for removal of secretion. Intubation is convenient for emergencies and short-term use. For long-range rehabilitation, we prefer a tracheostomy.

Technique of Tracheostomy
Equipment. In preparation for tracheostomy the patient's bed area should be organized to permit efficient nursing care including aspira-

tion of secretions from the nose, the mouth and the tracheobronchial tree. Often, the operation is done in the ward or room, thus avoiding loss of time and the hazards of transportation to the operating room. Wherever the operation is performed, the surgical tray should be readily available and should contain the following:

No.	INSTRUMENT
2	B.P. Knife Handle #3
	B.P. Blades #10, #11, #15
1	Scissors, curved Mayo
1	Scissors, straight Mayo
1	Scissors, Metzenbaum
1	Tissue forceps—teeth
1	Dressing forceps
4	Kelly-Murphy hemostatic forceps, curved
4	Halsted mosquito forceps, straight
4	Halsted mosquito forceps, curved
1	Rochester-Pean hemostatic forceps, curved
2	Allis tissue forceps
2	Blunt double ended retractors, Farabeuf or Parker
2	U.S. Army or Mathieu retractors
1	Blunt hook
1	Tracheal dilator
1	Needle holder
1	Robinson catheter #10
1	Robinson catheter #12
2	Sims' tips
1	Tracheostomy tube #7
1	Tracheostomy tube #4

(Additional tracheostomy tubes of various diameters, curves and sizes available in individually sterilized packets)

1   Killian nasal speculum, 3 in. (7.62 cm.) (for spreading cuff to receive tracheostomy tube if cuff is separate from tube)
1   Packet sterile talc
Double walled cuffs, assorted sizes, low pressure type, for tracheostomy tubes

No.	ITEM
1	Medicine glass
1	Syringe 10 ml., Luer-lok
1	Syringe, 2 ml.

Needles, hypodermic
  25 g., ⅝ in. (1.59 cm.)
  22 g., 1 in. (2.54 cm.) and 1½ in. (3.81 cm.)
  20 g., 1 in. (2.54 cm.)
  18 g., 1½ in. (3.81 cm.)

1	Sponge stick
1	Prep. cup
6	Prep. sponges
6	Gauze pads, 4″ x 4″
1	Eye drape

Sutures:
  Plain 000
  Chr. 000
  Silk 000
  Dermalon 000 with needle

Needles:
  Assorted round and cutting

Gloves
Suction tubing
Tape for tracheostomy tubes (bias, hernia tape)

Procedure. In performing the tracheostomy, the following outline should be used:

1. Anesthesia
   a. General
   b. Local
   c. None, in unconscious patient

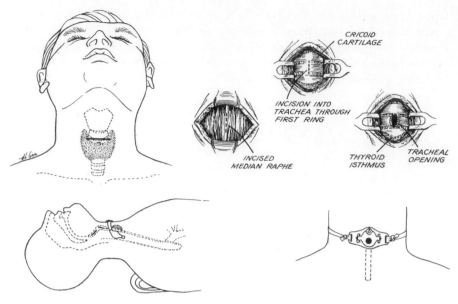

Fig. 17-9. Tracheostomy procedure.

2. Airway

    a. Endotracheal catheter, for ventilation prior to and during operation, with or without general anesthesia

    b. Bronchoscope, used for emergency diagnosis or treatment; in place during operation, in lieu of endotracheal catheter

    c. Normal airway

3. Position and preparation

    a. Extend head on neck in back-lying position by placing a rolled-up sheet under scapulae.

    b. Cleanse area and drape; do not obscure chest and abdomen; allow opportunity to observe respiratory excursion.

    c. Maintain artificial respiration without interruption in the patient with respiratory paralysis or marked respiratory depression.

    d. Prepare appropriate tracheostomy tubes according to the purpose for which the operation is performed.

       (1) For artificial respiration, the largest tube which the trachea will tolerate, up to size No. 8, should be used. More than one size tube should be readied.

4. Surgical procedure (Fig. 17-9)

    a. Incision: Transverse, or vertical, through skin and platysma muscle at the level of the cricoid cartilage. Tie off skin bleeders.

    b. Dissection: Expose median raphe with minimal trauma.

Split the fascia of the sternohyoid muscles in the median raphe and retract the muscles laterally. Pick up the pretracheal fascia with tooth forceps, open the fascia and separate to expose the trachea. Identify the cricoid cartilage by measuring it and the cartilage below it with the end of a closed hemostat. The cricoid is about twice as wide as the cartilage below it.

c. Opening trachea and intubation: Using No. 11 knife blade, cut across the first tracheal cartilage *below* the cricoid, in the midline. *Never incise the cricoid!* Spread the tracheal opening with a tracheal dilator and pass the tracheal cannula with obturator in place, and cuffed or uncuffed as the situation requires, into the trachea. Remove the obturator, aspirate blood or secretions from airway, using the precautions described under "Tracheobronchial Aspiration" (p. 443), then insert inner cannula and secure the tube with tape ties.

5. Dressing

a. Tape ties, previously attached to the cannula, should be long on one side, short on the other. The tapes should be tied long enough to avoid neck vein constriction and short enough to prevent the cannula from being pulled or coughed out. The knot should be easily accessible on one side of the neck.

b. Use no sutures in the wound closure. The only ligatures needed are about four to tie off superficial vessels in the skin and platysma. The wound is left open for the following reasons:

(1) It heals from the extremes toward the center.

(2) The scar is less prominent than when sutured; there is no

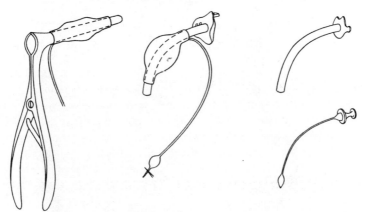

Fig. 17-10. Tracheal tube and cuff. Use of long nasal speculum to place rubber cuff on trachea tube. The cuffed trachea tube is shown with the cuff inflated. The inner cannula and the obdurator are shown separately.

Disabling Conditions Due to Respiratory Impairment 435

danger of leaving sutures in place too long; unsightly vertical suture scars, almost impossible to remove by plastic repair, are avoided.

(3) Infection is not sealed in.

(4) Subcutaneous emphysema is prevented.

c. A small gauze pad, placed on either side between the flange of the cannula and the skin, is the only dressing required.

Tracheostomy Tubes and Cuffs

Tracheostomy tubes are made of metal or plastic. They come in different widths, lengths and shapes. Some have an inner cannula which can be removed easily for cleaning. An obturator is used for insertion of the tube. A plug is available to close the opening in the tracheostomy tube. An inflatable cuff should surround the tube to

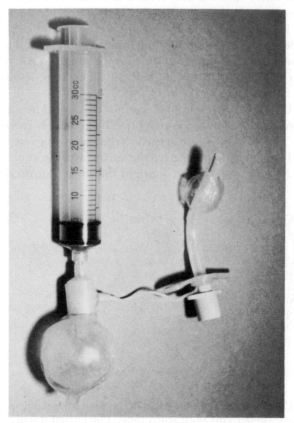

Fig. 17-11. Lanz tube with soft cuff and outside bag to indicate cuff pressure.

TABLE 17-6. CHARACTERISTICS AND INDICATIONS OF SOME COMMONLY USED TRACHEOSTOMY TUBES

NAME	MATERIAL	INNER CANNULA	CUFF	SPECIAL FEATURES	ADVANTAGES	INDICATIONS
Jackson	Metal	Yes	No	None	Thin walled	Persons who cannot tolerate plastic
Hollinger	Metal	Yes	No	Initial curve, then straight	Less danger of pressure against anterior wall of trachea	Patients with small and straight trachea
Gabriel Tucker	Metal	Yes	No	Valve on inner cannula channels expired air into larynx	Assists speech	Vocal cord paralysis
Vail	Plastic	Yes	No	Choice of 3 lengths	Choice of length	Special length required
Lanz	Plastic	No	Yes	1. Universal adaptor 2. Soft cuff with outside bulb within bulb	Adapts to most positive pressure apparatus Well controlled cuff pressure	Emergency and long-term use

block off the tracheal space. This prevents aspiration of material from the mouth and pharynx into the lungs. The cuff also prevents air, oxygen and medication delivered to the lung via the tracheal tube from escaping around the tube.

Some tubes have a permanently attached cuff; others come without cuff, so that a separate cuff has to be slipped over the tube prior to use. This is the case for the Jackson tracheal tube (Fig. 17-10).

It has been demonstrated that the high pressure, hard cuff when inflated can produce erosion of the tracheal mucous membrane, especially when high pressures are used for breathing. There are cases on record of air embolism as a result of cracks in the tracheal mucosa with air entering the venous system under pressure and causing cerebral air embolism. To prevent such complications, there are now cuffs which are soft and low pressure and which can be deflated from time to time. Cuffs are connected to a fine tube with a dilatation or small balloon outside the airway which shows whether the cuff is distended.

The Lanz tracheostomy tube has a balloon within a balloon (Fig. 17-11). As long as the walls are not touching, one can be assured that the pressure in the cuff is not excessive. Furthermore, the degree of pressure can be palpated on the inner balloon, making it possible to determine that this balloon is soft.

Characteristics of and indications for some of the most commonly used tracheostomy tubes are listed in Table 17-6.

Care of the Tracheostomy

Usually, the tract formed by tracheostomy is sealed over within 2 or 3 days at which time the tracheal tube may be easily changed if necessary. When artificial respiration is no longer required, the tube size can be reduced. The need for the cuff depends on such considerations as danger of aspiration, intact swallowing mechanism, amount of nasopharyngeal secretion and tolerance of the cuff. In general, a cuffed tube should be used for as long as possible. On rare occasions the presence of the cuff itself induces marked secretion which stops when an ordinary tube is placed in the trachea.

If there is an inner cannula it should be removed and cleansed at least three times daily. It may be soaked in hydrogen peroxide solution and cleaned with a pipe cleaner; never with a wood applicator!

The tracheal tube should normally be changed about once weekly and more often if it is crusted with secretions or causing discomfort. There should always be a reserve, complete tracheostomy tube of proper size at the patient's bedside.

The secretion withdrawn from the tracheal stoma should be cultured every time the tube is changed. In all probability, the area will prove to be infected, usually with gram negative bacilli or benign contaminants. Occasionally, Staphylococcus aureus, coagulase positive, is present.

The rubber cuff should be inflated by means of a Luer syringe attached to a blunt cannula of appropriate size to fit the narrow rubber tubing of the cuff. Approximately 3 to 7 ml. of air is necessary to close off the airway around the tube. The amount needed is determined by listening to air escape from the mouth and stopping the inflation at the point when no air can be heard with a stethoscope placed over the open mouth. If the patient is conscious, the point of adequate inflation will be determined by loss of voice. It is essential to explain the purpose and effects of the cuffed tube to the conscious patient. He should be provided at once with alternative methods of communication and should be informed that the cuff will be deflated periodically. When the cuff is inflated, the catheter used for the aspiration of secretions must allow air space; if the opening is filled with the catheter, the airway is totally occluded. To avoid this, the cuff should be deflated prior to the aspiration of secretions.

Most cuffs must be deflated for at least 10 minutes every 4 hours. Failure to deflate may lead to ulceration of the tracheal mucosa, tracheitis and hemorrhage. If artificial respiration is done by means of a pressure or flow-regulated, intermittent positive pressure machine, the flow rate or pressure must be increased to the extent needed to maintain respiration while the cuff is deflated.

The presence of a tracheal tube, especially when cuffed, calls for the most meticulous care. Improper aspiration, excessive pressure due to overinflation of the cuff and failure to decompress the cuff at intervals may seriously compromise the patient's prognosis.

Treatment of Lower Airway Obstruction

The principal difficulty in the lower airway is the accumulation of secretions which may increase because of the disease itself or because of secondary complications such as bronchitis and pneumonitis. At times, secretions are excessive because of the presence of a tracheostomy tube and will not be diminished until it is safely removed.

If a tracheostomy or endotracheal tube is present, it will be extremely difficult to cough up secretions because the tube prevents closure of the larynx. Cough is dependent upon the Valsalva maneuver whereby the glottis is closed off and pressure is developed in the chest prior to an expulsive effort. In paralysis of respiratory muscles, crushed chest and ventilatory insufficiency, there is little ability to

1. APICAL SEGMENTS

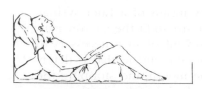

LEFT AND RIGHT ANTERIOR
Sitting — lean back against pillow; clap in front on both sides just above collar bones, between neck and shoulder.

2. APICAL SEGMENTS

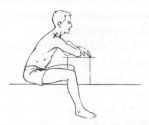

LEFT AND RIGHT POSTERIOR
Sitting — lean forward onto pillow; clap on both sides on the back above shoulder blades. Fingers usually go a little over shoulder.

3. LEFT POSTERIOR SEGMENT

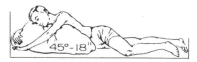

Lie on right side with head and shoulders elevated on pillows. Make 1/4 turn forward; clap over left shoulder blade.

4. APICAL SEGMENTS

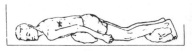

LEFT AND RIGHT (LOWER LOBE)
Lie flat on stomach; place pillow under stomach area for added comfort and clap just below the shoulder blade.

5. RIGHT POSTERIOR SEGMENT

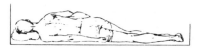

Lie on left side — place pillow in front from shoulder to hips and roll slightly forward onto it; clap over right shoulder blade.

6. ANTERIOR SEGMENTS

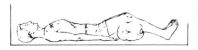

LEFT AND RIGHT
Lie flat on back with pillow under knees for comfort; clap on both sides just below collar bones and above the nipple line.

Fig. 17-12. Postural Drainage. (Karen Struebing Swigert, N. Illinois Chap, National Cystic Fibrosis Research Foundation).

7. RIGHT MIDDLE LOBE

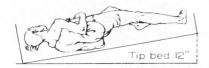

Lie on left side. Place pillow behind from shoulders to hips and roll slightly back onto it; clap over right nipple. For girls developing breast tissue, clap to the right of the nipple and below the armpit.

8. RIGHT LATERAL BASAL SEGMENT

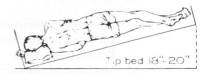

Lie on left side; clap at lower ribs. A pillow under the waist may help to keep the spine straight.

9. POSTERIOR BASAL SEGMENT

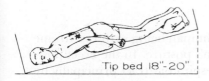

LEFT AND RIGHT
Lie on stomach and place pillow under hips; clap at lower ribs on both sides.

10. LEFT LATERAL BASAL SEGMENT

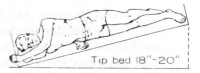

Lie on right side; clap at lower ribs. A pillow under the waist may help to keep spine straight.

11. LEFT LINGULA

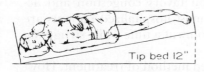

Lie on right side. Place pillow behind from shoulder to hips and roll slightly back onto it; clap over left nipple. For girls developing breast tissue, clap to the left of the nipple and below the armpit.

12. ANTERIOR BASAL SEGMENT

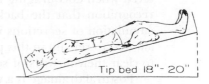

LEFT AND RIGHT
Lie on back and place pillow under knees; clap at lower ribs on both sides.

expel secretions by cough. In addition, there are times when secretions are so viscid that they cannot be expelled.

The following measures are used to help remove secretions:
1. Increase in the fluidity of the secretions
2. Postural drainage
3. Mechanical measures applied to the chest wall
4. Assisted cough
5. Tracheobronchial aspiration

Fluidity of Secretions

Fluidity of secretions can be increased by adequate fluid intake, by medications and by humidification of the inspired air. Bronchodilating and mucolytic agents may be added to the inspired mist. In the tracheostomized patient, instillation of a few drops of normal saline solution may be helpful.

Postural Drainage (Fig. 17-12)

Bronchopulmonary drainage in the human being suffers extreme mechanical disadvantage because of man's posture. In the erect position, secretions are removed from the respiratory tract principally by means of ciliary action of bronchial mucosa, assisted by mechanical forces such as cough. In the recumbent position, bronchial drainage is still uphill when the person lies on his back and is uphill for one lung when he lies on either side. Only the face-lying position slants the majority of the bronchi in a direction that favors gravitational flow. Except for a few areas in the lower anterior lungs, all of the bronchial tree drains downward when a patient lies face down in bed. The infrequency of such positioning of patients and the difficulty encountered when encouraging its use are hard to understand. Despite the recognition that the back-lying position favors congestion and accumulation of secretions in the lungs, most hospitalized patients are allowed to remain in this position for hours at a time while struggling to clear their airways of secretions.

Postural drainage is a well-established method of treatment. However, it is sometimes difficult to carry out because patients with severe impairment may be too short of breath to permit adequate positioning for satisfactory drainage. In such instances, the use of positive pressure respiratory assistance prior to bronchial drainage and intermittently during the course of repeated postural drainages may be helpful.

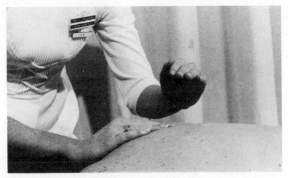

Fig. 17-13. Cupping. (From Wood, E. C.: Beard's Massage: Principles and Techniques, 2nd Ed. Philadelphia, W. B. Saunders Co., 1974.)

Mechanical Measures Applied to the Chest Wall

It would seem logical that percussion of the chest wall at the time of postural drainage may be helpful in loosening secretions from the bronchial wall. With this rationale in mind a number of massage motions have been applied to the chest wall. They are frequently described under the term "Percussion and Vibration." Percussion is a generic term and even in the narrow field of massage it includes several procedures such as "hacking," "beating" and "cupping" (or "clapping"). It is the latter procedure which is commonly used for chest physical therapy and we prefer the specific term "cupping" to the generic term percussion.

Cupping is the application of percussion with cupped hands, fingers and thumbs together, the wrists and arms very relaxed and loose (Fig. 17-13). The hands rhythmically and alternately strike the chest wall at the rate of 100 to 150 beats per minute with emphasis on the area of the lung being drained. The patient must be in a position which drains the cupped area. Each site is cupped for 3 to 5 minutes. The total treatment usually takes 20 minutes. During and after the procedure the patient is encouraged to cough. While coughing, he should be in a face-down position and if possible in a postural drainage position.

Two other massage movements are "Vibration" and "Shaking." Both procedures are carried out by pressure of the flat hand against the chest wall while the therapist produces a tremor with his arm. The procedures are technically difficult and strenuous for the therapist. We do not use them routinely in respiratory rehabilitation.

Controlled studies of the usefulness of cupping, vibration and shaking are not available. Nevertheless, we use cupping routinely since it assures at least an organized program of postural drainage. The attention to the patient at a regular schedule, the change of position and the coughing associated with the "cupping ritual" may be as useful as the percussion itself.

Assisted Cough

There are several ways of assisting the patient to cough, the simplest being the application of manual pressure on the abdomen during expiration. For patients with respiratory paralysis, a widely used device is the Cof-Flater which relies on a positive pressure pump which forcefully inflates the lung, then reverses its flow and assists in expiration or cough. For patients in a tank respirator, the negative pressure within the tank can be rapidly released by forcibly opening the bedpan opening at the height of a deep inspiration, thereby causing an expiratory surge of air into the airway.

Tracheobronchial Aspiration

In a patient without tracheostomy it is possible to remove thick secretions by bronchoscopy or through an endotracheal tube. However, when there is a need for prolonged control of bronchial secretions a tracheostomy is indicated. The tracheostomized patient can benefit from fluidity of secretions, postural drainage and assisted cough but the most effective measure is the aspiration of bronchial secretions at regular intervals. The principle is similar to that of a vacuum cleaner. A tube attached to a suction pump is inserted into the bronchial tree through the tracheostomy opening. One danger of this procedure is damage to the tracheobronchial mucosa. Another is the introduction of pathogenic bacteria. Good technique can minimize these dangers. Therefore we shall describe this procedure in detail.

Equipment. Assemble the following equipment before beginning the procedure:

1. A source of negative pressure (suction); either a portable apparatus (Gomco, Chaffin-Pratt, Sklar or other) or an outlet to a central unit with a control valve.

2. Sterilized rubber or plastic tubing.

3. A collecting bottle and connections.

4. "Y" tubes.

5. Bronchial catheters, F-8 to F-14, opening at the tip. A sufficient number of catheters should be available to permit the use of a fresh sterilized catheter for each aspiration session.

6. Sterile gloves.

Solutions.   The following solutions should be available before beginning the procedure:

1. Sterile water.
2. Sterile isotonic saline solution.

Setting Up and Checking the Equipment.   The following steps should be taken to prepare the equipment for the procedure:

1. Connect the tubing from the suction apparatus or outlet to the stem of the "Y" tube.

2. Connect one branch of the "Y" tube to a bronchial catheter, using sterile technique. The other branch of the "Y" tube permits the control of the suction by occluding it with a finger tip (suction on) or leaving it open (suction off).

3. With the negative pressure control turned on, clamp off the tube between the "Y" tube and the collecting bottle and read the pressure gauge. Most portable units have gauges which register 0-30 and indicate inches of mercury. Most new central unit outlets are equipped with gauges which register 0-200 and indicate millimeters of mercury. When a portable suction apparatus is used, the negative pressure with the tube clamped off on the patient side of the collecting bottle should be about 4 inches of mercury and should never exceed 8 inches of mercury. When a central outlet is used the pressure should be set at 100 mm. Hg and should not exceed 200 mm. Hg. Instead of turning the negative pressure apparatus off and on during the procedure, the "Y" tube is occluded or opened with the finger tip while the apparatus remains on.

Procedure.   The following procedure should be used for the aspiration of bronchial secretions:

1. Wash hands thoroughly and put on sterile gloves.

2. Lubricate the catheter with sterile normal saline solution.

3. Insert the catheter well into the bronchial tree, with the free branch of the "Y" tube *open* to avoid suction while the catheter is being inserted.

4. Have the patient turn his head to the left so that the catheter can enter the right main stem bronchus.

5. Enter promptly, close off the open end of the "Y" tube to activate suction, then withdraw the catheter slowly. Stop for a moment whenever the sound of the aspirating stream changes, an indication that secretion is entering the catheter. Slowly remove the catheter.

6. Have the patient turn his head to the right so that the catheter can enter the left main stem bronchus and aspirate as above.

7. Repeat aspiration until the airway is free of secretion. Discard the catheter.

Disabling Conditions Due to Respiratory Impairment   **445**

8. If the secretions are thick and difficult to aspirate, apply a medicine dropper's contents of normal saline solution into the tracheal cannula and aspirate again.

Oral and Pharyngeal Aspiration

In paralyzed and comatose patients there may also be accumulation of oral and pharyngeal secretions. These may be aspirated at the same time that tracheobronchial aspiration is carried out. However, a separate catheter should be used in the nose and mouth to aspirate pharyngeal secretions.

Mechanical Ventilation

The simplest form of *inspiratory assistance* is emergency mouth-to-mouth breathing. It is the most primitive form of intermittent positive pressure breathing. Mechanical inspiration can also be accomplished by negative pressure, i.e., by the old fashioned "Iron Lung." *Expiratory assistance* is used only in selected cases of respiratory paralysis.

Mechanical Inspiratory Assistance

Positive Pressure Respirators. This method consists of pumping air into the lung by positive pressure via the airway and allowing the patient to breathe out by the elasticity of the lung. The positive pressure is therefore applied intermittently during inspiration and ceases during expiration. There are two types of positive pressure apparatus available: pressure controlled and volume controlled. The pressure controlled apparatus can be used with a mask or with an adaptor to a tracheal tube. The volume controlled apparatus requires a tracheal tube with cuff.

Pressure Controlled Devices. The intermittent positive pressure breathing (IPPB) apparatus is now an essential part of the armamentarium of virtually all health facilities. These machines are derivatives of aviation medicine when their prototypes were used to administer an augmented oxygen supply under pressure to personnel flying at altitudes where ambient air was inadequate to maintain needed pO_2. In medicine, the IPPB units are used in a variety of ways, including artificial respiration at times. Some administer ambient air and are powered by pumps (Bennett AP-5; Bird with auxiliary pump), others are powered by the pressure of oxygen or compressed air in tanks (Bennett TV-2P; Bird attached to oxygen tank, Emerson); some by mixtures of oxygen and air regulated by mixing valves and other devices. All of them have nebulizing devices used both to humidify the air stream and to deliver medications.

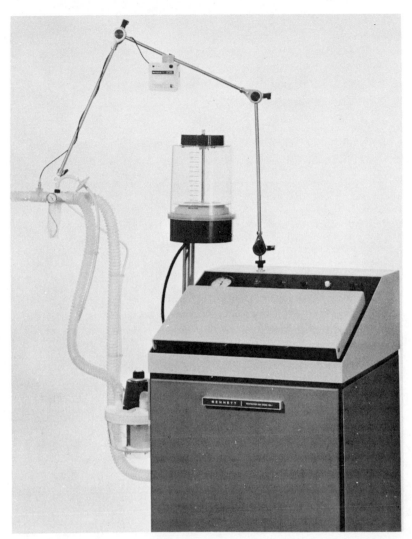

Fig. 17-14. MA-1 Respirator. (Bennett Respiration Products, Inc.)

Intermittent positive pressure devices are used for short periods to treat emphysema, bronchial asthma, and a variety of other respiratory disorders; to prevent atelectasis postoperatively; and to treat pulmonary edema. They are also used for prolonged periods as respirators, especially in emergencies. They are tripped by the shifts in the patient's respiratory pressure thus supplementing the patient's respiratory force, i.e., they are demand respirators.

Volume Controlled Devices.   A pressure sensitive apparatus is difficult to control and is not subject to the finesse of the more modern volume controlled respirators. Of these, the Engstrom respirator (Swedish) is the forerunner while the Emerson unit is considered the simplest and is relatively trouble-free. The Bennett MA-1 volume controlled respirator (Fig. 17-14) is in wide use and permits control of many parameters of respiration. Since it is the one with which we have had the greatest experience, reference will be made largely to it. Other volume controlled respirators are the Ohio 560, the Monaghan 225 Ventilator, the Air Shields Respirator and the new Searle Adult Volume Respirator.

All of these volume controlled respirators require a closed system. Therefore, the trachea must either be intubated with a cuffed endotracheal tube, or a tracheostomy tube with cuff.

The advantage of the volume controlled respirators is that a person with a cuffed tube in his trachea, either nasotracheal, orotrachreal or tracheostomy, can be set up with a specific mixture of oxygen in the inspired air with a set pressure limit beyond which the machine will not go. The rate of respiration can be adjusted to either control respiration in time with the patient's cycle, or to assure adequate respiration with the patient using it as a demand respirator and breathing at his own rate with supplemental breaths from the machine. This requires that the rate on the panel be set lower than the patient's normal rate but sufficiently increased in volume to avoid hypoxia. There are good safeguards and signals to indicate any failure by the apparatus. The spirometer of the MA-1 machine indicates the tidal volume with reasonable accuracy, provided one makes adjustment for extension of tubing. A heated mist, which is delivered to the air stream, is controllable.

Provision is also made for periodic deep respirations, or sighs, to help keep the alveoli open. Repair is relatively simple especially when a company repairman is nearby.

The disadvantages of this apparatus are the very high cost, the requirement of a cuffed endotracheal or tracheostomy tube and the relative difficulty of maintenance, requiring an established program in every hospital where such a machine is set up.

Negative Pressure Respirators. *The Tank Respirator.*   The names Emerson and Drinker have been associated with the modern tank respirator since their inventions. While there are reports of prior negative pressure respirators, they are medical curiosities. Both varieties of the tank respirator consist of tanks with large openings for bellows which, when expanded, produce negative pressures within

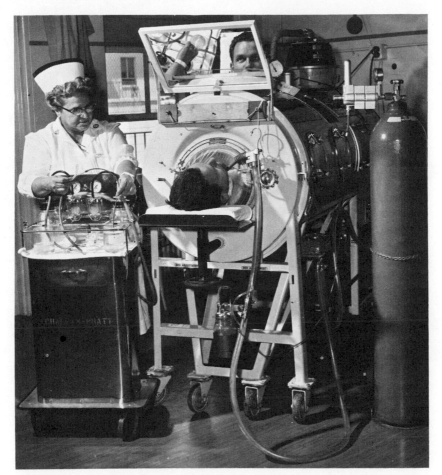

Fig. 17-15. Tank respirator and accessories. This Emerson respirator has an adjustable mirror which greatly facilitates communication and adds to patient comfort. Attached to the respirator (above) is an Emerson deep-breathing attachment which can be adjusted to provide deep inspirations at regular intervals controlled by a timing mechanism. On the right, attached to the respirator leg, is the manifold of a Monaghan positive pressure attachment. The tygon tubing shown leads from a small bellows which operates reciprocally with the tank bellows and supplies positive pressure via the tracheal tube. The positive pressure air stream is kept moist by means of an aerosol produced by flow of oxygen through a nebulizer shown at the front and below the tank. The nurse is holding catheter properly connected for aspiration of secretion from the patient's airway.

the interior of the tanks. There is one large, closable porthole at one end of the tank for the patient's neck and two small ones on each side for the entry of arms. Attendants can enter the tank with their arms without disrupting the cycle of the respirator, particularly if they pay attention to the gauge on top or side of the tank and make entry at a time when the pointer is at zero. The respirator is also equipped with a bedpan door.

The negative pressure on the inside of the tank can be varied by means of adjustments which will allow for a maximum negative pressure of from 15 to 24 cm. of water. Positive pressure can be created or prevented by means of escape areas which can be closed to produce the positive pressure or left open to avoid it. The positive pressure can be adjusted to produce anything from zero to somewhat less positive pressure than the negative pressure generated by the bellows.

There is a small bellows attachment which acts reciprocally with the main bellows and produces positive pressure which is transmitted through a manifold to either a tracheostomy tube or a mask. Use of this device makes it possible to respire the patient when the tank is open. The Emerson respirator (Fig. 17-15) also has a dome attachment over the patient's head which makes it possible to maintain a cycle of intermittent positive pressure when the tank is open. In addition, the Emerson tank can be fitted with a device that has an internal clock mechanism to trigger deep sighing respirations at intervals each hour. Intravenous tubes can be introduced through a stopcock at the head of the tank.

These respirators have wheeled, padded carts which constitute the beds of the respirators. They are locked in place, and a tight gasket assures airtightness when the head is closed. By means of a jack, the Trendelenburg position can be obtained. There are also adjustment wheels which can turn the bed up or down slightly on one side or the other. Usually, there is a thin foam rubber mattress conforming to the size of the tray on the cart portion of the tank.

It is possible to maintain patients for long periods of time in the tank respirator. There are people living now who contracted poliomyelitis as early as 1948 and still depend upon the tank respirator for breathing, sometimes throughout the day and night.

Fig. 17-16. *(Top)* Chest-abdomen cuirass respirator. Changeover to battery is automatic if power fails. In the back-lying position, the patient may use this respirator for sleep or for activities. The patient is shown during physical therapy. *(Bottom)* The same patient is shown in a wheel chair equipped with arm sling and lap board, using the cuirass respirator while working as a bookkeeper. (The Thompson-Hyxley Respirator)

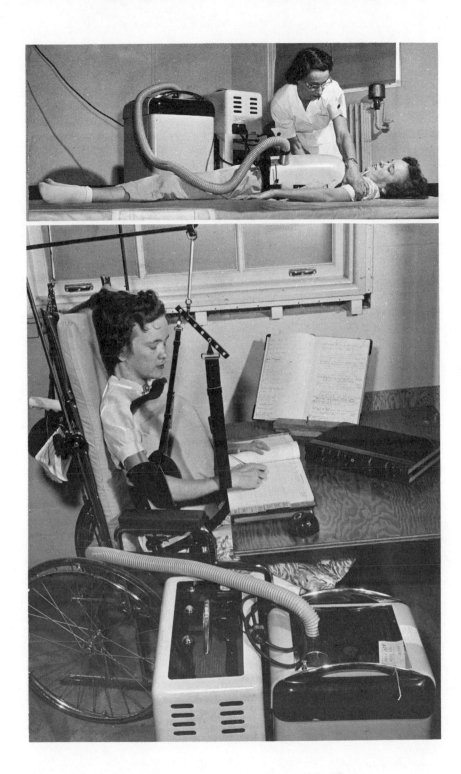

Cuirass Respirator. This type of respirator consists of a cover or plastic cuirass which fits over the chest or the chest and abdomen. A large tube leads from the cuirass to the respiratory unit which has a variable pressure and variable rate. Commonly used respirators of this type are the Huxley (now Thompson-Huxley), the Monaghan, and more recently, the Thompson respirators (Fig. 17-16).

Mechanical Expiratory Assistance

A common example of expiratory assistance is the method of resuscitation which is frequently used following drowning. In this procedure, the chest wall is compressed to press air out of the lungs. Inspiration is caused by the elastic expansion of the chest wall until it reaches the end-expiratory position.

A mechanical device to give expiratory assistance is known as a pneumobelt. The pneumobelt is a corset-like device which covers the abdomen and lower chest. Within it, in front, is an inflatable bag intermittently inflated by a pump. The pneumobelt is a useful device for expiratory assistance only in patients with severe respiratory paralysis including the abdominal muscles. It must be used while the patient is in a sitting or standing position. In this position, the weight of the abdominal viscera lowers the diaphragm during inspiration.

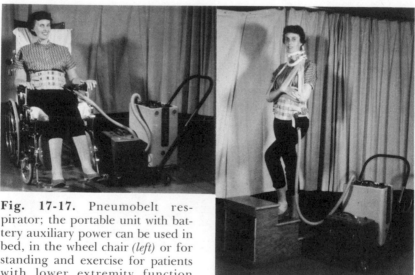

Fig. 17-17. Pneumobelt respirator; the portable unit with battery auxiliary power can be used in bed, in the wheel chair *(left)* or for standing and exercise for patients with lower extremity function *(right)*. The trunk must be upright or inclined at an angle of 30° or more from the horizontal.

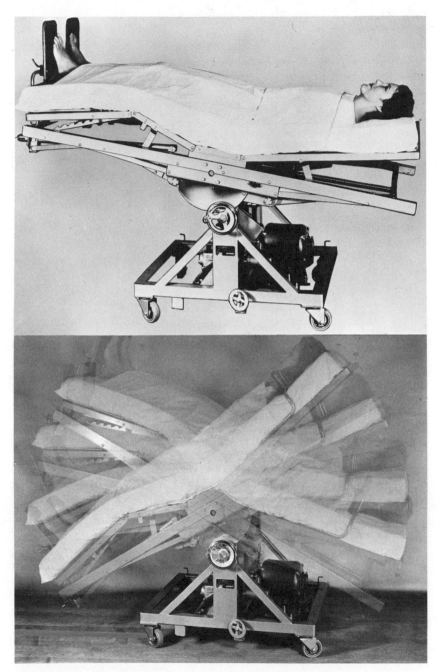

Fig. 17-18. *(Top)* Emerson rocking bed. *(Bottom)* The rocking bed in motion. Inspiration occurs during the footdown phase; expiration during the head-down phase. (J. H. Emerson Co.)

When the bag is inflated inside the abdominal corset, the abdomen is compressed and the viscera and the diaphragm are elevated causing expiration (Fig. 17-17).

Combined Expiratory and Inspiratory Assistance

An interesting device for mechanical respiration and resuscitation is the rocking bed. It is based upon the principle of rhythmically alternating the patient's position from a head-down position to a foot-down position. The upward thrust of the viscera in the head-down (or flat) position has an expiratory effect, while the downward thrust of the viscera in the foot-down position has an inspiratory effect. A patient with complete respiratory paralysis can be adequately ventilated by the rocking bed (Fig. 17-18).*

Another device which combines expiratory and inspiratory assistance is the multilung. This device uses the pneumobelt for expiratory assistance, while the same pump alternatingly gives the patient inspiratory assistance by positive pressure breathing.

Improvement of Ventilatory Ability

If the patient has become independent of mechanical ventilation, he must improve his own ventilatory ability. In the paralyzed patient, where strengthening of respiratory muscles cannot be expected, glossopharyngeal breathing is helpful. Other helpful measures include the improvement of chest compliance, breathing exercises and aerobic exercises.

Glossopharyngeal Breathing

This learned technique allows the patient to distend his lungs forcibly and to maintain flexibility of the thorax despite muscle weakness. The technique of glossopharyngeal breathing is illustrated in Figure 17-19.

Methods to Improve Compliance

In many conditions, particularly in respiratory paralysis, the thorax and lungs have a tendency to become stiff. A good method of stretching the lungs and chest is through "maximum" glossopharyngeal breathing, whereby inspiration is continued to a maximum effort of 100 breaths of 50 cc. each, as opposed to 10 breaths in simple glossopharyngeal breathing. In order to maintain

---

*The generally beneficial effect of the rocking bed has only been partially investigated. M. T. F. Carpendale, M.D. (personal communication) has used the rocking bed principle in his study of "A bed to prevent the pathology of recumbency."

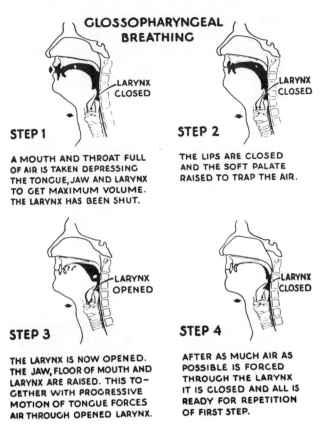

GLOSSOPHARYNGEAL BREATHING

STEP 1

LARYNX CLOSED

A MOUTH AND THROAT FULL OF AIR IS TAKEN DEPRESSING THE TONGUE, JAW AND LARYNX TO GET MAXIMUM VOLUME. THE LARYNX HAS BEEN SHUT.

STEP 2

LARYNX CLOSED

THE LIPS ARE CLOSED AND THE SOFT PALATE RAISED TO TRAP THE AIR.

STEP 3

LARYNX OPENED

THE LARYNX IS NOW OPENED. THE JAW, FLOOR OF MOUTH AND LARYNX ARE RAISED. THIS TO-GETHER WITH PROGRESSIVE MOTION OF TONGUE FORCES AIR THROUGH OPENED LARYNX.

STEP 4

LARYNX CLOSED

AFTER AS MUCH AIR AS POSSIBLE IS FORCED THROUGH THE LARYNX IT IS CLOSED AND ALL IS READY FOR REPETITION OF FIRST STEP.

Fig. 17-19. Glossopharyngeal breathing.

this compliance, maximum glossopharyngeal breathing must be practiced at least 3 times each day.

Another means of improving compliance is provided by the built-in "deep sighing" respiratory effort of the MA-1 and tank respirators. Rib cage compliance may be improved by manipulating and mobilizing the ribs and by aerobic exercise.

Breathing Exercises

The prescription of specific breathing exercises requires skillful appraisal of the nature of respiratory impairment and selection of exercises that are likely to prove beneficial. Ineffective exercises are discarded very quickly by most patients. Objective studies with adequate controls are very much needed to determine the value of procedures in the treatment of chronic pulmonary disorders. A large proportion of disabled persons with emphysema secondary to chronic bronchitis can be rehabilitated for self-care and employment by means of a program of breathing exercises, bronchodilation with drugs administered under intermittent positive pressure and postural drainage.

Many systems of breathing exercises have been proposed for the treatment of pulmonary emphysema. The effectiveness of these exercises is difficult to demonstrate, and the rationale for their use is often obscure. Simple techniques of breathing, which the patient with emphysema usually discovers on his own, can be helpful. Obstruction to the outflow of air in emphysema results, in part, from narrowing of the poorly supported bronchial airways during the expiratory phase. If air can be allowed to escape slowly, there is less tendency to trap the air within the lungs. Therefore, the patient with emphysema usually learns to purse his lips and to expire slowly over a period of several seconds in order to exhale better and completely. Air trapping, which results from attempts to breathe rapidly, increases the residual air in the lungs and leads to reduction of the percentage of oxygen in the alveoli. There is great advantage in adequate expiration and marked disadvantage in air trapping, which causes the lungs to remain in an inspiratory or inflated state.

In an attempt to assist development of adequate expiratory force, exercises have been developed which strengthen the abdominal muscles and presumably improve the expiratory effect of the intercostal muscles. Unfortunately, many of the exercises are not based on complete understanding of the physiologic difficulties in respiratory impairment. The abdominal muscles are useful expiratory adjuncts principally in the erect position. A week diaphragm works more effectively when the patient is recumbent. A flat diaphragm, such as that found in very pronounced emphysema, cannot be strengthened to do anything because diaphragmatic excursion is impossible. Induction of pneumoperitoneum to restore the arch of the diaphragm is sometimes of benefit in assisting breathing, and this maneuver also helps diminish the residual volume of gas in the lungs.

Among the various measures that assist in maintaining satisfactory respiratory function in people with handicapping disorders, specific respiratory exercises seem to be less important than maneuvers for emptying the lungs, such as breathing out through pursed lips, applying pressure on the abdomen while bending the trunk forward to express air manually, and spontaneous physiologic adaptations such as the development of slow deep breathing which is often encountered in emphysema. While patients with emphysema feel subjectively better with breathing exercises, laboratory studies have shown no improvement in ventilatory ability.

Aerobic Exercises

K. H. Cooper, M.D., a former medical officer in the Air Corps, has popularized a system of "aerobic" exercises which gradually increase the demand for oxygen. In his highly popular books he has set up systems of graduated exercises for nonimpaired individuals of all ages. A similar plan is certainly applicable to persons with respiratory impairment, but the plan must be tailored to each individual and also must be subject to change.

We have long applied Dr. Cooper's principles to patients with respiratory impairment, starting them on stand-up exercises while they receive augmented oxygen by mask through extra-long plastic tubes. After strengthening by this means, they proceed to the inclined treadmill and may continue to breathe 24 to 36 per cent oxygen. They gradually achieve the ability to breathe ambient air only while they gradually increase the exercise. Some patients become independent by this means.

REFERENCES

1. Bendixen, H. H., et al.: Respiratory Care. St. Louis: The C. V. Mosby Co., 1965.
2. Cherniak, R. M., Cherniak, L. and Naimark, A.: Respiration in Health and Disease, 2nd Ed. Philadelphia: W. B. Saunders Co., 1972.
3. Comroe, J. H., et al.: The Lung, 2nd Ed. Chicago: Year Book Medical Publishers, 1962.
4. Comroe, J. H.: Physiology of Respiration, 2nd Ed. Chicago: Year Book Medical Publishers, 1974.
5. Cooper, K. H.: Aerobics. New York: Bantam Books, Inc., 1972.
6. Cooper, K. H.: The New Aerobics. New York: Bantam Books, Inc., 1974.
7. Ganong, W. F.: Review of Medical Physiology, 7th Ed. Los Altos, Ca.: Lange Medical Publications, 1975.
8. Wood, E. C.: Beard's Massage—Principles and Techniques. Philadelphia: W. B. Saunders Co., 1974.

Rehabilitation of Cardiac Disabilities

INTRODUCTION

It is common knowledge that cardiac disease is both the most prominent killer of man and the most significant cause of disability. In this connection, both strokes and coronary artery attacks are grouped with cardiovascular disorders for statistical purposes.

It is true that every cardiac disability is probably amenable to some aspect of rehabilitative care. Basically, this means that the common causes of disuse phenomena should be avoided as much as possible, activity should be restored early, and a confident attitude toward recovery should be promoted.

At present the rehabilitation of cardiac disease is the rehabilitation of individuals with ischemic disease of the heart. It may well be that in the future there will be many institutions where all manner of cardiac disorders are treated with rehabilitation in mind, but such is not the case now.

Most cardiac rehabilitation is carried out by cardiologists in connection with hospital departments devoted to cardiac and vascular disease. Rehabilitation centers, in general, have not been the principal locations of facilities for cardiac rehabilitation.

In this brief chapter, we shall limit discussion to diagnosis and management of coronary artery disease by graduated exercise. We shall be concerned with (1) diagnostic methods, particularly stress tests, and (2) exercise programs for patients with ischemia, especially those convalescing from myocardial infarction.

STRESS TESTS*

Tests of cardiac function have long been with us. Until recently, most of the tests were relatively static, although they did involve exer-

*Whenever stress tests are administered or exercise programs for cardiacs are carried out, all necessary equipment for cardiac and respiratory resuscitation must be immediately available.

458

Contra Costa County Medical Services

T R E A D M I L L   T E S T

Date_____   Time_____

DIGITALIS: Yes No TOBACCO: _____

OTHER DRUGS:_____

HT:_____ WT:_____ AGE:_____

BD:_____ ETHNIC_____

SPECIFIC DIAGNOSIS:_____

Trained ☐   Untrained ☐
Masimum Pulse_____ ____% max._____

DIAGNOSTIC DATA
ETIOLOGIC   PHYSICAL ACTIVITY
1. No heart disease 1. Very active
2. Rheumatic   2. Normal
3. Congenital   3. Limited
4. Hypertension   4. Very limited
5. CAD   6. Other

ELECTROCARDIOGRAM   RHYTHM
1. Normal   1. Sinus
2. Dig. effect only 2. Atrial fib.
3. Abnormal   3. Other
4. Infarct

TEST DATA   Resting B.P._____ P._____

STAGE (mph, grade)	Blood Pressure 1½' 3'		Heart Rate	RECOVERY	Blood Pressure	Heart Rate
REST/ Hyper- ventilation				0 Recovery		
I 1.7, 10%				30 sec. rec.		
II 2.5, 12%				1 min. rec.		
III 3.4, 14%				2 min. rec.		
IV 4.2, 16%				3 min. rec.		
V 5.0, 18%				min. rec.		
VI 5.5, 20%				min. rec.		
VII 6.0, 22%				min. rec.		

TEST ANALYSIS
A. SYMPTOMS, Reasons for stopping:

B. EKG CHANGES FROM BASELINE
1. ST segment depression 1mm.
2. ST "J" depression 1.5 mm.
3. Significant arrhythmia
4. Significant conduction change
5. Other and comments

C. SIGNS - significant findings:
1. Exertional hypotension
2. Cyanosis
3. Pallor, diaphoresis
4. Syncope
5. Increased J-V pressure
6. Pulmonary congestion
7. Poor motivation
8. Gallop
9. Other   10. None

DURATION:_____seconds in Stage_____=_____seconds total or_____minutes.

INTERPRETATION: 1. Normal   3. Diagnostic of ischemia
                2. Equivocal evidence of ischemia 4. Other

TEST REQUESTED BY:_____ DONE BY_____

Fig. 18-1. Treadmill Test. (Modified from form used at Pacific Medical Center.)

Rehabilitation of Cardiac Disabilities   **459**

cise. In the Master test, for example, a person climbs over a two-step test stairs and back at a certain rate for a number of excursions, determined by his age and weight. Electrocardiographic tracings are then made of several leads immediately after exercise and after varying intervals following exercise. Search is made for ST-T changes or arrhythmias, and an estimate of the severity of the ischemic or arrhythmic disease is made.

With the development of interest in progressive exercise, various stress tests have been improvised which are much more dynamic in nature. Devices used for exercising the patient vary from a one step step-up device to a very sophisticated treadmill apparatus (Fig. 18-1), as well as the stationary bicycle, the complexity of which also varies greatly.

Equipment

We have used the Quinton treadmill with control unit and monitors and have applied electrodes for a single lead tracing. The left upper extremity electrode is applied to the left chest wall and the right upper extremity electrode to the manubrium sterni. The ground is applied to the right upper abdomen and a precordial electrode is placed in the V-4 or V-5 position. Sites for applying electrodes vary from institution to institution; the most important thing is that a nearly representative output be obtained and that the peaks of the R-wave be sufficiently high to trigger the pulse recorder. T-waves should not be high enough to do so.

The cardiac monitor attached to the control box provides a continuous observable trace in which abnormalities of rhythm and ST-T changes can be identified. The pulse rate is shown continuously on a meter.

Precautions

Before the patient is subjected to a test, a maximum pulse rate is established, based upon a chart, such as that shown in Table 18-1. This shows maximum pulse rates for individuals, trained and untrained according to age, and it also gives 90 and 75 per cent values. We usually use the 75 per cent limit initially because most of the subjects are, of course, untrained. Prior to testing, the individual is apprised of the fact that he should be on the lookout for anginal pain, either direct or referred, and should call attention to marked dyspnea, leg cramps, or marked fatigue. Any of these symptoms is sufficient reason to discontinue the test. At the time of discontinuation, it is very important to obtain an electrocardiographic strip to see

AGE	20	25	30	35	40	45	50	55	60	65	70	75	80	85	90
Max H.R. Untrained	197	195	193	191	189	187	184	182	180	178	176	174	172	170	168
90% MHR	177	175	173	172	170	168	166	164	162	160	158	157	155	153	151
75% MHR	148	146	144	143	142	140	138	137	135	134	132	131	129	128	126
60% MHR	118	117	115	114	113	112	110	109	108	107	106	104	103	102	101
Max. H.R. Trained	190	188	186	184	182	180	177	175	173	171	169	167	165	163	161
90% MHR	171	169	167	166	164	162	159	158	156	154	152	150	149	147	145
75% MHR	143	141	140	138	137	135	133	131	130	128	127	125	124	122	121
60% MHR	114	113	112	110	109	108	106	105	104	103	101	100	99	98	97

Patients are categorized as "trained" or "untrained." The maximum pulse allowable (maximal heart rate or M.H.R.) for the trained is always less than for the untrained, an indication of better conditioning. Maximum heart rates should not be exceeded in the exercise test. Most cardiac patients are poorly conditioned when first seen, and pulse rates of somewhere between 75 and 90% of the maximum heart rate is set as a limit. From: Cardiac Laboratory, Pacific Medical Center, San Francisco.

whether there are objective criteria of angina. A 12-lead electrocardiogram should be made promptly.

Table 18-2 discloses the various exercise phases which may be carried out in a single test. These, of course, may vary and this particular schedule is not routinely followed even in our institution.

TABLE 18-2. Test Data

STAGE (MPH, GRADE)	BLOOD PRESSURE	HEART RATE	RECOVERY	BLOOD PRESSURE	HEART RATE
REST/ Hyperventilation			0 Recovery		
I 1.7, 10%			30 sec. rec.		
II 2.5, 12%			1 min. rec.		
III 3.4, 14%			2 min. rec.		
IV 4.2, 16%			3 min. rec.		
V 5.0, 18%			min. rec.		
VI 5.5, 20%			min. rec.		
VII 6.0, 22%			min. rec.		

From the Test Data Report Sheet used at Contra Costa County Hospital, Martinez, California; Modified from the report sheet used at the Pacific Medical Center, San Francisco.

Test Procedure

A standard 12 lead electrocardiogram is first recorded and compared to prior tracings, then the electrodes are applied to the patient's chest, as described. These are attached to a preamplifier which is worn around the waist, with a line plugged into the recording device. The monitor is observed and checked before the test is done to see that it is functioning properly. The person being tested then sits on the edge of the bed and hyperventilates to the point of symptoms. This is a means of determining whether dyspnea alone or hyperventilation will induce electrocardiographic changes. If this test is negative, the patient is then asked to stand on the platform of the treadmill or to mount the stationary bicycle. At the word "Go" and with the machine on, he steps on the treadmill and starts to walk, holding the railing in front of him. If he rides the stationary bicycle, he is to begin to pedal at the prescribed resistance and rate indicated for the test.

Each stage of the treadmill test is carried out at a certain rate in miles per hour and a certain inclination of the treadmill belt. It is gradually elevated to a greater angle and is made to go faster in each succeeding stage of the test. The patient carries out as many stages as possible.

Obviously short, obese persons who are in poor condition cannot do any treadmill exercises. For them, the Master two-step test is reserved as a means of determining whether they have any signs of coronary insufficiency. The average person completes three stages of the treadmill exercise test, and some people begin the fourth, but very few go beyond. The pulse rate and blood pressure are monitored. A falling blood pressure with exercise is an indication to stop the test. Extreme tachycardia is limited by the pulse rate accepted as maximum, and the test is stopped when this pulse is reached.

REHABILITATION PROGRAM

Progressive Exercise

In many medical centers at this time, the individual who survives a coronary occlusion (myocardial infarction) is discharged to his home after he survives 2 or 3 weeks of hospitalization and is told, "Take it easy. Don't do anything which causes pain," etc. Such a patient is hard pressed to know exactly what he may do. It is much wiser to prescribe a specific activity, such as walking a certain distance and increasing it daily by a certain amount; or first climbing three stairs and then five, then seven, etc., until at the end of 3 months the patient has achieved some success in walking a mile or climbing a flight of stairs several times daily. At this point, he should be subjected to his first stress test. There is no fixed rule about the time since it may vary with the individual's progress, but one should be sure that the test will not be harmful when it is performed.

When the stress test is performed, the patient's cardiac status can be assessed by the duration of the test, and evidence of myocardial damage or coronary insufficiency can be determined by the presence or absence of ST-T changes. An attempt can then be made to prescribe an exercise program which will fall short of producing ST-T changes and which will be symptomatically tolerable.

For those patients who have a facility available and who can afford it, the method is to visit a rehabilitation area daily or three times a week where exercises, preceded by a warm-up period, may be carried out. The exercises are usually done for a maximum of an hour with rest intervals every ten minutes. They may consist of walking or jogging, or they may be quite liberalized to permit the person to do what he pleases, such as swimming, playing games or engaging in any other type of activity. A common method of control is to have available a large, 10-second floor clock, which permits the individual to count his pulse rate either at the carotid artery, the heart, or wrist for ten seconds and multiply by six. Each person has a prescribed limit of pulse rate, after which he is to stop and rest. The reasons for stopping exercises are similar to the reasons for discontinuing the treadmill test; angina, leg cramps, fatigue, etc. are common causes for modifying the exercise program.

Progressive exercise may be carried on for 3 months or more, depending upon the individual's response. At intervals, he is retested on the treadmill. Successful rehabilitation is usually based upon his ability to resume normal activities without angina or dyspnea.

Cardiac Evaluation for Work

The object of work assignment is matching a worker to a job. In cardiac patients it is now possible to determine work capacity fairly accurately. Work has been studied by determining oxygen consumption, which can be transposed mathematically to Kcal/min. Since O_2 consumption has been determined for various exercises as well as work, it is possible to equate the two and give reasonable work prescriptions. These may be in terms of caloric expenditure or in METS. (A MET is the energy expenditure at rest, approximately 3.5 ml. O_2/kg. body wt./min.)

The literature on work evaluation is extensive. The reader is referred to Chapter 39 of Smith and Germain, Care of the Adult Patient, 4th ed. J. B. Lippincott, 1975 for a concise presentation of rehabilitation, testing and work prescription.

Sometime in the future, people with cardiac disease will have access to careful evaluations of function and, where applicable, will be given the opportunity for progressive exercise with the object of improving function. Meanwhile, rehabilitation medicine has much to offer in preventive care, avoiding the damage which can result from prolonged bed rest and insufficient activity. It goes without saying that social workers, psychologists, and psychiatrists have a large role to play in relation to heart disease. Fear of invalidism and hypochondriasis are very common in disorders of the heart. Much of the resulting disability is reversible on the basis of counseling alone.

REFERENCES

1. Allgood, L.: "Physical Activity After Myocardial Infarction—Changing Concepts." Southern Med. J., 62:525, 1969.
2. Altekrose, J. M.: "Exercise in Cardiovascular Conditioning." J. Occup. Med., 10:296, 1968.
3. Bruce, R. A., et al.: "Cardiovascular Function Tests." Heart Bulletin, 14:9, 1965.
4. Bruce, R. A. and McDonough, J. R.: "Coronary Disease and Exercise." Texas Med., 65:73, 1969.
5. Brusis, O. A.: "Rehabilitating Coronary Patients Through Exercise." Postgrad. Med., 44:131, 1968.
6. Cantwell, J. D.: "Post-Infarction Cardiac Rehabilitation." AFP, 77:137, 1973.
7. Cooper, K. H.: Aerobics. New York: Bantam Books, Inc., 1972.
8. Cooper, K. H.: The New Aerobics. New York: Bantam Books, Inc., 1974.
9. Germain, C. P.: "Exercise Makes the Heart Grow Stronger." Amer. J. Nurs., 72:2169, 1972.
10. Gooch, A. S. and McConnell, D.: "Analysis of Transient Arrhythmias and Conduction Disturbances Occurring During Submaximal Treadmill Exercise Testing." Prog. Cardio. Dis., 13:293, 1970.
11. Heller, E. M.: "Four-Year Experience with a Guided Exercise Program for Postcoronary Patients." Appl. Thera., 11:386, 1969.
12. Heller, E. M.: "Graded Exercise Program After Myocardial Infarction." Arch. Phys. Med. & Rehab., 50:655, 1969.
13. Kellermann, J. J., et al.: "Functional Evaluation of Cardiac Work Capacity by Spiro-Ergometry in Patients with Rheumatic Heart Disease." Medicine, 50:189, 1969.
14. Kellermann, J. J.: "Physical Conditioning in Patients After Myocardial Infarction." Schweiz. Med. Wschr., 103, No. 2:73, 1973.
15. Long, C.: "Concept of Key Pulse Rates in Coronary Rehabilitation." Arch. Phys. Med. & Rehab., 55:255, 1974.

16. Manelis, G., et al.,: Physical Activity at Work; Lipoproteins and the Incidence of Angina Pectoris, Myocardial Infarction and Deaths Due to Ischemic Heart Disease. Proceedings of the 4th Asian-Pacific Congress of Cardiology. New York: Academic Press, 1969.
17. Simonson, E.: "Electrocardiographic Stress Tolerance Tests." Prog. Cardio. Dis., 13:269, 1970.
18. Saltin, B., et al.: "Response to After Bed Rest and After Training." Circulation, 38, No. 5: Suppl. VII, l, 1968.
19. Stuart Pharmaceuticals: Angina Pectoris; Heart in Jeopardy. New York: IntraMed Communications, Inc.
20. University of California, Los Angeles: "Multi-Stage Method: Exercise Capacity Testing by Graded Treadmill Walking." Los Angeles: UCLA.
21. Wenger, N. K.: "Benefits of a Rehabilitation Program Following Myocardial Infarction." Geriatrics, 7:64, 1973.
22. Zohman, L. R.: "Chapter XX" in Licht, S.: Rehabilitation and Medicine. New Haven: Elizabeth Licht, 1968.
23. Zohman, L. R. and Tobis, J. S.: Cardiac Rehabilitation. New York: Grune and Stratton, 1969.

Index

Bed mobility
 and hemiplegic, 221-226
 and paraplegic, 272-278
 and quadriplegic, 293-294
 methods of promoting, 70-73
 problems related to, 69-70
Bed positioning, 71-73
 and disuse, 34
 and lumbar disc lesion, 366-367
 for amputee, 384-385
 for hemiplegic, 248
 for paraplegic, 272-276
Bed rest
 and lumbar disc lesion, 365-372
 prolonged, disadvantages, 31
Beds
 and facilities design, 157-158
 for hemiplegic, 223
 for paraplegic, 272
Bed transfer, 75-76
Bladder capacity, measurement, 321
Bladder function, 24-26
Bladder incontinence, 25-26, 137,
 322-325
Bladder paralysis, 311-312, 314-322
 and quadriplegic, 294
Bladder training, for hemiplegic, 249
Blindness, and communication
 disability, 112
Blood pressure regulation, and
 quadriplegic, 295-296
Board and care homes, 152, 181
Body heat regulation, and
 quadriplegic, 294-295
Bowel function, 20-24
Bowel incontinence, 137, 322-325
Bowel paralysis, 311-313
Bowel training, 22-23
 for hemiplegic, 249
 for paraplegic, 313
Braces, leg, 86-89, 353
 for hemiplegic, 230
 for paraplegic, 280-281
Bracing, and rehabilitative process, 61
Brain
 and communication disability,
 121-122
 structure and function, 203, 205
Brain damage, 262-267
 and aphasia, 122-123, 136-138

Breathing, *see* Pulmonary;
 Respiration; Respiration
 disabilities
Bronchial secretions, removal,
 439-446
Bronchitis, 423
Bulbar paralysis, 303-304, 304-311

Calcium balance maintenance, 12
Cane walking, 234-236
Canes, 93
Cardiac disabilities, 9, 461-463
Cardiac function, 457-461
Casting, and treatment of
 contractures, 338
Catheter, indwelling, and patient
 management, 324-325
Cerebellum, structure and function,
 203
Cerebral embolism, 124
Cerebral hemispheres, structure and
 function, 203
Cerebral hemorrhage, 124
Cerebral palsy, 261-262
Cerebral thrombosis, 124
Cerebral vascular accident. *see also*
 Hemiplegia
 and aphasia, 123, 136-138
 and visual disability, 111
Chairs, and facilities design, 158
Charting, 173
Chloroquine, and arthritis, 341
Chorea, 215
Chronic brain syndrome, 262-267
CircOlectric bed, 73
Circulation
 and disuse, 31-32
 pulmonary, 419-421
Collagen system diseases, 331
Coma
 and bulbar paralysis, 310
 and organic mental impairment,
 265
Communication
 and urinary incontinence, 25
 definition, 100
 evaluation of ability, 104-109
 importance, between staff and
 patient, 59-61
 process, 101-104

Lip reading, 115-117
Locomotion. *see also* Ambulation
   definition and types, 76-77
   wheelchair, 78-85, 230-231,
     279-280, 295-300
Long leg braces, 88
Low back disabilities. *See also* Lumbar
   disc lesions
   causes of pain, 358-360, 365-368
Lumbar disc lesion, 360-363
   and ambulation, 372-380
   and bed rest, 365-372
   treatment, 367-368
Lung disabilities, *see* Pulmonary;
   Respiratory disabilities
Lung volume, measurement, 409-410.
   see also Pulmonary

Malum coxae senilis, 347-348, 349-350
Mattresses, and prevention of pressure
   sores, 35-36
Mechanical ventilation, 445-453
Mental impairment, organic, 262-267
Metabolism, and disuse, 30-31
Misuse syndromes, 27, 28-29, 37-38
Mobility, *see* Bed mobility; Locomotion
Motivation, and rehabilitation, 55-63
Motor deprivation, 52
Motor function, and neurologic
   disability, 198-199
Multiple sclerosis, 209-210
Muscle coordination, physiology,
   208-209
Musculoskeletal disabilities, 7, 9, 29.
   See also specific types, e.g. Arthritis
Myocardial infarction, 461-463
Myopia, 110-111

Nervous system, structure and
   function, 119-209
Neurogenic bladder, 314-322
Neurologic disabilities, 7, 198-199. *See
   also specific types, e.g.* Hemiplegia
   and bladder function, 314-322
   and bowel function, 312-313
   causes, 197, 209-215
   prognosis, 215-217
Neuropathies, toxic, 304-305
Nurse, role in rehabilitative process,
   193

Nursing care, for disabled, 68
Nursing homes, 148-149
   and discharge planning, 181-182
   suggestions for reform, 150-151
Nutrition management, 11-20

Obesity management, 13-19, 254
Oral apraxia, 108
Organic mental impairment, 262-267
Orthostatic hypotension, 31
Osteoarthritis, 329-331, 343
   of hip, 347-348, 349-350
Osteoporosis, 13, 30
Outpatient care, for disabled, 183
Overweight management, 13-19, 254
Oxygen therapy, 428-432

Pads, and prevention of pressure
   sores, 35-36
Pain
   and arthritis, 332, 334-337,
     341-343
   and low back disability, 358-360,
     365-368
Painful shoulder, 37, 247
Palatopharyngeal paralysis, 309
Palsy, 247, 248, 260-262, 305
Paralysis, 208, 211-214. *see also specific*
   types of paralysis
   and back knee deformity, 37-38
   and communication disability,
     119-121
Paraplegia
   and bladder function, 315-318
   and bowel function, 313
   causes, 211-212, 213, 268-269
   prognosis, 165, 217, 269-270
   rehabilitative treatment, 270-271,
     286-290
   mobility, 76, 271-284
   self-care, 284-285
Parkinsonism, 215, 260-261
Passive positioning, *see* Bed positioning
Perception, sensory, and
   communication disability, 105,
     106-107
Phlebothrombosis, 31
Phonation disabilities, 118
Physical conditioning, and self-care,
   96, 98